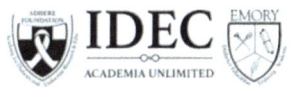

Textbook of
Obesity and Diabetes

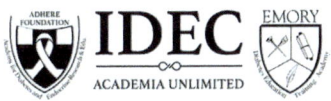

Textbook of
Obesity and Diabetes

Editors

Sanjay Agarwal MD FACE FACP FRSSDI
Organising Chairperson—IDEC
Secretary General—RSSDI
Director, Aegle Clinic—Diabetes Care
Head, Department of Medicine and Diabetes
Ruby Hall Clinic
Head, Department of Diabetes, Obesity &
Metabolic Diseases
Super Speciality Hospital
Pune, Maharashtra, India

Guillermo Umpierrez MD CDCES FACE MACP
Organising Chairperson—IDEC
President, Medicine and Science
American Diabetes Association
Professor of Medicine
Emory University
Atlanta, Georgia, USA

Neeta Deshpande MD (Medicine) FRCP (Edinburgh)
PG Endo (London) ASBP Cert Obesity (USA)
Scientific Chairperson—IDEC
Consultant Diabetologist and Obesity
Physician, Belgaum Diabetes Centre
Children's Diabetes Centre and Weight Watch Centre
Professor and Head, Department of Medicine
MM Dental College
Associate Professor, Department of Medicine
USM-KLE International Medical Program
Belgaum, Karnataka, India

Nitin Kapoor MD (Medicine) DM (Endocrinology)
ABBM (USA) Post Doc Fellowship (Endocrinology)
PhD (University of Melbourne)
Jt. Organising Secretary—IDEC
Professor and Head (Unit 1)
Department of Endocrinology, Diabetes and
Metabolism
Christian Medical College
Vellore, Tamil Nadu, India
Honorary Scientist, Baker Heart and
Diabetes Institute
Melbourne, Victoria, Australia

Associate Editors

Archana Sarda MD (Medicine)
Organising Secretary—IDEC
Consultant Diabetologist
Sarda Centre for Diabetes and
Self-care
Founder: UDAAN, An NGO for
Children with Diabetes
Aurangabad, Maharashtra, India

Shilpa Joshi MSc RD
Chairperson Nodal Update—IDEC
Consultant Dietitian
Mumbai Diet and Health Centre
Mumbai, Maharashtra, India

Anjali Bhatt MD Postdoctoral
Fellow (Diabetes) Diploma and
MSc (Endocrinology)
Founder and Chief Consultant
Diabetes and Metabolic Centre
Pune, Maharashtra, India

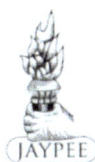

JAYPEE BROTHERS MEDICAL PUBLISHERS
The Health Sciences Publisher
New Delhi | London

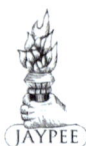 **Jaypee Brothers Medical Publishers (P) Ltd**

Headquarters
EMCA House
23/23-B, Ansari Road, Daryaganj
New Delhi 110 002, India
Landline: +91-11-23272143, +91-11-23272703
+91-11-23282021, +91-11-23245672
E-mail: jaypee@jaypeebrothers.com

Corporate Office
Jaypee Brothers Medical Publishers (P) Ltd.
4838/24, Ansari Road, Daryaganj
New Delhi 110 002, India
Phone: +91-11-43574357
Fax: +91-11-43574314
E-mail: jaypee@jaypeebrothers.com

Overseas Office
JP Medical Ltd.
83, Victoria Street, London
SW1H 0HW (UK)
Phone: +44-20 3170 8910
Fax: +44(0)20 3008 6180
E-mail: info@jpmedpub.com

Website: www.jaypeebrothers.com
Website: www.jaypeedigital.com

© 2024, Jaypee Brothers Medical Publishers

The views and opinions expressed in this book are solely those of the original contributor(s)/author(s) and do not necessarily represent those of editor(s) or publisher of the book.

All rights reserved. No part of this publication may be reproduced, stored or transmitted in any form or by any means, electronic, mechanical, photocopying, recording or otherwise, without the prior permission in writing of the publishers.

All brand names and product names used in this book are trade names, service marks, trademarks or registered trademarks of their respective owners. The publisher is not associated with any product or vendor mentioned in this book.

Medical knowledge and practice change constantly. This book is designed to provide accurate, authoritative information about the subject matter in question. However, readers are advised to check the most current information available on procedures included and check information from the manufacturer of each product to be administered, to verify the recommended dose, formula, method and duration of administration, adverse effects and contraindications. It is the responsibility of the practitioner to take all appropriate safety precautions. Neither the publisher nor the author(s)/editor(s) assume any liability for any injury and/or damage to persons or property arising from or related to use of material in this book.

This book is sold on the understanding that the publisher is not engaged in providing professional medical services. If such advice or services are required, the services of a competent medical professional should be sought.

Every effort has been made where necessary to contact holders of copyright to obtain permission to reproduce copyright material. If any have been inadvertently overlooked, the publisher will be pleased to make the necessary arrangements at the first opportunity.

Inquiries for bulk sales may be solicited at: jaypee@jaypeebrothers.com

Textbook of Obesity and Diabetes / Sanjay Agarwal, Guillermo Umpierrez, Neeta Deshpande, Nitin Kapoor

First Edition: 2024

ISBN: 978-93-5696-336-8

Printed at Repro India Limited

Preface

Diabetes and obesity have reached pandemic proportions globally and even in India. However, many times, they coexist during clinical evaluation. At times, obesity may precede the occurrence of diabetes. Furthermore, presence of obesity can also be associated with multiple other metabolic disorders. Despite several textbooks on diabetes, there are very few books that highlight the evaluation and management of obesity. Moreover, the South Asian phenotype of obesity is very different from other ethnicities. The complications of obesity in the Indian setting arise at a much lower threshold and tend to affect at a relatively younger age. To address these knowledge gaps, the International Diabetes Experts Consortium (IDEC) study group has composed this book.

This book comprises several sections covering the epidemiology, pathophysiology, and clinical management of obesity. These have been written by experts in the field in a very simple yet clinically relevant manner. A special highlight on the genetics of human obesity has been mentioned, which is very relevant in countries which have a higher prevalence of consanguineous marriages. The evaluation and assessment tools that have been highlighted are clinically relevant and validated in previously large studies. A special section has also been dedicated to the prevention of obesity.

Not only the recent most up-to-date information on the nutrition aspects and pharmacotherapy has been mentioned but also those in the pipeline and likely to be available in the near future are covered in detail.

We acknowledge the role played by Jaypee Brothers Medical Publishers and all the contributions by each author for this book.

Team IDEC
Sanjay Agrawal, Guillermo Umpierrez, Neeta Deshpande,
Nitin Kapoor, Archana Sarda, Shilpa Joshi, and Anjali Bhatt

Contents

Chapter 1: Introduction: Obesity and Diabetes   1
- Overview of Obesity and Diabetes   *1*
- Prevalence and Epidemiology   *3*
- Causes and Risk Factors   *10*

Chapter 2: Obesity and Diabetes Pathophysiology   22
- Insulin Signaling, Insulin Resistance in Obesity, and Type 2 Diabetes Mellitus   *23*
- Role of Adipose Tissue and Inflammation   *29*
- Metabolic Dysregulation and Hormonal Imbalances   *35*
- Mechanism of Action of Gut Microbiota in Obesity   *48*
- Endocrine Cause of Obesity and Diabetes   *48*
- Endocrine Cause of Diabetes   *49*

Chapter 3: Genetics of Human Obesity   54
- Heritability and Familial Clustering of Obesity   *56*
- Heritability Reported in Adoptee Studies   *59*
- Monogenic and Polygenic Forms of Obesity   *62*
- Genetic Markers and Variants Associated with Obesity   *69*

Chapter 4: Clinical Manifestations and Diagnosis   74
- Symptoms and Signs of Obesity and Diabetes   *75*
- Diagnostic Criteria for Diabetes and Prediabetes   *81*
- Assessment of Obesity and Comorbidities   *83*

Chapter 5: Prevention and Lifestyle Interventions   97
- Dietary Strategies for Weight Loss and Glycemic Control   *99*
- Physical Activity and Exercise Recommendations   *105*
- Behavioral Modification and Psychological Support   *108*

Chapter 6: Nutrition and Obesity/Diabetes   115
- Nutrition Transition and Global Dietary Trends   *116*

Chapter 7: Pharmacotherapy for Diabetes and Obesity   138
- Oral Antidiabetic Agents and Insulin Therapy   *140*
- Weight Loss Medications and Bariatric Surgery   *153*
- Combination Therapy and Novel Approaches   *162*
- Weight Impact of Endocrinotropic Drugs   *165*

Chapter 8: Management of Diabetes and Obesity Complications   168
- Cardiovascular Disease and Hypertension *170*
- Neuropathy, Nephropathy, and Retinopathy *174*
- Metabolic Dysfunction-associated Steatotic Liver Disease *188*
- Osteoarthritis *192*
- Obstructive Sleep Apnea *196*
- Malignancies *201*

Chapter 9: Special Populations and Issues   206
- Pediatric and Adolescent Obesity and Diabetes *206*
- Weight Management of Gestational Diabetes and Pregnancy Management *216*
- Diabetes and Obesity In the Elderly and Geriatric Patients *222*
- Sarcopenic Obesity *228*
- Polycystic Ovary Syndrome *233*
- Menopause *236*

Chapter 10: Future Directions and Research   242
- New Therapeutic Targets and Approaches *245*
- Personalized Medicine and Precision Health *258*
- Public Health Strategies and Policy Recommendations *263*

Chapter 11: Conclusion   267
- Summary and Implications for Clinical Practice *267*
- Challenges and Opportunities for the Future *270*

Index   273

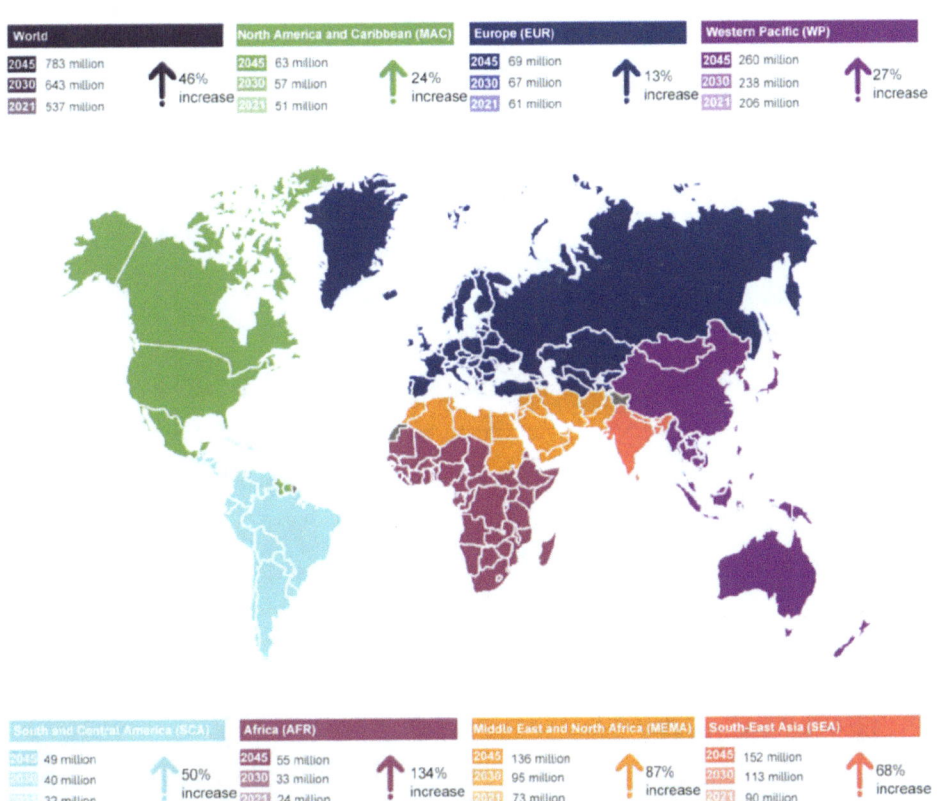

FIG. 1: Number of people with diabetes worldwide as per the International Diabetes Federation (IDF) region in 2021–2045 (20–79 years). *(Chapter 1)*

Plate 2

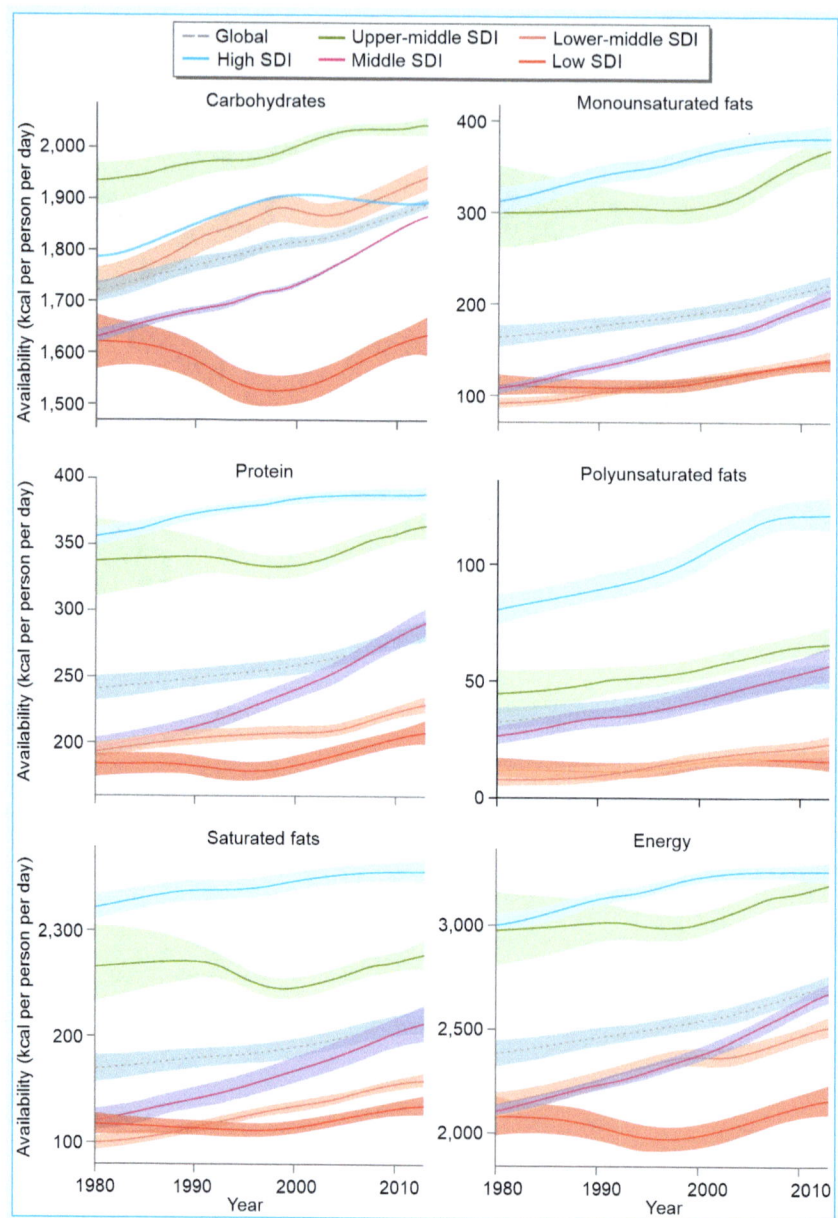

FIG. 4: Trend of energy and macronutrients availability at global and regional level, 1980–2013. *(Chapter 6)*

(SDI: sociodemographic index)

TABLE 1: Profiles of type 2 diabetes mellitus (T2DM) therapy. (Chapter 7)

	Metformin	DPP-4 inhibitor	GLP-1 RA	SGLT-2 inhibitor	TZD	SU and GLN	Pramlintide
Hypoglycemia	Neutral	Neutral	Neutral	Neutral	Neutral	Mild/Moderate	Neutral
Weight	Slight loss	Neutral	Loss	Loss	Gain	Gain	Loss
Renal/GU	Contraindicated if eGFR <30 mL/min/1.73 m²	Dose adjustment is necessary (except linagliptin). Effective in reducing albuminuria	Exenatide not indicated CrCl <30; Possible benefit of liraglutide	Not indicated for eGFR <45 mL/min/1.73 m²; Genital mycotic infection; Possible benefit of empagliflozin	Neutral	More hypo risk	Neutral
GI	Moderate	Neutral	Moderate	Neutral	Neutral	Neutral	Moderate
Cardiac	Neutral	Possible increase in hospitalization with alogliptin and saxagliptin	Liraglutide prevents MACE events	Empagliflozin reduces CV mortality; Canagliflozin reduces MACE events	Moderate risk for CHF; May reduce stroke risk	Possible ASCVD risk	Neutral
Bone	Neutral	Neutral	Neutral	Mild fracture risk	Neutral	Neutral	Neutral
Ketoacidosis	Neutral	Neutral	Neutral	DKA can occur in various stress settings	Neutral	Neutral	Neutral

Possible benefit | Use with caution | Possible adverse effects

(ASCVD: atherosclerotic cardiovascular disease; CHF: congestive heart failure; CrCl: creatinine clearance; CV: cardiovascular; DKA: diabetic ketoacidosis; DPP-4: dipeptidyl peptidase-4; eGFR: estimated glomerular filtration rate; GI: gastrointestinal; GLN: glinide; GU: genitourinary; MACE: major adverse cardiac events; SGLT-2: sodium-glucose cotransporter-2; SU: sulfonylurea; TZD: thiazolidinedione)

Plate 4

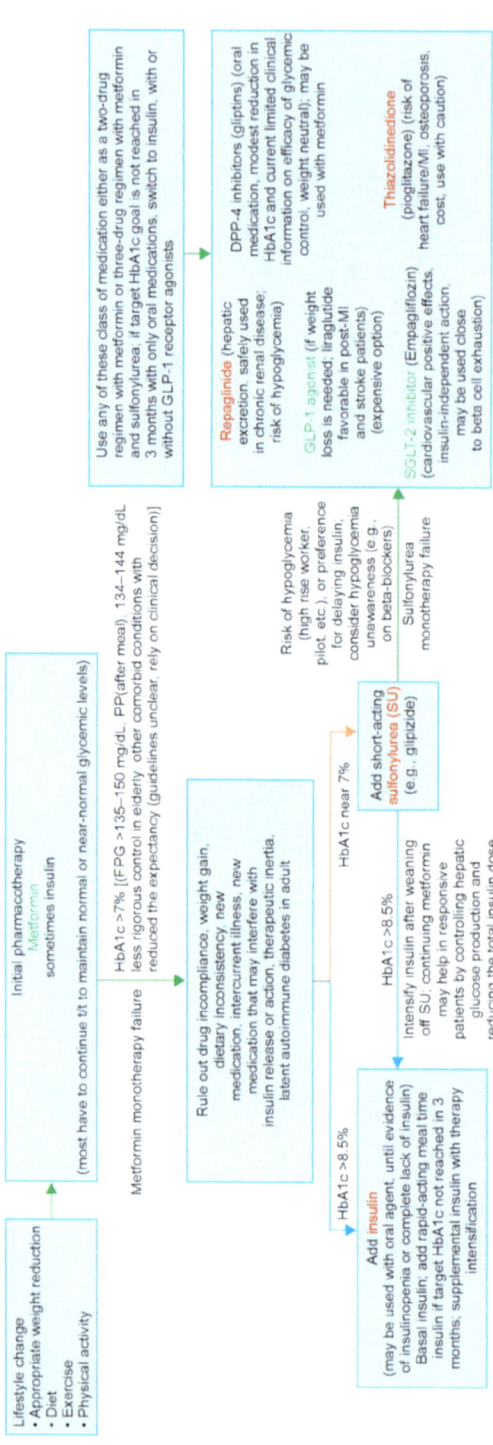

FLOWCHART 1: An algorithm for use of drug regimen in treating diabetes mellitus. *(Chapter 7)*

(DPP-4: dipeptidyl peptidase-4; GLP-1: glucagon-like peptide-1; HbA1C: glycated hemoglobin; SGLT-2: sodium-glucose cotransporter-2)

Note: Several concepts presented here are adapted from American Diabetes Association/European Association for the study of diabetes. Medication in green causes weight loss, in red causes weight gain.

Plate 5

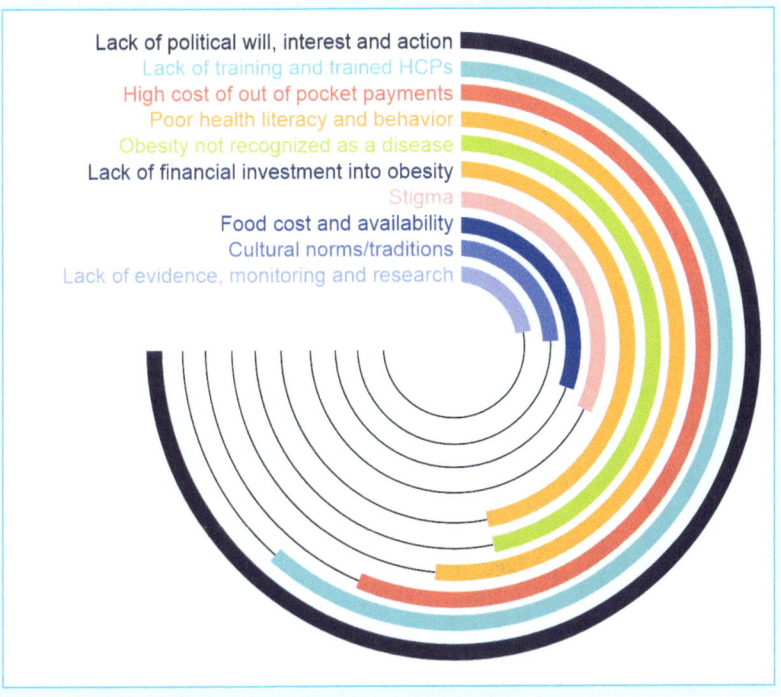

FIG. 1: Based on findings from over 274 obesity specialists from 68 countries. *(Chapter 10)*
(HCPs: healthcare professionals)
Source: With permission from Leach RJ, et al. (2020).[4]

CHAPTER 1

Introduction: Obesity and Diabetes

> **Key Highlights**
> - The term "diabesity" is often used to highlight the interconnection between diabetes and obesity because they are both characterized by impairment in insulin action.
> - As of 2021, it is estimated that 537 million people have diabetes, and it will reach to 783 million by 2045 whereas 1.9 billion adults worldwide were overweight accounting 39% of global population.
> - The World Health Organization (WHO) and the National Institute for Health and Care Excellence (NICE) both recommend a body mass index (BMI) cutoff of 27.5 kg/m^2 to define obesity in South Asian and Chinese populations, aiming to initiate lifestyle interventions.
> - Several risk factors contribute to the prevalence of diabetes, such as sleep quality and quantity, smoking, depression, cardiovascular disease (CVD), dyslipidemia, hypertension, aging, ethnicity, family history of diabetes, physical inactivity, and obesity.

OVERVIEW OF OBESITY AND DIABETES

As per the World Health Organization (WHO) definition, overweight and obesity are defined as abnormal or excessive fat accumulation that may impair health. Body mass index (BMI) is a straightforward measurement that relates an individual's weight to their height, i.e., a person's weight in kilograms divided by the square of his height in meters (kg/m^2) and it is commonly used to classify overweight and obesity in adults. For adults, WHO defines overweight (BMI ≥ 25) and obesity (BMI ≥ 30). The BMI is a valuable tool for measuring overweight and obesity at a population level since it is applicable to all adult ages and sexes. Nonetheless, its utility is limited as it may not accurately reflect the degree of adiposity across all individuals. When evaluating overweight and obesity in children, it is essential to take into account their age. For children under 5 years of age, overweight is defined as weight-for-height that exceeds 2 standard deviations above the median of the WHO Child Growth Standards. Obesity, on the other hand, is defined as weight-for-height that exceeds 3 standard deviations above the median of the WHO Child Growth Standards. For children aged between 5 and 19 years, overweight is defined as BMI-for-age that is above 1 standard deviation from the median of the WHO Growth Reference. Obesity is defined as a BMI-for-age that exceeds 2 standard deviations from the median of the WHO Growth Reference. These criteria help assess and classify weight status in children within this age range.[1]

While excess energy consumption, or an imbalance between dietary intake and energy expenditure, is a common cause of obesity, the underlying causes of obesity are multifaceted and involve various genetic, physiological, environmental, psychological, social, economic, and political factors. These factors interact in complex ways and contribute to the development of obesity.[2] The primary influences of obesity are increased caloric intake and decreased energy expenditure (physical activity). The food environment, also known as the "built" environment, has undergone changes that encourage overeating. High-calorie and high-fat foods are not only cost-effective but also readily available, with numerous fast-food restaurants and vending machines offering energy-dense options in schools and workplaces. Additionally, these foods are often highly palatable and served in large portions, leading to an increased daily calorie intake.[2] In recent decades, physical activity levels have significantly declined, with <50% of US adults estimated to engage in recommended levels of physical activity in 2005. This trend is also observed among adolescents, with a decrease in physical activity levels. Contributing factors include reduced access to physical activity due to fewer sidewalks, decreased physical education in schools, and increased time spent on sedentary behaviors such as watching television, browsing the internet, and playing video games.[2] Though a reduction in diet and increased physical activity can result in weight loss, such behaviors are often biologically driven and cannot be solely blamed to the deliberate wrong choices of a given individual. In addition to the primary influences, Keith et al. identified ten other contributing factors to the obesity epidemic which will be discussed latter in this chapter (**Box 1**).[3]

Obesity is linked to >45 comorbidities, including a cluster of atherogenic disorders that comprise the metabolic syndrome. The metabolic syndrome is recognized by the International Diabetes Federation (IDF) guidelines as a progressive condition that contributes to the development of diabetes, increases the risk of adverse cardiovascular events, and overall mortality. Despite intensive research, the causes of obesity remain unclear, with data suggesting a complex interaction between genetic, cultural, and environmental-behavioral factors. These factors have varying impacts, with genetics accounting for 30%, cultural factors for 10%, and environmental-behavioral factors for 60% of the underlying causes of obesity. Ultimately, an imbalance between energy intake and expenditure results in excess energy storage in the form of fat. The prevalence of diabetes has also experienced a sharp and unexpected increase in recent years, with large epidemiological studies revealing a parallel escalation of the obesity and diabetes epidemics. Metabolic disorders such as diabetes and obesity share a close relationship, as they are both characterized by impairments in insulin action. The term "diabesity" is often used to highlight this interconnectedness between the two conditions. Despite several

> **BOX 1: Contributing factors to the obesity epidemic.[3]**
>
> *Contributing factor:*
> - The food environment
> - Decreases in physical activity
> - Sleep debt
> - Drug-induced weight gain
> - Decline in cigarette smoking
> - Endocrine disruptors
> - Reduction in variability of ambient temperature
> - Changes in distribution of ethnicity and age
> - Increasing gravida age
> - Intrauterine effects
> - Greater reproductive fitness of higher body mass index (BMI)
> - Individuals yielding the selection for obesity-predisposing genotypes
> - Assortative mating and floor effects
> - Changes in policy
> - Infections

theories linking different pathogenic mechanisms that make obese individuals resistant to insulin and lead to pancreatic beta cell failure, resulting in frank diabetes, a unifying hypothesis remains elusive.[3]

PREVALENCE AND EPIDEMIOLOGY

Global Trend of Diabetes

The global crisis of twin obesity and diabetes has reached epidemic proportions. Numerous epidemiological studies have demonstrated the parallel increase in both conditions, and they are closely related to each other due to their shared characteristics of insulin action defects.[4] As per the findings of current IDF atlas edition confirm that diabetes is a rapidly growing global health crisis in the 21st century **(Fig. 1)**. As of 2021, it is estimated that 537 million people have diabetes, and this figure is anticipated to reach 643 million by 2030, and 783 million by 2045. Furthermore, it is estimated that 541 million people have impaired glucose tolerance in 2021. In 2021, >6.7 million people aged 20–79 years are expected to die due to diabetes-related causes. The number of children and adolescents (i.e., those under 19 years of age) living with diabetes increases each year. As of 2021, >1.2 million children and adolescents have type 1 diabetes mellitus (T1DM).[5] Type 2 diabetes mellitus (T2DM) accounts for around 90% of all diabetes cases and is as prevalent as obesity.[6]

Regional Prevalence of Diabetes

In 2021, the Middle East and North Africa (MENA) region had the highest relative prevalence of diabetes, with 18.1% of people aged 20–79 years affected. This prevalence is expected to continue to rise, with the MENA region projected to

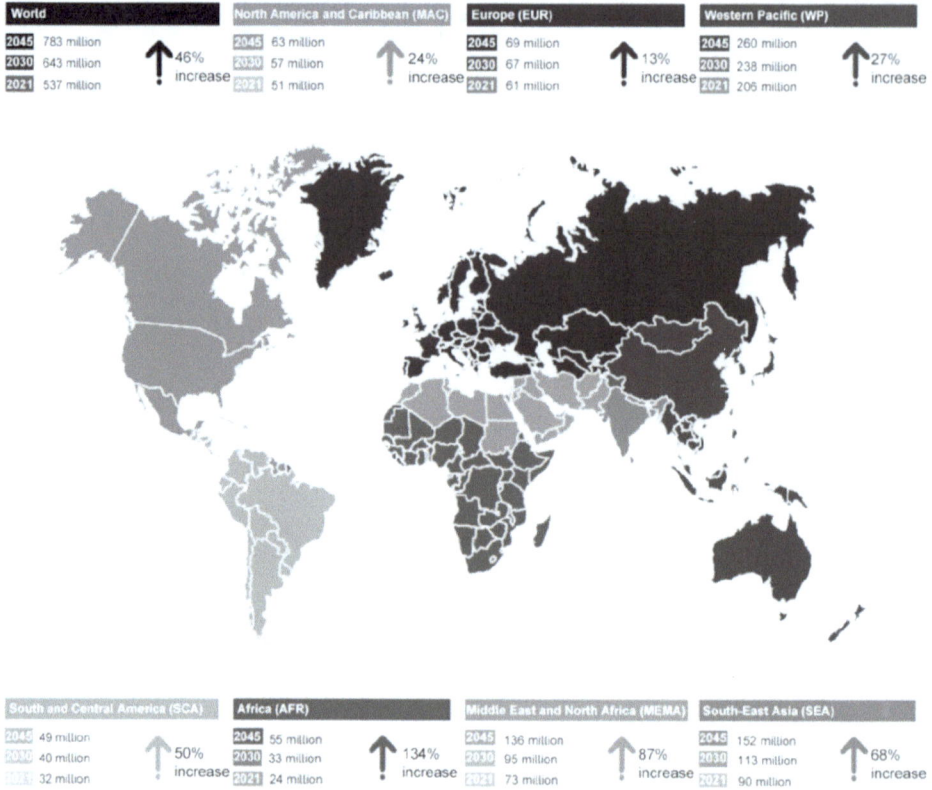

FIG. 1: Number of people with diabetes worldwide as per the International Diabetes Federation (IDF) region in 2021–2045 (20–79 years). *(For color version, see Plate 1)*

maintain the highest relative prevalence in 2045 at 20.4%. In contrast, the Africa region currently has the lowest relative prevalence of diabetes at 5.3%, which may be due in part to low levels of urbanization and lower prevalence of overweight and obesity. However, its prevalence is estimated to increase slightly from 4.5% in 2021 to 5.2% in 2045, which is a smaller increase compared to other regions. The countries with the highest numbers of adults with diabetes aged 20-79 years in 2021 are China, India, and Pakistan, and they are predicted to remain so in 2045. Pakistan, French Polynesia, and Kuwait had the highest relative diabetes prevalence rates in 2021, with Pakistan projected to reach 33.6%, Kuwait 29.8%, and French Polynesia 28.2% in 2045, indicating that these countries will continue to face significant challenges with diabetes.[5]

Global Trend of Overweight and Obesity

In 2016, it was estimated that 1.9 billion adults worldwide were overweight, and an additional 650 million were considered obese, equating to approximately 39% and 13% of the global population.[1] Among young adults (20–44 years old), the prevalence of overweight was lower in women than in men, but this trend was reversed after age 45-49 years, which may coincide with menopause in women. Across all age groups, the prevalence of obesity tends to be higher in women compared to men. The greatest disparities between the sexes are observed between the ages of 50–65 years. Both overweight and obesity rates increased with age, peaking between 50 and 65 years old and declining slightly thereafter. Between 1980 and 2015, the age-standardized prevalence of overweight has increased from 26.5 to 39.0%, which represents a nearly 50% rise in the past 35 years. Additionally, the prevalence of obesity witnessed a nearly 80% increase, rising from 7% in 1980 to 12.5% in 2015.[7]

Regional Prevalence of Overweight and Obesity

The prevalence of overweight and obesity was highest in the American and European regions, according to **Figures 2 and 3**. The US and Mexico had the highest rates in both categories. Prevalence rates were consistent across countries within each region. In the European and American regions, Turkey and the US had the highest rates, respectively, while France and Colombia had the lowest. In the African region, overweight and obesity rates approximately doubled from 1980

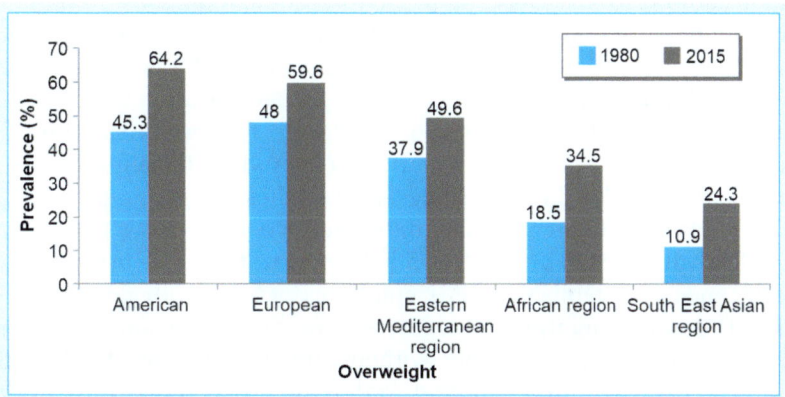

FIG. 2: Region-wise prevalence trend in overweight.

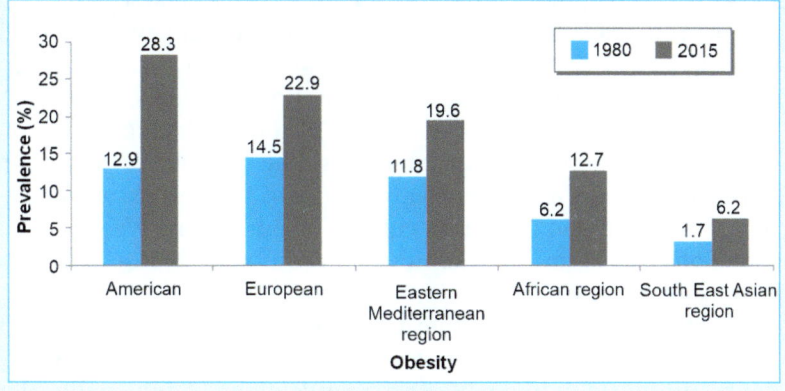

FIG. 3: Region-wise prevalence trend in obesity.

to 2015, with Iraq and Pakistan showing different trends. In South Africa, rates of overweight increased from 49.4 to 57.8%, while in Ethiopia they increased from 7.1 to 15.9%. The West Pacific region had the lowest rates of overweight and obesity but still experienced an increase in prevalence over the past 35 years. Overweight prevalence in China tripled from 7.8 to 29.9%, with similar trends in the Southeast Asian region. Overall, all regions experienced a rising trend in prevalence rates of overweight and obesity over the past 35 years, with some regions showing evidence of leveling off but not all **(Figs. 2 and 3)**. Variability in absolute prevalence rates of overweight and obesity was five- to six-fold among regions.[7]

Race and Ethnic Differences in Prevalence of Diabetes and Obesity

The current BMI cutoff of ≥30 kg/m^2 used to define obesity was derived from observational studies conducted in Europe and the USA, primarily involving White populations, focusing on the relationship between BMI and mortality. However, there is increasing evidence indicating a higher prevalence of T2DM among Asian populations at lower BMI levels compared to White populations. In light of these emerging findings, the WHO recommended a reduction in the BMI cutoffs for defining obesity in south Asian populations to better identify cardiometabolic risks in this group. This recommendation, which originated from a 2004 WHO expert consultation, suggested a BMI cutoff of 27.5 kg/m^2 for south Asian and Chinese populations to trigger the implementation of lifestyle interventions. The expert consultation reevaluated BMI cutoffs based on studies measuring percentage body fat, which tends to be higher in Asian individuals compared to White individuals, conducted in various Asian countries.[8-10] However, it is noteworthy that despite the significance of establishing BMI cutoffs associated with adverse outcomes such as T2DM and generating clinically relevant guidelines for patient care, the WHO made these recommendations without sufficient data on the BMI-diabetes association in Black, South Asian, and Arab populations. Preventing or delaying the onset of T2DM can be achieved through dietary modifications, increased physical activity, or the use of medications like metformin. Early utilization of other antihyperglycemic therapies also helps reduce the long-term complications associated with T2DM by improving glycemic control. In a population-based cohort study, the electronic health records of approximately 1.5 million individuals were analyzed, including 97,823 diagnosed with T2DM over a median follow-up period of 6.5 years, the findings have identified new BMI thresholds for obesity that can trigger interventions aimed at lowering the risk of developing T2DM in Black, South Asian, Chinese, and Arab populations residing in England. In comparison to White populations, where an equivalent incidence of T2DM is observed at a BMI of 30.0 kg/m^2, the study found lower BMI cutoffs for south Asian, Black, Chinese, and Arab populations 23.9 kg/m^2, 28.1 kg/m^2, 26.9 kg/m^2, and 26.6 kg/m^2, respectively after adjusting for age and sex.[11]

The WHO and the National Institute for Health and Care Excellence (NICE) both recommend a BMI cutoff of 27.5 kg/m^2 to define obesity in south Asian and Chinese populations, aiming to initiate lifestyle interventions. Additionally, the NICE suggests using this lower BMI threshold to take preventive measures against T2DM among Black populations.[9,10] The earlier mentioned study findings demonstrate that the risk of developing T2DM among South Asian individuals occurs at a significantly lower BMI of 23.9 kg/m², indicating a considerable deviation from the recommended ethnicity-specific cutoff of 27.5 kg/m², and supporting previous research that suggests the need to lower the cutoffs recommended by the WHO and NICE for non-White populations.[12-15] For instance, in the Southall and Brent Revisited (SABRE) cohort study involving Europeans, South Asians, and African-Caribbeans, we observed age- and sex-adjusted BMI cutoffs of 25.2 kg/m² for south Asians and 27.2 kg/m² for African-Caribbeans to define obesity.[15] The population-based study further revealed that the incidences of T2DM among south Asian subpopulations were equivalent to those in the White population but occurred at consistently lower BMI values. However, among Black ethnic subgroups, including Black Africans, Black Caribbean, Black British, and other Black individuals, the incidences of T2DM were comparable to the White population but at lower BMI values specifically observed in Black Caribbean individuals and Black individuals of other ethnic origins. Moreover, the study indicated that BMI cutoffs for overweight, based on the risk of T2DM, were lower for south Asian, Black, Chinese, and Arab populations compared to White populations, highlighting the need to lower the recommended BMI cutoff for overweight in these groups to effectively mitigate the risk of T2DM **(Fig. 4)**.[11]

In a retrospective cross-sectional study conducted in the United States, data from 283,110 White, 33,263 Chinese, 38,766 Filipino, and 17,959 South Asian adults aged 45–64 years were examined. These individuals were members of a Northern California health plan in 2016 and had their height and weight measured. The study concluded that Chinese, Filipino, and South Asian adults had a higher prevalence of prediabetes and diabetes compared to White adults in all weight categories, despite using lower BMI thresholds for weight classification in Asian groups. Filipino and South Asian adults had particularly higher diabetes prevalence compared to Chinese adults within the Asian ethnic groups.[16]

The findings revealed that diabetes prevalence was higher among Asian adults compared to White adults across all weight categories, with Filipino and South

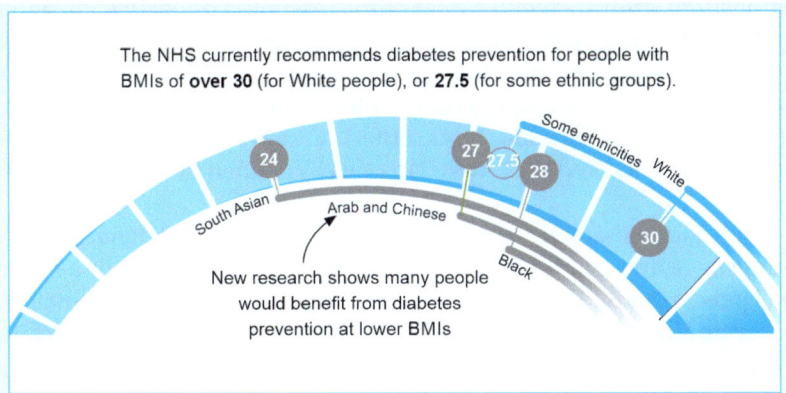

FIG. 4: The National Health Service (NHS) recommendation for body mass Index (BMI) in different ethnic groups.

Asian adults having the highest rates. When comparing prediabetes and diabetes prevalence ratios (PRs) for Asian groups to White adults within each weight category, adjusted for age and BMI, South Asian men/women at a healthy BMI had PRs of 1.8/2.8 for prediabetes and 5.9/8.0 for diabetes, respectively. Filipino men/women at a healthy BMI had PRs of 1.8/2.6 for prediabetes and 5.0/7.5 for diabetes, respectively. Chinese men/women at a healthy BMI had similar PRs for prediabetes (2.1/2.9) compared to Filipino and South Asian groups but lower PRs for diabetes (2.1/3.4).[16]

The prevalence of prediabetes among Asian groups (across all weight categories) was much higher than that among White adults. For White men, the prevalence of prediabetes by healthy weight, overweight, and obesity categories was 18%, 23%, and 27%, respectively, while for men in Asian groups, it ranged from 29 to 35%, 33 to 39%, and 33 to 36%. Among women, the prevalence of prediabetes in the respective weight categories was 11%, 17%, and 24% for White women and 26–28%, 30–33%, and 29–34% for women in Asian groups. The age-standardized prevalence of diabetes followed a similar pattern, with lower rates among White men (5%, 9%, and 23%) compared to Chinese men (10%, 15%, and 28%) and Filipino and South Asian men (25–28%, 29–30%, and 38%). Similar trends were observed among women, with lower prevalence for White women (2%, 6%, and 17%) compared to Chinese (6%, 10%, and 24%), Filipina (13%, 21%, and 36%), and South Asian (14%, 18%, and 29%) women. Overall, the prevalence of diabetes increased with higher weight categories. However, even in the healthy weight range, Asian adults had a significantly higher burden of prediabetes compared to healthy weight White adults. For example, approximately 56% of Filipino and South Asian, 45% of Chinese, and 23% of White men had either diabetes or prediabetes in the healthy weight range.[16] These findings align with previous research that has consistently demonstrated a significantly higher prevalence of diabetes at lower BMI levels among US, South Asian, Filipino, and Chinese adults when compared to White adults.[17-22] Another population-based cohort study utilizing primary care records from the UK Clinical Practice Research Datalink, linked with secondary care and death registry records, has provided evidence that the risk of developing T2DM is higher in overweight and obese individuals from Asian and Black ethnic populations compared to White populations. The study included a total of 193,528 obese or overweight adults (BMI of 25 or greater) without preexisting T2DM, identified between January 1, 1995, and April 20, 2018. The three ethnic groups evaluated in the study were Asian (including Bangladeshi, Chinese, Indian, Pakistani, and Asian Other), Black (including Black African, Black Caribbean, and Black other), and White (including White Irish, White Gypsy/Traveler, and White other) as clearly defined by the Office for National Statistics.[23]

The study found that individuals of Asian ethnicity were diagnosed with T2DM at a younger age and had the highest incidence rate of T2DM, with a rate of 35.33 per 1,000 person-years. This was followed by individuals of Black ethnicity with an incidence rate of 21.20, while the lowest prevalence was observed in the White ethnic group with a rate of 19.67 **(Figs. 5 and 6)**. When compared to White overweight and obese adults, the incidence rate ratio for T2DM was 1.08 for Black overweight and obese adults and 1.80 for Asian individuals. Over a median follow-up period of 9.8 years, the risk of developing T2DM was 2.2-fold higher in Asians [hazard ratio (HR)

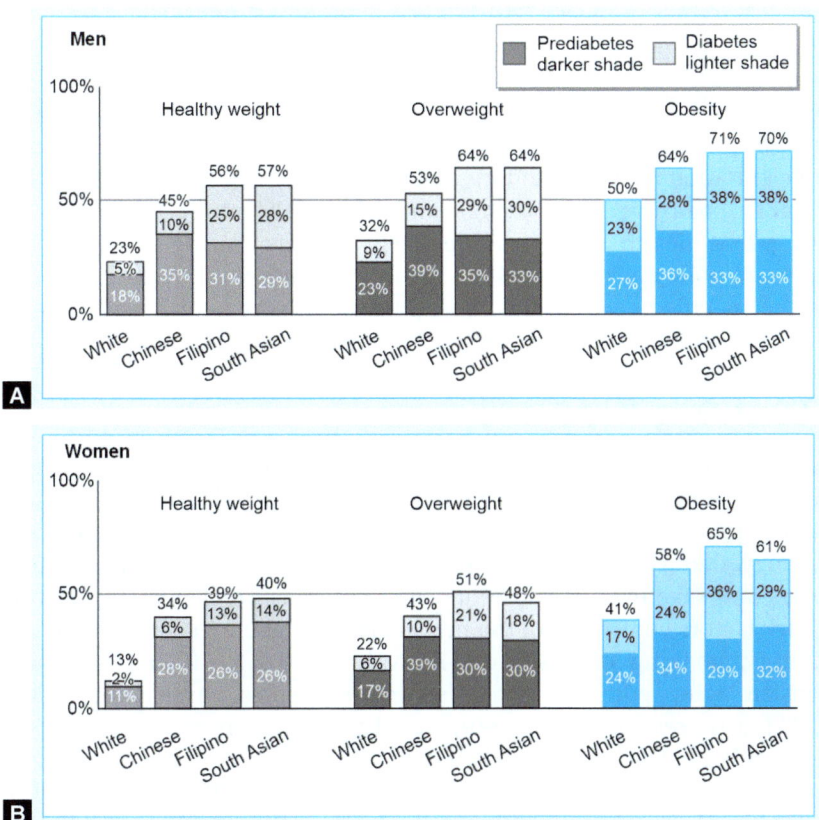

FIGS. 5A AND B: Age-standardized prevalence of diabetes and prediabetes by race/ethnicity and weight category in men and women.

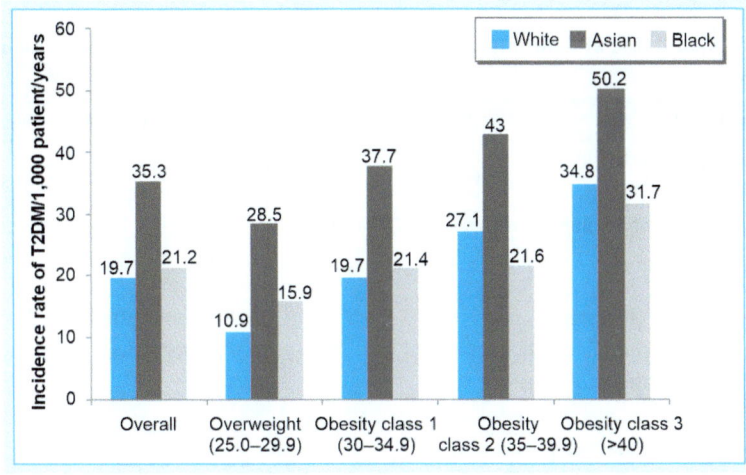

FIG. 6: Incidence of type 2 diabetes mellitus (T2DM) in adults who are overweight or obese (*n* = 193,528).

2.19] and 30% higher in Blacks (HR 1.34) compared to Whites. However, adjusted HRs for mortality were significantly lower in Asians (HR 0.70) and Blacks (HR 0.71) when compared to Whites.[23]

These studies highlights the impact of ethnicity on the risk of developing T2DM and the significant disparities in mortality risk associated with T2DM among obese or overweight adults. Understanding and acknowledging these ethnic variations are crucial for healthcare professionals and policymakers in setting priorities and directing public health strategies effectively. By recognizing these disparities, clinicians and policymakers can develop targeted interventions and initiatives to address the specific needs of different ethnic populations, ultimately improving outcomes and reducing the burden of T2DM within these communities.

CAUSES AND RISK FACTORS

Diabetes presents a global crisis fueled by rapid urbanization, evolving lifestyles, and inconsistent dietary patterns. The surge in obesity and T2DM worldwide can be attributed to multiple factors, including changes in the economy, demographics, epidemiology, dietary habits, and physical activity patterns. To mitigate the risk of diabetes and save lives, it is essential to predict its prevalence in individuals. Several risk factors contribute to the prevalence of diabetes, such as sleep quality and quantity, smoking, depression, cardiovascular disease (CVD), dyslipidemia, hypertension, aging, ethnicity, family history of diabetes, physical inactivity, and obesity. Extensive research has investigated the association between each of these risk factors and the development of T2DM.[24]

Risk factors for T2DM can be classified into nonmodifiable and modifiable factors **(Table 1)**. Notably, sleep quantity and quality, smoking, dyslipidemia, hypertension, ethnicity, family history of diabetes, obesity, and physical inactivity are strongly linked to the development of T2DM.[24-27] Relative risk (RR) for T2DM risk factors are mentioned in **Table 2**.[28-31] According to data from the Global Burden of Disease Study 2017, the primary contributors to deaths and disability-

TABLE 1: Modifiable and nonmodifiable risk factors associated with type 2 diabetes mellitus.

Modifiable risk factors	Nonmodifiable risk factors
• Overweight and obesity • Sedentary lifestyle • Previously identified glucose intolerance (IGT and/or IFG) • Hypertension • Decreased HDL cholesterol • Increased triglycerides • Dietary factors and alcohol use • Smoking • Ambient particulate matter pollution • Inflammation	• Ethnicity • Family history of type 2 diabetes mellitus • Age • Gender • Previous gestational diabetes • Polycystic ovary syndrome
(IFG: impaired fasting glycemia; IGT: impaired glucose tolerance)	

TABLE 2: Relative risk associated with type 2 diabetes mellitus risk factors.

Risk factor	Relative risk
Age ≥45 years	7.5×
Obesity: Body mass index ≥30 kg/m^2	5.2×
Overweight: Body mass index ≥25 kg/m^2 and <30 kg/m^2	5.4×
Hypertension	2–2.5×
Hyperlipidemia	4–6×
Family history	
Moderate familial risk	2.3×
High familial risk	5.5×
Genetic variant carrier	
Heterozygous	1.1–1.4×
Homozygous	Up to 10×

Note: Relative risk estimates of overweight and obesity are compared with those with body mass index, 25 kg/m^2.

adjusted life years (DALYs) in diabetes were metabolic risks (high BMI) and behavioral factors (inappropriate diet, smoking, and low physical activity). The three leading risk factors were high BMI, dietary risks, and ambient particulate matter pollution. High BMI accounted for 30.8% of deaths and 45.8% of DALYs, dietary risks accounted for 24.7% of deaths and 34.9% of DALYs, and ambient particulate matter pollution accounted for 13.4% of deaths and 15.4% of DALYs. When examining the burden of diabetes attributable to all risk factors, measured by age-standardized mortality and DALYs rates, the highest burden was observed in regions with low, low-middle, and middle socio-demographic index. In low and low-middle socio-demographic index regions, a major risk factor was low fruits consumption. Additionally, regions with low, low-middle, and middle socio-demographic index regions experienced a higher risk of deaths and DALYs from household air pollution caused by solid fuels.[25]

Obesity is a diverse collection of conditions with various causes. Body weight results from a complex interplay of genetic, environmental, and psychosocial factors, which influence the physiological mechanisms governing energy intake and expenditure. While genetics certainly play a role, the substantial increase in obesity rates can be primarily attributed to behavioral and environmental shifts driven by technological advancements. While excessive energy intake compared to expenditure is a primary cause of obesity, its origins are intricate and involve genetic, physiological, environmental, psychological, social, economic, and sometimes political factors that interact to varying extents in fostering its development.[2,32]

Sleep Quantity and Quality

The quality and quantity of sleep are influenced by various cultural, social, behavioral, psychological, and environmental factors. Individuals in the working profession often experience fatigue, tiredness, and daytime napping due to irregular working hours and shifts. Research indicates that the average amount of sleep per night for individuals today, which is 6.8 hours, is 1.5 hours less than it was a century ago. The reasons for sleep loss are multifaceted. For example, 45% of adults report sleeping fewer hours to accomplish more work, 43% mention watching television or using the Internet as a factor, and 22% report suffering from insomnia. Disturbed and reduced sleep has been associated with glucose intolerance.[24]

Mallon et al. conducted a study examining the impact of gender on the link between sleep and diabetes. The study concluded that in men, a shorter sleep duration increases the risk of developing diabetes, while in women, longer sleep duration is dominant. Results demonstrated that a higher percentage of men who developed diabetes reported short sleep duration (≤5 hours per night) (difference—10.1%; 16.0% vs. 5.9%, $p < 0.01$), difficulties initiating sleep (16.0% vs. 3.1%, $p < 0.001$), and difficulties maintaining sleep (difference—21.7%; 28.0% vs. 6.3%, $p < 0.001$) compared to men who did not develop diabetes. On the other hand, women who developed diabetes reported long sleep duration (≥9 hours per night) more frequently at baseline than women who did not develop diabetes (difference—5.5%; 7.9% vs. 2.4%, $p < 0.05$).[33] Xu et al. investigated the association between daytime napping and T2DM, revealing that individuals who nap for >1 hour during the day are 1.5 times more likely to develop diabetes compared to those who do not nap. When compared to 7-8 hours of night sleep, the individuals who sleeps for 5 hours, 5-6 hours, and 9 hours have 1.46 times, 1.11 times, and 1.11 times higher risk to develop diabetes.[34] Concerning sleep quality, the risk of developing T2DM is higher in individuals who have difficulty initiating sleep (DIS), and this risk increases with the frequency of DIS. Moreover, this association is more pronounced in women with DIS compared to men.[33,35] Both sleep duration and quality have a profound impact on the risk of developing T2DM, with women sleeping longer hours and men sleeping fewer hours displaying a stronger association.

Insufficient sleep can compromise both mental and physical functions, potentially leading to cognitive impairments and metabolic disturbances. Numerous research has illuminated the detrimental impacts of sleep deprivation on both mental and physical well-being, encompassing alterations in cognitive functions such as memory, emotional regulation, and appetite control. Moreover, inadequate or disrupted sleep has been linked to compromised immune function and an increased susceptibility to metabolic disturbances. Numerous studies have underscored how reduced sleep duration and quality can influence glucose metabolism and disrupt the secretion of anabolic hormones such as growth hormone (GH), prolactin, and testosterone. Furthermore, it can perturb the quantity and timing of catabolic hormones such as glucocorticoids and catecholamines, along with changes in dietary regulation. Numerous epidemiological studies have consistently demonstrated that reduced sleep duration and poorer sleep quality, typically in the range of 6-7 hours per night, are closely linked to a higher incidence of obesity.[36]

An observational study led by Bonanno et al. revealed that both the quantity and quality of sleep can serve as risk factors for overweight and obesity. Sufficient sleep plays a pivotal role in maintaining a healthy weight. Individuals, both adults and children, who experience insufficient sleep, are at a heightened risk of obesity and overweight. This increased risk is associated with disrupted eating patterns, reduced physical activity, and alterations in metabolic processes.[36]

Smoking

Smoking is responsible for >8 million deaths annually, including both active smokers and nonsmokers exposed to secondhand smoke. Smokers have a 30-40% higher likelihood of developing T2DM compared to nonsmokers. The act of smoking increases nicotine levels in the body, which leads to reduced muscle glucose intake, insulin resistance, and ultimately the development of T2DM.[24]

Research findings indicate that the association between smoking and diabetes becomes stronger with an increase in the number of cigarettes smoked per day. Studies conducted by Will et al. and Jee et al. support the notion that the association between cigarette smoking and T2DM is more pronounced in men than in women.[37,38] Furthermore, Wannamethee et al. demonstrated that individuals who smoke pipes or cigars are 2.15 times more likely to develop T2DM, while those who smoke cigarettes are 1.6 times more likely compared to nonsmokers. According to the US Health Professional Study, which followed participants for a period of 6 years, there was a dose-response relationship between smoking and the risk of developing certain health conditions. Specifically, the study found that as the amount of cigarettes smoked per day increased, the risk also increased. The study reported an odds ratio (OR) of 1.37 for light smokers (1-14 cigarettes per day), indicating a higher risk compared to nonsmokers. For heavier smokers (25 or more cigarettes per day), the OR was even higher at 1.94, indicating a further increased risk compared to both nonsmokers and light smokers.[39] Kowall et al. found that the risk of developing T2DM is significantly higher in active or passive smokers with prediabetes compared to active or passive smokers without prediabetes. This suggests that smoking, both active and passive, has an even greater impact on diabetes risk among individuals who already have prediabetes.[40] Incidence and prevalence studies have shown that the risk of developing T2DM increases by 17-60% among individuals who have quit smoking.[24] Smoking is identified as a significant risk factor for T2DM, affecting both active and passive smokers. Furthermore, individuals who have quit smoking still face a heightened risk of developing T2DM for the first 5-10 years after cessation.

The relatively recent decrease in cigarette smoking rates may also have played a role in the obesity epidemic. Research has indicated that weight gain is a common outcome after quitting smoking. Additionally, individuals who smoke generally have lower body weights compared to those who do not smoke.[2] In a cross-sectional study involving 499,504 middle-aged adults, it was observed that former smokers had a higher likelihood of being obese compared to both current smokers, with an adjusted OR of 1.33, and never smokers, with an adjusted OR of 1.14. Among individuals who smoked, the risk of obesity was found to rise with the quantity of cigarettes smoked, and former heavy smokers had a greater likelihood of obesity than former light smokers, with an adjusted OR of 1.60 ($p < 0.001$).[41]

Dyslipidemia

In dyslipidemia, imbalances in lipid levels, specifically elevated low-density lipoproteins (LDLs) and lowered high-density lipoproteins (HDLs), can lead to beta cell dysfunction, inhibiting insulin secretion and ultimately contributing to the development of T2DM. The role of dietary fats is significant in the development of T2DM, particularly those that raise total cholesterol and LDL levels.[24] To mitigate the risk of T2DM, it is recommended to substitute saturated fatty acids with polyunsaturated fatty acids and animal fats with vegetable fats. This dietary change can help lower blood cholesterol levels, ultimately reducing the risk of T2DM.[42]

Both polyunsaturated fatty acids and vegetable fats have an inverse relationship with the risk of developing T2DM, with a RR of 0.84 and RR of 0.78, respectively, for the highest quintile of intake.[42] Tajima et al. also confirmed the association between a high cholesterol diet (intake >273 mg/day) and T2DM, with an RR of 1.25 compared to a low cholesterol diet (intake <185 mg/day).[43] Individuals with familial hypercholesterolemia, a genetic disorder resulting in high LDL levels, are actually less likely to develop T2DM compared to individuals with high LDL levels due to dietary patterns.[44] Zhang et al. conducted an analysis and found that the ratio of non-HDL to HDL levels is an independent risk factor for developing T2DM. They observed that an individual with a ratio of 3.1 has a 40% increased risk of developing diabetes [OR 1.4; 95% confidence interval (CI) 1.1–1.8] compared to an individual with a ratio of 1.4. Elevated levels of non-HDL and lowered levels of HDL are significantly associated with the incidence of T2DM.[45] Dyslipidemia, characterized by elevated non-HDL and reduced HDL cholesterol levels, is strongly associated with T2DM.

Around 60–70% of individuals classified as obese exhibit dyslipidemia, a condition characterized by abnormal lipid levels in the bloodstream. Similarly, approximately 50–60% of individuals categorized as overweight also present with dyslipidemia. Dyslipidemia often involves imbalances in cholesterol and triglyceride levels, which are risk factors for CVD and other health complications.[46]

Cross-sectional data, as well as findings from the Coronary Artery Risk Development in Young Adults (CARDIA) Study, support the notion that increasing body weight is linked to elevated plasma triglycerides. Additionally, longitudinal data from studies lasting at least 1 year have consistently demonstrated significant reductions in triglyceride levels following weight loss. Obesity also appears to be associated with reductions in HDL cholesterol. Data from the second National Health and Nutrition Examination Survey (NHANES II), involving white men and women, have shown a decline in HDL levels as BMI increases across all age groups. This decline can amount to around 10 mg/dL in HDL levels between normal-weight and obese men, with even more pronounced decreases in HDL observed in obese women. Long-term weight loss studies have consistently reported an increase in HDL levels.[47]

In contrast, the effect of obesity on LDL concentrations has been less consistent. NHANES II data indicate that young white men (aged 20–44 years) experience a significant rise in LDL concentration as their BMI increases, with obese young men showing LDL levels roughly 30 mg/dL higher than their normal-weight counterparts. The primary dyslipidemia associated with obesity is characterized by elevated triglycerides, reduced HDL levels, and alterations in LDL composition. This obesity-related dyslipidemia is a key contributor to the development of atherosclerosis and CVD in obese individuals.[47]

Hypertension

Hypertension, characterized by elevated blood pressure (BP), can lead to increased activity of the sympathetic nervous system, which in turn results in decreased glucose uptake by the body. This condition, known as insulin resistance, ultimately contributes to the development of T2DM. Additionally, hypertension impairs vasodilation in skeletal muscles, leading to reduced glucose uptake by the muscles and further contributing to the development of T2DM.[24]

Hayashi et al. conducted a study to examine the association between high-normal BP (130 to <140 mm Hg systolic or 85 to <90 mm Hg diastolic) and hypertension (≥140 mm Hg systolic or ≥90 mm Hg diastolic) with the incidence of T2DM in men. The authors concluded that both high-normal BP (RR 1.39) and hypertension (RR 1.75) are associated with an increased risk of T2DM.[48] This association is influenced by obesity and the use of hypertension medications. The type of medication used to treat hypertension can also impact the risk of developing diabetes. For example, individuals taking thiazide diuretics and angiotensin-converting enzyme medications have a lower risk of diabetes compared to those not taking any medication. However, individuals taking beta blockers are at a 28% higher risk of developing T2DM (HR 1.28).[49] The association between hypertension and the incidence of T2DM is also significant in women. Women with hypertension are at a twofold increased risk of developing diabetes (HR 2.03) compared to women with normal BP (<120/75 mm Hg).[50] This association is more pronounced in overweight and obese women. Regardless of gender, prehypertension (HR 1.27) and hypertension (HR 1.51) are associated with an increased risk of developing T2DM.[51] Hypertension, particularly in obese individuals, is a significant risk factor for T2DM.

While obese subjects are prone to hypertension, hypertensive subjects also appear to be prone to weight gain. Both the Framingham and Tecumseh studies have indicated that individuals with hypertension tend to experience more substantial future weight gain compared to those with normal BP levels. This suggests that even individuals with a normal weight who have hypertension are at a heightened risk of developing obesity. Achieving lasting weight loss requires sustained modifications in dietary choices, calorie intake, and physical activity levels. Weight loss efforts have been associated with a noteworthy decrease in BP and also offer advantageous effects on related risk factors.[52]

Family History

Family history of diabetes plays a crucial role in both prognosis and diagnosis, as well as in public health efforts. It encompasses genetic and environmental factors and provides valuable insights for predicting the development of T2DM beyond genetic or environmental factors alone. When combined with other risk factors such as age, gender, and CVDs, a parental history of diabetes increases the risk of developing T2DM.[24]

Research conducted by Tsenkova et al. demonstrated a strong association between a family history of diabetes and the incidence of diabetes (OR 2.77).[53] Another study found that a parental history of diabetes is an independent risk factor for diabetes (OR 1.73).[54] Rodríguez-Moran et al. showed that having a family history of diabetes among first-degree relatives (parents, offspring, and siblings) is a significant and independent risk factor for the prevalence of impaired fasting glucose (prediabetes) in children and adolescents (OR 11.7; 95% CI 9.5–21.2).[55] Additionally, Valdez et al. demonstrated that a family history of diabetes in at least two first-degree relatives or one first-degree relative and at least two second-degree relatives is a significant factor in the prevalence of T2DM.[56]

Importantly, the presence of a family history of diabetes can further strengthen the association between obesity and diabetes.[57] It highlights the interaction between genetic susceptibility and lifestyle factors, such as obesity, in the development of T2DM. The presence of a family history of diabetes, particularly in first-degree relatives, is strongly associated with the development of T2DM. Additionally, family history of diabetes underscores the relationship between obesity and T2DM.

In a comprehensive study led by van der Sande et al., the researchers delved into the profound impact of family history in high-risk groups for major noncommunicable diseases (NCDs) on the development of these conditions among family members. The study took into account the influential role of strong community and family coherence as critical determinants that needed consideration when advocating for lifestyle changes aimed at preventing these diseases. The research findings unveiled compelling insights into the relationships between family history and various health conditions.[58]

The study revealed that a family history of hypertension, obesity, diabetes, or stroke was indeed a significant risk factor for the onset of obesity among family members. It was discovered that individuals with a family history of obesity faced an elevated risk of becoming obese themselves. Furthermore, those with a family history of hypertension exhibited higher diastolic BP and elevated BMI, coupled with increased cholesterol and uric acid concentrations. These findings underscored the heightened susceptibility to obesity in individuals with a family history of hypertension. Additionally, the study delved into the correlation between family history and stroke. Subjects with a family history of stroke displayed an elevated BMI, along with increased levels of cholesterol, triglycerides, and uric acid. These findings collectively emphasized the far-reaching impact of family history on health outcomes, particularly in the context of obesity and related health conditions.[58]

In another case-control study conducted in Spain, it was found that a family history of obesity is a significant predictive factor for childhood obesity. The study reported an OR of 4.18 indicating a strong association between a family history of obesity and the likelihood of a child developing obesity. This finding underscores the considerable influence of familial factors in shaping the risk of childhood obesity and highlights the importance of considering family history when addressing and preventing obesity in children.[59]

Physical Inactivity

Over the past two decades, numerous prospective studies have provided strong evidence supporting the association between daily physical activity and a decreased risk of developing T2DM. These studies, conducted in various countries such as the UK, Japan, Finland, and Germany, have consistently demonstrated a reduction in the RR of developing T2DM ranging from 15 to 60% with increased levels of daily physical activity **(Table 3)**.[60-65]

In addition to these observational studies, clinical trials focusing on lifestyle modifications have further reinforced the positive impact of physical activity on T2DM prevention. These trials have shown that incorporating physical activity along with dietary modifications can effectively reduce the incidence of T2DM. The combined approach of regular exercise and healthy eating has been found to be particularly beneficial in lowering the risk of developing this metabolic disorder.[60-65]

The cumulative evidence from both prospective studies and clinical trials underscores the importance of daily physical activity in mitigating the risk of T2DM. These findings highlight the potential of lifestyle interventions, including increased physical activity and improved dietary habits, in preventing the onset of T2DM and promoting overall health and well-being.[2] Physical activity is a highly variable component of total energy expenditure, accounting for approximately 20–50% of the total. Interestingly, when analyzing physical activity levels across groups with different BMI ranges (<20, 20–25, and 25–35), there appear to be similar levels of habitual physical activity. Measurements of energy expenditure within home environments, using doubly labeled water, also indicate comparable values when adjusted for differences in body size between obese and lean individuals. Cross-cultural studies examining the relationship between physical activity and BMI have revealed a striking finding: those with a low physical activity level ratio (total energy expenditure/RMR) of <1.8 have a seven-fold increased risk of being overweight (BMI > 25). In developed countries, a clear link exists between low physical activity levels and obesity.[2]

A longitudinal study conducted in Finland further emphasized the importance of physical activity. It revealed that individuals who engaged in physical exercise three or more times per week had, on average, experienced weight loss since a

TABLE 3: Prospective studies associate physical inactivity as a risk factor in type 2 diabetes mellitus patients.

Author; year; country	Participants (n)	Comments
Helmrich et al. 1991; USA[60]	5,990 men	Decreased in risk by 6% with every 500 kcal of leisure time physical activity
Perry et al. 1995; UK[62]	7,735 men	Decreased in risk by 60% in moderately active men versus inactive men
Hu et al. 1999; USA[61]	70,102 women	Decreased in risk by 26% in upper quintile versus lower of physical activity
Nakanishi et al. 2004; Japan[63]	2,924 men	Decreased in risk by 59% in upper quintile versus lower of physical activity
Hu et al. 2004; Finland[64]	2,017 men and 2,352 women	Decreased in risk by 15 and 57% in moderate and high versus low physical activity
Meisinger et al. 2005; Germany[65]	4,069 men and 4,034 women	Decreased in risk by 13, 30, and 76% in low, moderate, and high versus no physical activity

previous survey. In contrast, those with minimal physical activity gained weight and had double the risk of gaining 5 kg or more. Notably, Finland has seen a decline in physical activity at work and during transportation over the past decade, which has coincided with a significant increase in leisure time. Among children in the United States, the risk of obesity is 5.3 times higher for those who watch television for 5 hours or more daily compared to children who watch <2 hours, even after adjusting for various socioeconomic factors.[2]

In a cross-sectional electronic health survey (E-MOVO) involving >35,000 Dutch adolescents, aged either 13-14 years (grade 2) or 15-16 years (grade 4) and attending secondary educational schools, the study found that physical inactivity was significantly associated with overweight. This association was particularly pronounced among younger adolescents, suggesting that the link between physical inactivity and overweight is more prominent in this age group compared to older adolescents.[66]

Two to Tango: Obesity and Type 2 Diabetes Mellitus

Obesity (specifically abdominal fat), contributes to inflammation and disrupts the function of beta cells, leading to decreased insulin sensitivity and insulin resistance, which is a key factor in the development of T2DM.[24]

Ishikawa-Takata et al. found that the risk of diabetes significantly increases in individuals with a BMI >29 kg/m^2. Subjects with BMI between 27 and 29 kg/m^2 had a two-fold higher RR than subjects with BMI < 18.5 kg/m^2, and the risk was dramatically increased to almost seven-fold in subjects with BMI of >29 kg/m^2.[67] Additionally, the association between obesity and the incidence of diabetes is influenced by gender. For every 2 kg/m^2 decrease in BMI, men have a 23% lower risk of diabetes (15–30%), while women have a 27% lower risk (23–32%). Ethnicity also plays a role, with Asians having a 37% lower risk (26–46%) and Australians having a 25% lower risk (21–29%) of diabetes for every 2 kg/m^2 decrease in BMI. Central obesity, which refers to excess fat around the abdomen, has been found to be strongly associated with the risk of T2DM compared to overall obesity.[68] Ohnishi et al. reported a higher risk of T2DM in individuals with central obesity (RR 2.07), particularly in elderly individuals over 60 years old (OR 3.8). The association between central obesity and diabetes is significant in both men and women, but women with central obesity have a higher risk (OR 2.875) compared to men (OR 2.308).[69-71] Furthermore, the prevalence of T2DM in individuals with central obesity is influenced by ethnicity. Non-Hispanic women with central obesity have a higher risk (OR 15.1) compared to Hispanic women (OR 1.6). Centrally obese Hispanic men also face a higher risk (OR 2.1), whereas no such association is observed in centrally obese non-Hispanic men. It should be noted that different studies use varying definitions of central obesity, such as waist circumference cutoffs, making it challenging to draw conclusive associations.[72]

In summary, obesity is a significant predictor of T2DM, but the association is influenced by gender and ethnicity. Women with a high BMI have a greater risk of diabetes compared to men, and the association is stronger in Asians compared to Australians. Central obesity is also strongly associated with the prevalence of T2DM, particularly in non-Hispanic women. However, further studies are needed to establish a consistent criterion for defining central obesity and examining its association with T2DM. Obesity is a prominent risk factor for the incidence of T2DM, with a stronger association observed in women compared to men.

REFERENCES

1. World Health Organization. (2021). Obesity and Overweight. [online] Available from https://www.who.int/news-room/fact-sheets/detail/obesity-and-overweight. [Last accessed October, 2023].
2. Wright SM, Aronne LJ. Causes of obesity. Abdom Imaging. 2012;37(5):730-2.
3. McAllister EJ, Dhurandhar NV, Keith SW, Aronne LJ, Barger J, Baskin M, et al. Ten putative contributors to the obesity epidemic. Crit Rev Food Sci Nutr. 2009;49(10):868-913.
4. Lois K, Kumar S. Obesity and diabetes. Endocrinol Nutr. 2009;56(Suppl 4):38-42.
5. Verma S, Hussain ME. Obesity and diabetes: An update. Diabetes Metab Syndr. 2017;11(1):73-9.
6. International Diabetes Federation. IDF Diabetes Atlas, 10th edition. Brussels, Belgium: International Diabetes Federation; 2021.
7. Pereira SS, Alvarez-Leite JI. Low-Grade Inflammation, Obesity, and Diabetes. Curr Obes Rep. 2014;3(4):422-31.
8. Chooi YC, Ding C, Magkos F. The epidemiology of obesity. Metabolism. 2019;92:6-10.
9. WHO Expert Consultation. Appropriate body-mass index for Asian populations and its implications for policy and intervention strategies. Lancet. 2004;363(9403):157-63.
10. National Institute for Health and Clinical Excellence. (2013). BMI: preventing ill health and premature death in black, Asian and other minority ethnic groups. [online] Available from https://www.nice.org.uk/guidance/ph46. [Last accessed October, 2023].
11. Caleyachetty R, Barber TM, Mohammed NI, Cappuccio FP, Hardy R, Mathur R, et al. Ethnicity-specific BMI cutoffs for obesity based on type 2 diabetes risk in England: a population-based cohort study. Lancet Diabetes Endocrinol. 2021;9(7):419-26.
12. Chiu M, Austin PC, Manuel DG, Shah BR, Tu JV. Deriving ethnic-specific BMI cutoff points for assessing diabetes risk. Diabetes Care. 2011;34(8):1741-8.
13. Ntuk UE, Gill JM, Mackay DF, Sattar N, Pell JP. Ethnic-specific obesity cutoffs for diabetes risk: cross-sectional study of 490,288 UK biobank participants. Diabetes Care. 2014;37(9):2500-7.
14. Razak F, Anand SS, Shannon H, Vuksan V, Davis B, Jacobs R, et al. Defining obesity cut points in a multiethnic population. Circulation. 2007;115(16):2111-8.
15. Tillin T, Sattar N, Godsland IF, Hughes AD, Chaturvedi N, Forouhi NG. Ethnicity-specific obesity cut-points in the development of Type 2 diabetes—a prospective study including three ethnic groups in the United Kingdom. Diabet Med. 2015;32(2):226-34.
16. Vicks WS, Lo JC, Guo L, Rana JS, Zhang S, Ramalingam ND, et al. Prevalence of prediabetes and diabetes vary by ethnicity among U.S. Asian adults at healthy weight, overweight, and obesity ranges: an electronic health record study. BMC Public Health. 2022;22(1):1954.
17. Jih J, Mukherjea A, Vittinghoff E, Nguyen TT, Tsoh JY, Fukuoka Y, et al. Using appropriate body mass index cut points for overweight and obesity among Asian Americans. Prev Med. 2014;65:1-6.
18. Oza-Frank R, Ali MK, Vaccarino V, Narayan KM. Asian Americans: diabetes prevalence across U.S. and World Health Organization weight classifications. Diabetes Care. 2009;32(9):1644-6.
19. Chan K, De Souza LR, Kobayashi K, Fuller-Thomson E. Diabetes and diabetes care among non-obese South Asian Americans: Findings from a population-based study. Diabetes Metab Syndr. 2019;13(1):96-102.
20. Hsu WC, Araneta MR, Kanaya AM, Chiang JL, Fujimoto W. BMI cut points to identify at-risk Asian Americans for type 2 diabetes screening. Diabetes Care. 2015;38(1):150-8.
21. Fuller-Thomson E, Roy A, Tsz-Kit Chan K, Kobayashi KM. Diabetes among non-obese Filipino Americans: Findings from a large population-based study. Can J Public Health. 2017;108(1):e36-42.
22. Gupta LS, Wu CC, Young S, Perlman SE. Prevalence of diabetes in New York City, 2002-2008: comparing foreign-born South Asians and other Asians with U.S.-born whites, blacks, and Hispanics. Diabetes Care. 2011;34(8):1791-3.
23. Iyen B, Vinogradova Y, Akyea RK, Weng S, Qureshi N, Kai J. Ethnic disparities in mortality among overweight or obese adults with newly diagnosed type 2 diabetes: a population-based cohort study. J Endocrinol Invest. 2022;45(5):1011-20.

24. Ismail L, Materwala H, Al Kaabi J. Association of risk factors with type 2 diabetes: A systematic review. Comput Struct Biotechnol J. 2021;19:1759-85.
25. Lin X, Xu Y, Pan X, Xu J, Ding Y, Sun X, et al. Global, regional, and national burden and trend of diabetes in 195 countries and territories: an analysis from 1990 to 2025. Sci Rep. 2020;10(1):14790.
26. Jaacks LM, Siegel KR, Gujral UP, Narayan KM. Type 2 diabetes: A 21st century epidemic. Best Pract Res Clin Endocrinol Metab. 2016;30(3):331-43.
27. Alberti KG, Zimmet P, Shaw J. International Diabetes Federation: a consensus on Type 2 diabetes prevention. Diabet Med. 2007;24(5):451-63.
28. Dallo FJ, Weller SC. Effectiveness of diabetes mellitus screening recommendations. Proc Natl Acad Sci U S A. 2003;100(18):10574-9.
29. Valdez R. Detecting undiagnosed type 2 diabetes: family history as a risk factor and screening tool. J Diabetes Sci Technol. 2009;3(4):722-6.
30. Malandrino N, Smith RJ. Personalized medicine in diabetes. Clin Chem. 2011;57(2):231-40.
31. Moltke I, Grarup N, Jørgensen ME, Bjerregaard P, Treebak JT, Fumagalli M, et al. A common Greenlandic TBC1D4 variant confers muscle insulin resistance and type 2 diabetes. Nature. 2014;512(7513):190-3.
32. Kopelman PG. Obesity as a medical problem. Nature. 2000;404(6778):635-43.
33. Mallon L, Broman JE, Hetta J. High incidence of diabetes in men with sleep complaints or short sleep duration: a 12-year follow-up study of a middle-aged population. Diabetes Care. 2005;28(11):2762-7.
34. Xu Q, Song Y, Hollenbeck A, Blair A, Schatzkin A, Chen H. Day napping and short night sleeping are associated with higher risk of diabetes in older adults. Diabetes Care. 2010;33(1):78-83.
35. Meisinger C, Heier M, Loewel H; MONICA/KORA Augsburg Cohort Study. Sleep disturbance as a predictor of type 2 diabetes mellitus in men and women from the general population. Diabetologia. 2005;48(2):235-41.
36. Bonanno L, Metro D, Papa M, Finzi G, Maviglia A, Sottile F, et al. Assessment of sleep and obesity in adults and children: Observational study. Medicine (Baltimore). 2019;98(46):e17642.
37. Will JC, Galuska DA, Ford ES, Mokdad A, Calle EE. Cigarette smoking and diabetes mellitus: evidence of a positive association from a large prospective cohort study. Int J Epidemiol. 2001;30(3):540-6.
38. Jee SH, Foong AW, Hur NW, Samet JM. Smoking and risk for diabetes incidence and mortality in Korean men and women. Diabetes Care. 2010;33(12):2567-72.
39. Wannamethee SG, Shaper AG, Perry IJ; British Regional Heart Study. Smoking as a modifiable risk factor for type 2 diabetes in middle-aged men. Diabetes Care. 2001;24(9):1590-5.
40. Kowall B, Rathmann W, Strassburger K, Heier M, Holle R, Thorand B, et al. Association of passive and active smoking with incident type 2 diabetes mellitus in the elderly population: the KORA S4/F4 cohort study. Eur J Epidemiol. 2010;25(6):393-402.
41. Dare S, Mackay DF, Pell JP. Relationship between smoking and obesity: a cross-sectional study of 499,504 middle-aged adults in the UK general population. PLoS One. 2015;10(4):e0123579.
42. Meyer KA, Kushi LH, Jacobs DR Jr, Folsom AR. Dietary fat and incidence of type 2 diabetes in older Iowa women. Diabetes Care. 2001;24(9):1528-35.
43. Tajima R, Kodama S, Hirata M, Horikawa C, Fujihara K, Yachi Y, et al. High cholesterol intake is associated with elevated risk of type 2 diabetes mellitus—a meta-analysis. Clin Nutr. 2014;33(6):946-50.
44. Besseling J, Kastelein JJ, Defesche JC, Hutten BA, Hovingh GK. Association between familial hypercholesterolemia and prevalence of type 2 diabetes mellitus. JAMA. 2015;313(10):1029-36.
45. Zhang N, Hu X, Zhang Q, Bai P, Cai M, Zeng TS, et al. Non-high-density lipoprotein cholesterol: High-density lipoprotein cholesterol ratio is an independent risk factor for diabetes mellitus: Results from a population-based cohort study. J Diabetes. 2018;10(9):708-14.
46. Feingold KR. Obesity and Dyslipidemia. South Dartmouth (MA): MDText.com, Inc.; 2023.
47. Howard BV, Ruotolo G, Robbins DC. Obesity and dyslipidemia. Endocrinol Metab Clin North Am. 2003;32(4):855-67.
48. Hayashi T, Tsumura K, Suematsu C, Endo G, Fujii S, Okada K. High normal blood pressure, hypertension, and the risk of type 2 diabetes in Japanese men. The Osaka Health Survey. Diabetes Care. 1999;22(10):1683-7.
49. Gress TW, Nieto FJ, Shahar E, Wofford MR, Brancati FL. Hypertension and antihypertensive therapy as risk factors for type 2 diabetes mellitus. Atherosclerosis Risk in Communities Study. N Engl J Med. 2000;342(13):905-12.
50. Conen D, Ridker PM, Mora S, Buring JE, Glynn RJ. Blood pressure and risk of developing type 2 diabetes mellitus: the Women's Health Study. Eur Heart J. 2007;28(23):2937-43.

51. Kim MJ, Lim NK, Choi SJ, Park HY. Hypertension is an independent risk factor for type 2 diabetes: the Korean genome and epidemiology study. Hypertens Res. 2015;38(11):783-9.
52. Narkiewicz K. Obesity and hypertension--the issue is more complex than we thought. Nephrol Dial Transplant. 2006;21(2):264-7.
53. Tsenkova VK, Karlamangla AS, Ryff CD. Parental History of Diabetes, Positive Affect, and Diabetes Risk in Adults: Findings from MIDUS. Ann Behav Med. 2016;50(6):836-43.
54. Burchfiel CM, Curb JD, Rodriguez BL, Yano K, Hwang LJ, Fong KO, et al. Incidence and predictors of diabetes in Japanese-American men. The Honolulu Heart Program. Ann Epidemiol. 1995;5(1):33-43.
55. Rodríguez-Moran M, Guerrero-Romero F, Aradillas-García C, Violante R, Simental-Mendia LE, Monreal-Escalante E, et al. Obesity and family history of diabetes as risk factors of impaired fasting glucose: implications for the early detection of prediabetes. Pediatr Diabetes. 2010;11(5):331-6.
56. Valdez R, Yoon PW, Liu T, Khoury MJ. Family history and prevalence of diabetes in the U.S. population: the 6-year results from the National Health and Nutrition Examination Survey (1999-2004). Diabetes Care. 2007;30(10): 2517-22.
57. Sargeant LA, Wareham NJ, Khaw KT. Family history of diabetes identifies a group at increased risk for the metabolic consequences of obesity and physical inactivity in EPIC-Norfolk: a population-based study. The European Prospective Investigation into Cancer. Int J Obes Relat Metab Disord. 2000;24(10):1333-9.
58. van der Sande MA, Walraven GE, Milligan PJ, Banya WA, Ceesay SM, Nyan OA, et al. Family history: an opportunity for early interventions and improved control of hypertension, obesity and diabetes. Bull World Health Organ. 2001;79(4):321-8.
59. Ochoa MC, Moreno-Aliaga MJ, Martínez-González MA, Martínez JA, Marti A; GENOI Members. Predictor factors for childhood obesity in a Spanish case-control study. Nutrition. 2007;23(5):379-84.
60. Helmrich SP, Ragland DR, Leung RW, Paffenbarger RS Jr. Physical activity and reduced occurrence of non-insulin-dependent diabetes mellitus. N Engl J Med. 1991;325(3):147-52.
61. Hu FB, Sigal RJ, Rich-Edwards JW, Colditz GA, Solomon CG, Willett WC, et al. Walking compared with vigorous physical activity and risk of type 2 diabetes in women: a prospective study. JAMA. 1999;282(15):1433-9.
62. Perry IJ, Wannamethee SG, Walker MK, Thomson AG, Whincup PH, Shaper AG. Prospective study of risk factors for development of non-insulin dependent diabetes in middle aged British men. BMJ. 1995;310(6979):560-4.
63. Nakanishi N, Takatorige T, Suzuki K. Daily life activity and risk of developing impaired fasting glucose or type 2 diabetes in middle-aged Japanese men. Diabetologia. 2004;47(10):1768-75.
64. Hu G, Lindstrom J, Valle TT, Eriksson JG, Jousilahti P, Silventoinen K, et al. Physical activity, body mass index, and risk of type 2 diabetes in patients with normal or impaired glucose regulation. Arch Intern Med. 2004;164(8): 892-6.
65. Meisinger C, Lowel H, Thorand B, Doring A. Leisure time physical activity and the risk of type 2 diabetes in men and women from the general population. The MONICA/KORA Augsburg Cohort Study. Diabetologia. 2005;48(1):27-34.
66. Croezen S, Visscher TL, Ter Bogt NC, Veling ML, Haveman-Nies A. Skipping breakfast, alcohol consumption and physical inactivity as risk factors for overweight and obesity in adolescents: results of the E-MOVO project. Eur J Clin Nutr. 2009;63(3):405-12.
67. Ishikawa-Takata K, Ohta T, Moritaki K, Gotou T, Inoue S. Obesity, weight change and risks for hypertension, diabetes and hypercholesterolemia in Japanese men. Eur J Clin Nutr. 2002;56(7):601-7.
68. Asia Pacific Cohort Studies Collaboration, Ni Mhurchu C, Parag V, Nakamura M, Patel A, Rodgers A, Lam TH. Body mass index and risk of diabetes mellitus in the Asia-Pacific region. Asia Pac J Clin Nutr. 2006;15(2):127-33.
69. Ohnishi H, Saitoh S, Takagi S, Katoh N, Chiba Y, Akasaka H, et al. Incidence of type 2 diabetes in individuals with central obesity in a rural Japanese population: The Tanno and Sobetsu study. Diabetes Care. 2006;29(5):1128-9.
70. Hadaegh F, Zabetian A, Harati H, Azizi F. The prospective association of general and central obesity variables with incident type 2 diabetes in adults, Tehran lipid and glucose study. Diabetes Res Clin Pract. 2007;76(3):449-54.
71. He YH, Jiang GX, Yang Y, Huang HE, Li R, Li XY, et al. Obesity and its associations with hypertension and type 2 diabetes among Chinese adults age 40 years and over. Nutrition. 2009;25(11-12):1143-9.
72. Bermudez OI, Tucker KL. Total and central obesity among elderly Hispanics and the association with Type 2 diabetes. Obes Res. 2001;9(8):443-51.

CHAPTER 2

Obesity and Diabetes Pathophysiology

> **Key Highlights**
> - The pathogenesis of obesity and type 2 diabetes mellitus (T2DM) is predominantly driven by the synergistic effects of genetic susceptibility and environmental factors, which intricately interplay to amplify the development of these conditions.
> - The metabolic microenvironment undergoes significant remodeling and reshaping in obesity, leading to a marked attenuation of insulin signaling and promoting the progressive elevation of blood glucose.
> - These alterations are driven by the detrimental accumulation of specific nutrients and metabolites, persistent low-grade inflammation, impaired autophagy, and disrupted energy balance, all of which stem from dysregulation of the microbiome–gut–brain axis.
> - The systemic reprogramming of immunometabolism and the local toxicity inflicted on the pancreas, leading to reduced functional beta cell numbers, primarily result from the extensive ectopic expansion of adipose tissue (AT).
> - Disruption of the normal physical interaction between beta and alpha cells in pancreatic islets is alleged to be a contributing factor in dysregulation of glucagon secretion in individuals with diabetes.
> - Increased expression of adipocytokines such as resistin, vaspin, apelin, and tumor necrosis factor alpha (TNF-α) has been associated with the development of insulin resistance, which is closely linked to obesity and T2DM.

INTRODUCTION

Obesity is strongly associated with glucose intolerance and type 2 diabetes mellitus (T2DM). Several studies have demonstrated the correlation between increasing body mass index (BMI) and the incidence of impaired fasting glucose and T2DM in both men and women.[1] The Coronary Artery Risk Development in

Young Adults study found that higher BMI was associated with an increased risk of T2DM in women. The study followed a cohort of over 100,000 nurses for 14 years and revealed that women with a BMI of 24.0–24.9 kg/m² had five times the risk of T2DM compared to women with a BMI of <22 kg/m². The risk of T2DM further increased to 40 times and 93 times in women with a BMI greater than 31 kg/m² and 35 kg/m², respectively.[2] Similar findings were observed in a study involving male health professionals. Men with a BMI greater than 35 kg/m² had 42 times the risk of developing T2DM compared to men with a BMI of <23 kg/m². This study also highlighted that BMI at age 21 years and absolute weight gain were independent risk factors for T2DM.[3] Another study conducted by Schienkiewitz et al. revealed that weight gain during early adulthood (between ages 25 and 40 years) was associated with a higher risk of T2DM compared to weight gain during late adulthood (between ages 40 and 55 years). Additionally, individuals who experienced weight gain in both early and late adulthood had a relative risk of T2DM greater than 14 times compared to those who maintained their BMI.[4] These findings emphasize the strong association between obesity, BMI, and the risk of developing T2DM in both men and women.

The consequences of obesity are not limited to simple weight gain but extend to various metabolic disorders, with T2DM being strongly associated with obesity. The development and progression of T2DM are characterized by hyperglycemia caused by reduced insulin sensitivity and a decline in functional beta cell mass. Obesity plays a significant role in driving these processes, contributing to genetic and epigenetic vulnerabilities, microenvironmental changes that impair insulin signaling, compromised beta cell function, and dysregulated microbiome-gut–brain axis (**Fig. 1**). However, it is important to note that T2DM can also manifest inversely, occurring before the onset of obesity in certain individuals who have inherent insulin resistance. In these cases, increased hepatic glucose production (HGP) and elevated insulin levels are the primary culprits behind obesity development. Therefore, the relationship between obesity and T2DM is complex, involving a bidirectional influence where obesity can contribute to T2DM development, but T2DM can also precede obesity in certain individuals with underlying insulin resistance.[5]

INSULIN SIGNALING, INSULIN RESISTANCE IN OBESITY, AND TYPE 2 DIABETES MELLITUS

Insulin Signaling

Insulin exerts its intracellular functions through the activation of insulin receptor tyrosine kinase (IRTK). Upon binding of insulin to the extracellular domain of IRTK, a conformational change occurs, leading to the autophosphorylation of tyrosine residues within IRTK. This autophosphorylation event triggers the activation of various phosphotyrosine-binding proteins, including insulin receptor substrate (IRS), growth factor receptor-bound protein-2 (GRB-2), GRB-10, SHC-transforming protein (SHC), and SH2B adapter protein-2 (SH2B-2).[6] The effects of insulin on glucose and lipid metabolism primarily rely on the phosphorylation of IRS by IRTK. This phosphorylation event enables IRS to

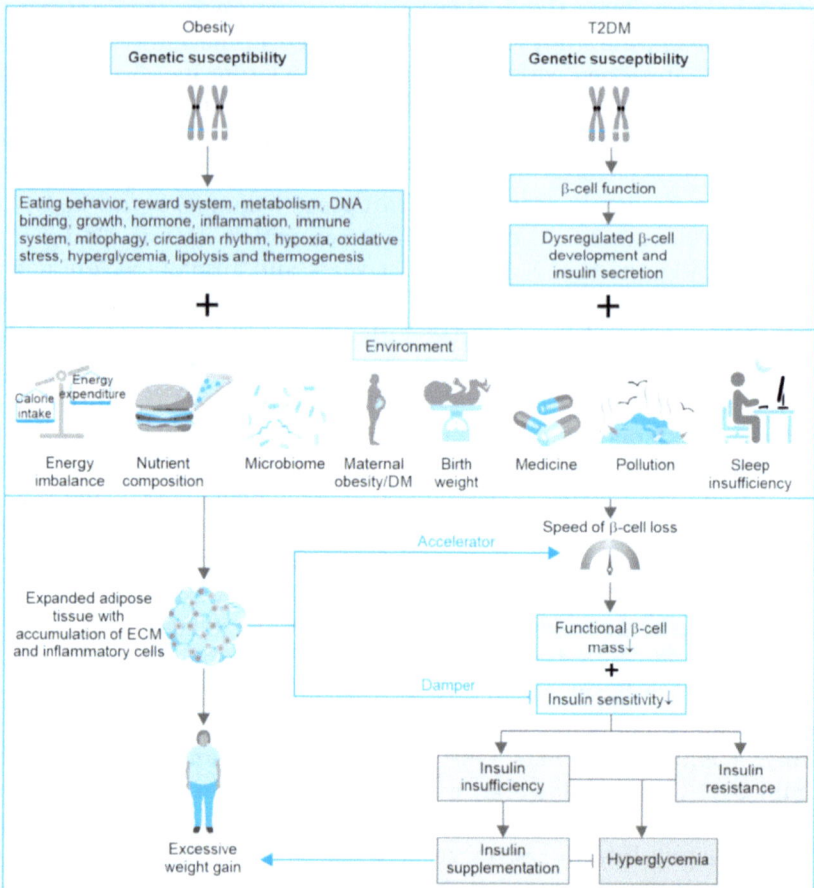

FIG. 1: Genetic and environmental factors affecting islet function and connecting obesity and type 2 diabetes mellitus (T2DM). Genetic and environmental factors play significant roles in the interplay between obesity and T2DM. Genetic factors primarily influence energy balance in obesity and impact the development and function of beta cells in T2DM. Environmental factors further contribute to the progression of obesity and exacerbate beta cell loss while impairing insulin signaling in T2DM. Additionally, the administration of insulin as a treatment for T2DM can potentially lead to weight gain. The colored arrows symbolize the dynamic interactions between obesity and T2DM, highlighting the complex relationship between these two conditions.

(ECM: extracellular matrix)

Source: With permission from Ruze et al. (2023).[5]

recruit phosphatidylinositol 3-kinase (PI3K), which catalyzes the conversion of phosphatidylinositol-4,5-bisphosphate (PIP2) to phosphatidylinositol-3,4,5-trisphosphate (PIP3). Subsequently, PIP3 recruits protein kinase B (Akt) to the plasma membrane, where it is phosphorylated and activated by 3-phosphoinositide-dependent kinase-1 (PDK1) and mechanistic target of rapamycin complex 2 (mTORC2). Akt then phosphorylates various downstream substrates in metabolic tissues, including skeletal muscle, liver, and adipose tissue (AT), leading to insulin-induced nutrient preservation in these tissues.[7]

In skeletal muscle, insulin signaling promotes glucose uptake and glycogen synthesis. Insulin enhances glucose transport activity through the coordinated translocation and fusion of glucose transporter type 4 (GLUT4) storage vesicles (GSVs) with the plasma membrane. Akt, when activated by insulin signaling, inactivates AS160 (TBC1D4), which controls vesicle trafficking by regulating small Rab GTPase protein switches. Additionally, insulin regulates glycogen phosphorylase activity by dephosphorylating phosphorylase kinase.[8,9]

In the liver, insulin activates IRTK, leading to the phosphorylation of IRS1 and IRS2 and subsequent activation of Akt2. This activation decreases HGP, promotes glycogen synthesis, and activates lipogenesis. The primary role of hepatic insulin signaling is to reduce HGP by inhibiting gluconeogenesis through Akt-mediated phosphorylation of forkhead box O1 (FOXO1). This phosphorylation excludes FOXO1 from the nucleus, preventing the transcriptional activation of gluconeogenic genes, such as glucose-6-phosphatase (*G6PC*) and phosphoenolpyruvate carboxykinase (*PEPCK*).[10,11] In addition to suppressing gluconeogenesis, insulin inhibits adipocyte lipolysis, reducing gluconeogenesis substrates in the liver.[12] Furthermore, insulin increases hepatic glycogen synthesis by regulating glycogen synthase (particularly GYS2 in the liver) and glycogen phosphorylase through glycogen synthase kinase 3 (GSK3) and PP1, similar to its actions in skeletal muscle.[13]

In AT, the primary physiological function of insulin is to inhibit lipolysis, thereby suppressing HGP by reducing gluconeogenic substrates **(Fig. 2)**. The

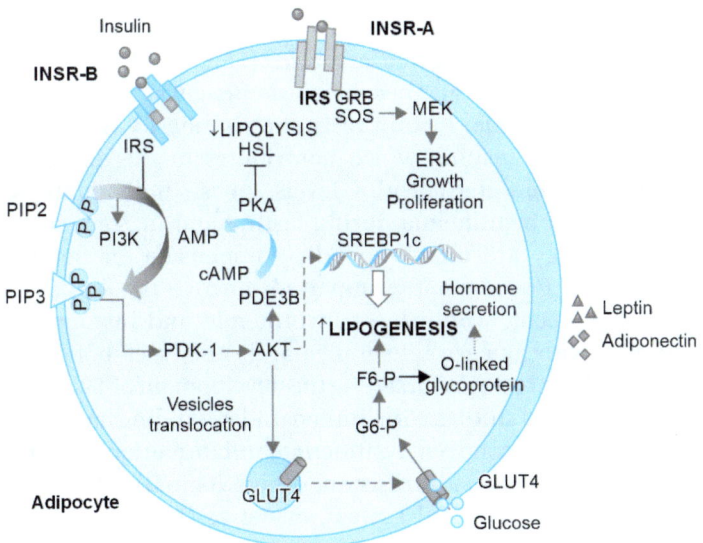

FIG. 2: Insulin action in adipocytes.

(AKT: protein kinase B; AMP: adenosine monophosphate; cAMP: cyclic adenosine monophosphate; ERK: extracellular signal-regulated kinase; F6-P: fructose 6-phosphate; GLUT4: glucose transporter type 4; GRB: growth factor receptor-bound protein; G6-P: glucose 6-phosphate; HSL: hormone-sensitive lipase; INSR-A: insulin receptor isoform A; INSR-B: insulin receptor isoform B; IRS: insulin receptor substrate; MEK: mitogen-activated protein kinase; PDE3B: phosphodiesterase 3B; PDK-1: phosphoinositide-dependent kinase 1; PIP2: phosphatidylinositol 4,5-bisphosphate; PIP3: phosphatidylinositol 3,4,5-triphosphate; PI3K: phosphatidylinositol 3-kinase; PKA: protein kinase A; SOS: son of sevenless protein; SREBP1c: sterol regulatory element-binding protein 1)

Source: With permission from Cignarelli et al. (2019).[14]

precise mechanism underlying insulin-induced lipolysis suppression is not yet fully elucidated, but it is thought to involve phosphodiesterase 3B (PDE3B) and decreased activity of cyclic adenosine monophosphate (cAMP)-dependent protein kinase A (PKA). Additionally, PP1 and PP2A are believed to mediate the PI3K-dependent insulin-induced suppression of lipolysis through dephosphorylation of lipolytic regulatory proteins.[23,24] While insulin promotes glucose transport by facilitating the phosphorylation of targets involved in vesicle tethering, docking, and fusion, its overall contribution to whole-body glucose disposal is relatively minor. Insulin also plays a role in promoting lipogenesis in white adipose tissue (WAT). It activates the transcription factor called sterol regulatory element-binding protein-1c (SREBP-1c), which leads to the translocation of glucose or fatty acid transport proteins (FATPs), promoting the uptake and esterification of fatty acids. Moreover, insulin stimulates adipogenesis, the process of generating new adipocytes, through the activation of the transcription factor peroxisome proliferator-activated receptor-γ (PPARγ).[14-16]

Obesity and Insulin Resistance

There is a strong association between obesity and insulin resistance, which is characterized by reduced responsiveness to insulin's effects. Obesity encompasses both subcutaneous and visceral adiposity, and the measurement commonly used to assess adiposity is BMI. In obese individuals, increased AT is closely related to elevated insulin levels and insulin resistance. It is proposed that greater lipolytic activity in the abdominal AT of individuals with increased abdominal adiposity leads to higher levels of circulating free fatty acids (FFAs).[17,18] Consequently, the liver increases triglyceride synthesis and becomes less efficient at breaking down insulin, resulting in hyperinsulinemia. Insulin resistance in obesity is also characterized by decreased binding of insulin, which contributes to the development of the condition.[19,20] Despite elevated insulin levels, obese individuals with insulin resistance exhibit hyperinsulinemia during fasting and in response to a glucose stimulus. However, they are unable to fully compensate for insulin resistance in peripheral tissues. Consequently, impaired glucose uptake and inadequate suppression of HGP occur.[21] Both hyperinsulinemia and insulin resistance are strongly associated with glucose intolerance and other metabolic abnormalities. Obesity plays a significant role in worsening the development of T2DM by promoting insulin resistance. Various studies with limited understanding have highlighted the connection between mitochondrial dysfunction, inflammation, hyperinsulinemia, and lipotoxicity in relation to insulin resistance **(Figs. 3A to D)**.[18] Additionally, factors such as endoplasmic reticulum (ER) stress, oxidative stress, genetic background, aging, hypoxia, and lipodystrophy have been implicated in the pathogenesis of T2DM by inducing insulin resistance.

Insulin resistance is characterized by the reduced responsiveness of certain tissues to normal insulin levels, necessitating higher insulin levels to maintain proper insulin function. In insulin-resistant tissues, the beneficial effects of insulin on glucose regulation, such as the inhibition of HGP, suppression of lipolysis, uptake of glucose into cells, and glycogen synthesis, are impaired even with normal levels of insulin in the bloodstream.[15] The balance between insulin and glucagon is crucial in the regulation of various metabolic pathways, as it determines the extent

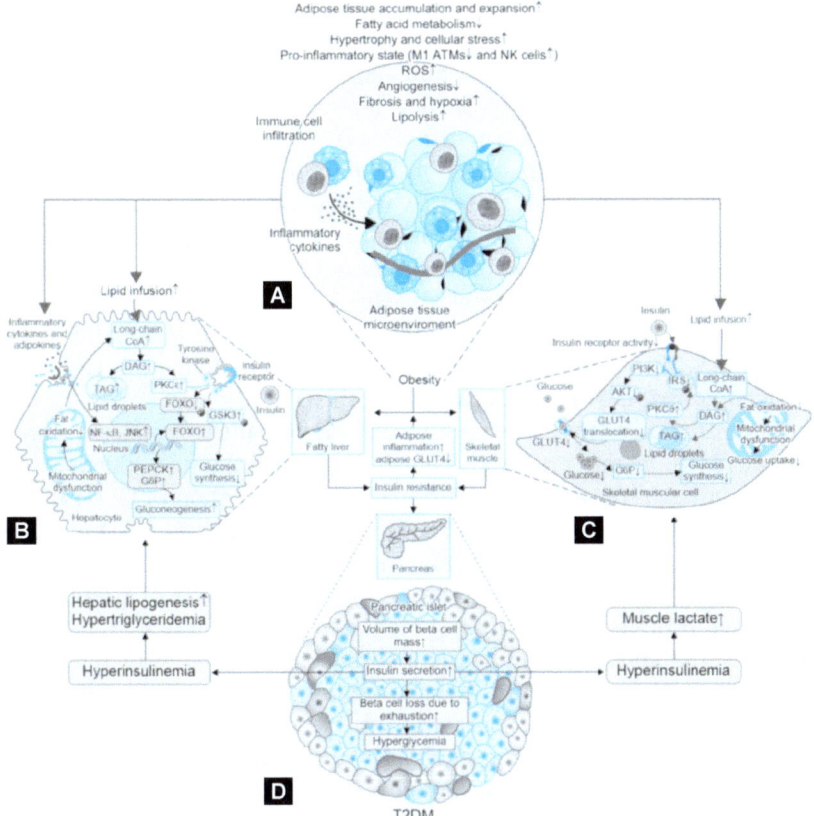

FIGS. 3A TO D: Obesity-induced insulin resistance contributes to a cascade of metabolic dysregulation. (A) In obesity, the abnormal accumulation and expansion of adipose tissue create a microenvironment characterized by impaired fatty acid metabolism, cellular stress, and inflammation. This leads to increased lipolysis, oxidative stress, and hypoxia due to fibrosis and inadequate blood vessel growth. (B) Within the liver, the excessive influx of fatty acids resulting from enhanced lipolysis in adipose tissue causes a temporary rise in diacylglycerol (DAG) levels. This occurs when DAG synthesis surpasses the capacity of mitochondrial long-chain CoA oxidation due to mitochondrial dysfunction. The elevated DAG is converted into triglycerides (TAG) and stored as lipid droplets. Additionally, DAG activates protein kinase C epsilon (PKCε), impairing insulin receptor signaling and reducing insulin-stimulated glycogen synthesis. It also inhibits glycogen synthase activity and promotes hepatic gluconeogenesis, further contributing to increased glucose production. (C) In skeletal muscle, increased lipid accumulation and reduced fat oxidation, attributed to mitochondrial dysfunction, lead to elevated intracellular long-chain CoA and DAG levels. Similar to the liver, DAG activates protein kinase C theta (PKCθ), which impairs insulin signaling and decreases glucose uptake and glycogen synthesis. These effects hinder the proper transport and utilization of glucose by skeletal muscle. (D) While obesity-induced insulin resistance exacerbates inflammation and impairs glucose transport in adipose tissue, the pancreatic beta cell mass expands to meet the increased demand for insulin secretion. However, the sustained elevation in insulin levels leads to hyperinsulinemia, which further exacerbates lipid accumulation in both the liver and systemic circulation. Hyperinsulinemia also stimulates lactate production in muscles, which is released into the bloodstream and used as a substrate for hepatic lipogenesis. Ultimately, the pancreatic beta cells become overwhelmed, leading to their dysfunction and insufficient insulin secretion, resulting in hyperglycemia.

[AKT: protein kinase B; ATM: adipose tissue macrophage; CoA: acetyl coenzyme A; FOXO: forkhead box subgroup O; G6P: glucose 6-phosphate; GLUT4: glucose transporter type 4; GSK3: glycogen synthase kinase 3; IRS-1: insulin receptor substrate 1; JNK: c-Jun N-terminal kinase; NF-κB: nuclear factor kappa B; NK: natural killer (cell); P: phosphorylation; PEPCK: phosphoenolpyruvate carboxykinase; PI3K: phosphatidylinositol 3-kinase; ROS: reactive oxygen species]

Source: With permission from Ruze et al. (2023).[5]

of phosphorylation of downstream enzymes involved in signaling pathways. While catecholamines promote lipolysis and glycogenolysis, glucocorticoids stimulate muscle breakdown, gluconeogenesis, and lipolysis. Therefore, excessive secretion of these hormones can contribute to the development of insulin resistance.[22] Insulin resistance or insulin-deficient conditions can be broadly classified into three categories: (1) reduced insulin secretion by pancreatic beta cells, (2) presence of insulin antagonists in the bloodstream, which can be counterregulatory hormones or nonhormonal factors that impair insulin receptors (IRs) or signaling, and (3) impaired insulin responsiveness in target tissues.[23] Among these categories, three key extrapancreatic organs—skeletal muscle, AT, and liver—play significant roles in the aforementioned processes and are highly sensitive to insulin. Defects in insulin action within these tissues often precede systemic insulin resistance and progressively contribute to the development of T2DM.

Insulin resistance in skeletal muscle significantly impacts whole-body metabolism as it is the primary site for insulin-stimulated glucose uptake.[24] Molecular studies have revealed that impaired translocation of GLUT4, a glucose transporter, to the plasma membrane is a key factor in insulin resistance affecting muscle glucose uptake. However, in individuals with T2DM, the translocation of GLUT4 and glucose transport can be stimulated by hypoxia or exercise through AMP-activated protein kinase (AMPK)-mediated regulation of GSV translocation. This suggests that abnormalities in the insulin signaling pathway, rather than the transport system itself, contribute to glucose transport defects in insulin resistance. Moreover, insulin resistance in skeletal muscle can result from defects at the proximal level of insulin signaling, such as impaired activities of IRTK, IRS1, PI3K, and Akt **(Fig. 3C)**.[5,15] Studies have shown reduced IRS1 tyrosine phosphorylation and diminished IRS1-associated PI3K activity in insulin-resistant skeletal muscle.[15]

Adipose tissue, a metabolically active tissue, plays a crucial role in regulating metabolic homeostasis at a systemic level. It participates in various biological processes including immunity, coagulation, angiogenesis, fibrinolysis, reproduction, vascular tone control, appetite regulation, body weight homeostasis, and glucose and lipid metabolism.[25,26] Impaired response to insulin stimulation in AT, known as adipose insulin resistance, leads to impaired suppression of lipolysis, reduced glucose uptake, and increased release of FFAs into the bloodstream, even in the presence of high insulin levels.[5,15] Among the signaling elements affected by adipose-insulin resistance, defective activation of Akt hinders GLUT4 translocation to the membrane and enhances the activity of lipolytic enzymes, further exacerbating hyperglycemia.[27] Adipose–insulin resistance is associated with glucose intolerance and elevated release of FFAs into the bloodstream, which can accumulate in other tissues like muscle or liver. In the case of the liver, increased FFA accumulation impairs insulin signaling, promotes hepatic gluconeogenesis, and disrupts the glucose-stimulated insulin response, ultimately contributing to the development of T2DM.[5,15] **Figure 3A** illustrates the effects of insulin stimulation on hypertrophic AT.

The liver plays a critical role in regulating postprandial carbohydrate levels by suppressing HGP and promoting the storage of glucose as glycogen. During fasting, the liver is the primary source of glucose production.[28] In patients with T2DM, insulin fails to regulate hepatic glycogen synthesis or glucose production, resulting in increased hepatic gluconeogenesis and fasting hyperglycemia.[29] Defective suppression of hepatic gluconeogenesis in insulin resistance is primarily associated with abnormalities in AT lipolysis and the derepression of the FOXO1 transcription factor in the liver **(Fig. 3B)**. Additionally, insulin resistance is linked to impaired insulin-induced stimulation of glycogen synthesis, as evidenced by lower fasting and postprandial hepatic glycogen content in T2DM patients.[28,30]

ROLE OF ADIPOSE TISSUE AND INFLAMMATION

Molecular Pathways Linking Obesity-induced Inflammation and Insulin Resistance

Systemic inflammation is characterized by elevated levels of inflammatory mediators in the bloodstream and the infiltration of immune cells into insulin-dependent tissues. The initiation of low-grade systemic inflammation primarily occurs in WAT, as discussed earlier in this chapter. In obesity, the accumulation of lipids in AT triggers an inflammatory response, leading to increased secretion of various inflammatory cytokines. These molecules can activate signaling pathways, such as c-Jun N-terminal kinase (JNK) and nuclear factor kappa B (NF-κB), in the liver and skeletal muscle, thereby inhibiting systemic insulin signaling. The inflammatory cascade initiated by obesity-induced inflammation originates in WAT and spreads to other tissues, causing low-grade systemic inflammation. Both the liver and skeletal muscle exhibit signs of local inflammation in the context of obesity **(Fig. 4)**.[31]

Studies in animals and humans have identified WAT as the main site where chronic inflammation associated with obesity is initiated and aggravated. Remodeling of AT during obesity generates numerous intrinsic and extrinsic signals capable of triggering an inflammatory response. Activation of the JNK and NF-κB signaling pathways enhances the production of pro-inflammatory cytokines, endothelial adhesion molecules, and chemotactic mediators, leading to the infiltration of monocytes into AT and their differentiation into pro-inflammatory M1 macrophages. These infiltrating macrophages secrete various inflammatory mediators that contribute to local and systemic pro-inflammatory conditions and impair insulin signaling **(Flowchart 1)**.[15,32,33]

The effects of these cytokines are mediated through the stimulation of inhibitor of κB (IκB) kinase beta (IKKβ) and *JNK1*, which are expressed in myeloid and insulin-targeted cells.[34-36] JNK has been extensively studied as a signal transducer in models of insulin resistance associated with obesity. It becomes activated in response to various inflammatory stimuli, including cytokines, FFAs, and activation of cellular pathways such as the unfolded protein response (UPR). Once activated, JNK initiates the transcription of pro-inflammatory genes and inhibits the insulin signaling pathway by serine–threonine phosphorylation of IRS-1, thereby reducing PI3K/PKB signaling.[34] Obesity is also linked to the activation of the NF-κB inflammatory pathway. Under normal physiological conditions, NF-κB proteins are retained in the cytoplasm of myeloid and insulin-targeted cells by a family of inhibitors known as inhibitors of κB. Activation of the IKK kinase complex (composed of IKKα and IKKβ subunits) leads to the degradation of IκBα

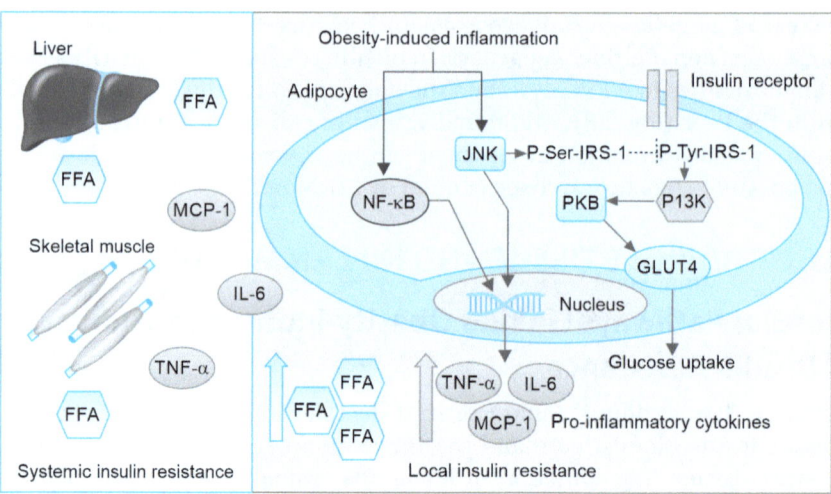

FIG. 4: Pathways linking local obesity-induced inflammation to systemic insulin resistance. The pathways connecting local obesity-induced inflammation to systemic insulin resistance involve the activation of inflammatory signaling pathways mediated by JNK and nuclear factor kappa B (NF-κB). In obesity, these pathways are triggered, leading to the production of pro-inflammatory cytokines in adipocytes, which contribute to insulin resistance and the infiltration of pro-inflammatory macrophages. The activation of the JNK signaling pathway initiates the transcription of pro-inflammatory genes and hinders the insulin signaling pathway by inhibitory serine phosphorylation of insulin receptor substrate-1 (IRS-1), thereby reducing the phosphatidylinositol 3-kinase (PI3K)/protein kinase B (PKB) signaling pathway. On the other hand, activation of the NF-κB signaling pathway results in the increased expression of several target genes, including tumor necrosis factor-α (TNF-α), interleukin-6 (IL-6), and monocyte chemotactic protein-1 (MCP-1), which leads to serine phosphorylation of IRS-1, ultimately impairing insulin signaling. These inflammatory mediators, such as free fatty acids (FFA), IL-6, TNF-α, and MCP-1, also circulate systemically and activate JNK and NF-κB signaling pathways in the liver and skeletal muscle, thereby inhibiting systemic insulin signaling.

(JNK: c-Jun N-terminal kinase; GLUT4: glucose transporter type 4; P-Tyr: tyrosine phosphorylation)

Source: With permission from Zatterale et al. (2020).[31]

via the proteasome, resulting in the nuclear translocation of NF-κB. This leads to increased expression of several NF-κB target genes, including interleukin-6 (IL-6), tumor necrosis factor alpha (TNF-α), interferon gamma (IFN-γ), transforming growth factor beta (TGF-β), monocyte chemotactic protein 1 (MCP-1), and IL-1β, which further exacerbate the progression of insulin resistance.[35] Macrophages play a significant role in mediating obesity-induced inflammation in AT. During obesity, macrophages infiltrate AT and secrete numerous pro-inflammatory cytokines. These mediators exert local effects on adipocytes and resident immune cells (such as neutrophils, B cells, and T cells) and circulate in the bloodstream, affecting insulin sensitivity in the liver and skeletal muscle.[36]

Obesity Induced at Inflammation Triggers

The precise mechanisms underlying obesity-induced inflammation in AT remain partially understood. However, several potential mechanisms have been identified,

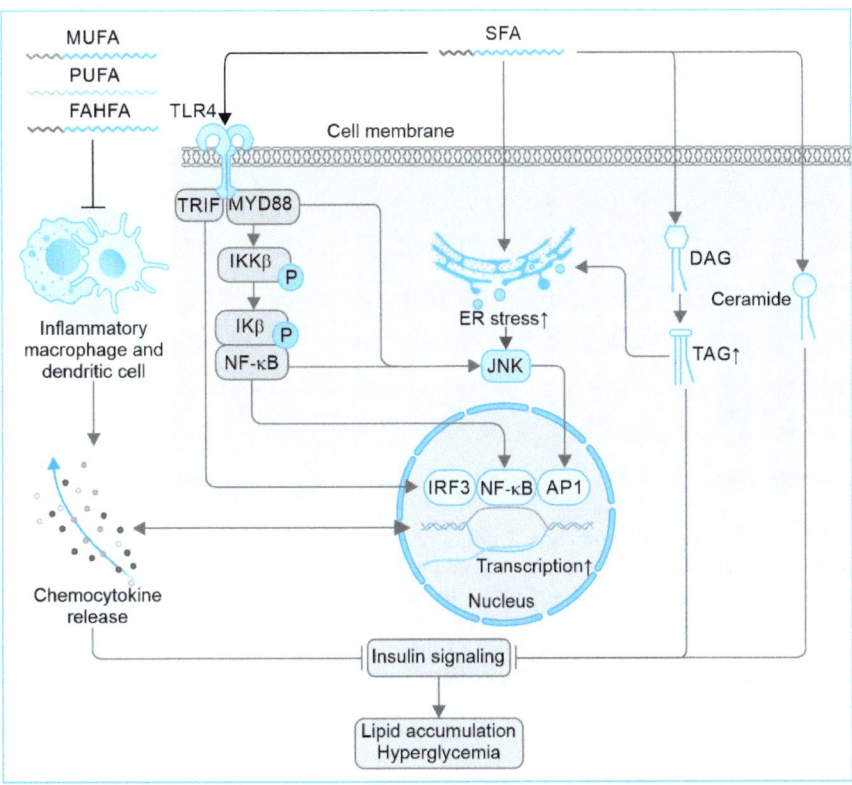

FLOWCHART 1: The mechanisms by which fatty acids affect insulin signaling and contribute to hyperglycemia. Contrary to the anti-inflammatory and insulin-sensitizing effects of PUFAs, MUFAs, and FAHFAs, SFAs hinder insulin sensitivity by promoting pro-inflammatory signaling through TLR4 and its adaptor proteins, such as TRIF and MYD88. This activation of TLR4 and its adaptors enhances the activity of pro-inflammatory pathways and transcription factors like IRF3, NF-κB, and AP1, resulting in increased expression of chemocytokines. Conversely, these pro-inflammatory chemocytokines can activate the same pro-inflammatory transcription factors, establishing a positive feedback loop that perpetuates an inflammatory environment detrimental to insulin signaling. Additionally, the accumulation of TAG, ceramides, and the induction of ER stress, triggered by activated NF-κB signaling and the inflammatory cascade, further exacerbate insulin resistance and contribute to the progression of hyperglycemia.

(AP1: activator protein 1; DAG: diacylglycerol; ER: endoplasmic reticulum; FAHFA: branched fatty acid esters of hydroxy fatty acid; IKKβ: inhibitor of NF-κB kinase subunit beta; IkB: inhibitor of NF-κB subunit beta; IRF3: interferon regulatory factor 3; JNK: c-Jun N-terminal kinase; MUFA: monounsaturated fatty acid; MYD88: myeloid differentiation primary response protein 88; NF-κB: nuclear factor kappa B; P: phosphorylation; PUFA: polyunsaturated fatty acid; SFA: saturated fatty acid; TAG: triglyceride; TLR4: toll-like receptor 4; TRIF: TIR-domain-containing adaptor-inducing interferon beta)

Source: With permission from Ruze et al. (2023).[5]

including dysregulation of fatty acid homeostasis, increased adipose cell size and death, local hypoxia, mitochondrial dysfunction, ER stress, and mechanical stress as depicted in **Figure 5**.[15,31] These mechanisms are considered crucial in establishing the connection between chronic caloric excess and inflammation in AT, and they may also contribute to the persistence of chronic tissue inflammation.[33]

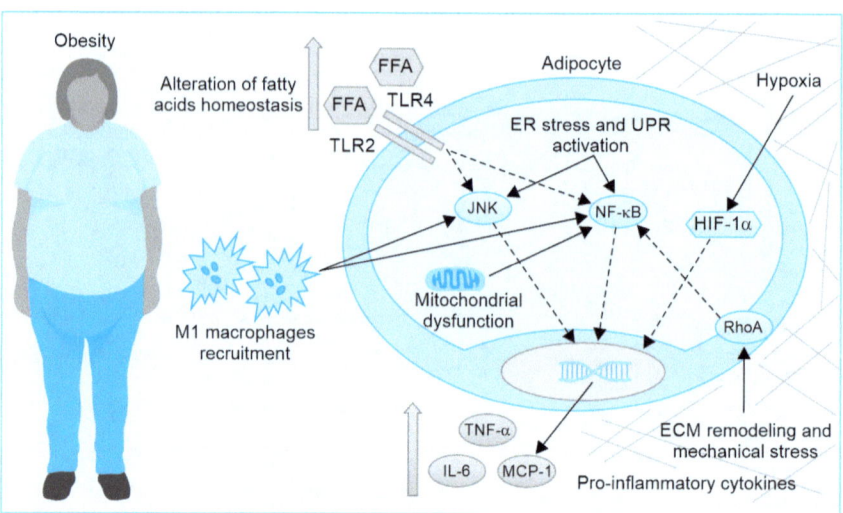

FIG. 5: Obesity triggers inflammation. Obesity gives rise to various intrinsic and extrinsic signals that can initiate an inflammatory response in adipose tissue (AT). These mechanisms serve as the link between prolonged caloric excess and inflammation in AT. Dysregulation of fatty acid homeostasis, increased adipose cell size and death, local hypoxia, mitochondrial dysfunction, endoplasmic reticulum (ER) stress, and mechanical stress are some of the mechanisms involved. These triggers converge on the activation of key signaling pathways, namely the c-Jun N-terminal kinase (JNK) and nuclear factor kappa B (NF-κB) pathways, which are considered central hubs for signaling. Activation of these pathways leads to heightened production of pro-inflammatory cytokines and facilitates the infiltration of pro-inflammatory M1 macrophages.

(ECM: extracellular matrix; FFA: free fatty acids; HIF-1α: hypoxia-inducible factor-1 alpha; MCP-1: monocyte chemotactic protein-1; IL-6: interleukin-6; RhoA: ras homolog gene family, member A; TLR2: toll-like receptor 2; TLR4: toll-like receptor 4; TNF-α: tumor necrosis factor alpha; UPR: unfolded protein response)

Source: With permission from Zatterale et al. (2020).[31]

Role of Adaptive and Innate Immunity in Obesity and Type 2 Diabetes Mellitus

In the current understanding, the development of insulin resistance in T2DM is intricately linked to both innate and adaptive immune factors. Epigenetic mechanisms governing the determination, function, and migration of immune cells have emerged as key players in the context of obesity and T2DM. The presence of obesity is associated with a state of chronic low-grade inflammation, triggering activation of the immune system in individuals affected by T2DM. The excessive accumulation of AT in obesity disrupts metabolic homeostasis and sets the stage for dysregulation. Notably, AT inflammation has emerged as a pivotal factor closely intertwined with the development of insulin resistance in the context of obesity. This inflammatory milieu within AT instigates abnormal activation and proliferation of both innate and adaptive immune components, further contributing to the pathogenesis of T2DM.[37-39] For instance, impaired function of natural killer (NK) cells, characterized by reduced expression of the NKG2D receptor, has been observed, displaying a negative correlation with glycated hemoglobin (HbA1c) levels.[40]

Additionally, there is a pronounced upregulation of pro-inflammatory M1 macrophage polarization and heightened activation of CD4$^+$ T lymphocytes within the visceral AT. These immune alterations signify the intricate interplay between immune dysregulation, AT inflammation, and the development of insulin resistance in T2DM.[31] Role of different immune cells activated after innate and adaptive immunity in AT and further associated with insulin resistance **(Fig. 6 and Box 1)**.[41,42]

Obesity triggers the accumulation of various innate and adaptive immune cell types within AT. Macrophages, constituting a substantial proportion of AT cells in obesity, are considered the primary source of pro-inflammatory cytokines, which contribute to insulin resistance. In obesity, the recruitment of M1-polarized macrophages is prominent, leading to the secretion of pro-inflammatory cytokines like TNF-α and IL-1β. This inflammatory milieu within AT is characterized by an overall increase in macrophage numbers and an elevated ratio of M1 to M2 (anti-inflammatory) macrophages, which coincides with obesity and is associated with the development of insulin resistance.[43,44]

Apart from adipose tissue macrophages (ATMs), other innate immune cell types contribute to the initiation and/or progression of AT inflammation in obesity. Neutrophils, a subset of leukocytes and granulocytes involved in innate immunity, play a role in AT inflammation by producing TNF-α and MCP-1. Moreover, neutrophils release elastase, which impairs glucose uptake in AT and promotes insulin resistance by degrading IRS-1.

Dendritic cells, specialized antigen-presenting cells bridging innate and adaptive immunity, accumulate in AT during high-fat diet feeding and in subcutaneous AT of obese individuals. These cells likely contribute to the pro-inflammatory environment by promoting macrophage recruitment and producing IL-6 which leads to insulin resistance.[44,45]

Mast cells, innate immune cells derived from hematopoietic stem cells, are present in AT and increase in number in both obesity and type 2 diabetes. Mast cells promote low-grade inflammation within AT and mediate macrophage infiltration. Notably, IL-6 and IFN-γ regulate mast cell function, and their dysregulation may contribute to obesity and diabetes. Immature mast cells infiltrating AT during the nonobese stage progress to a mature state and further promote obesity and diabetes progression.[44]

B cells, crucial components of adaptive immunity that produce antibodies, accumulate in AT and potentially contribute to AT inflammation by releasing pro-inflammatory cytokines and immunoglobulin G antibodies. The accumulation of B cells precedes that of T cells during the development of obesity.[46,47]

T cells can be classified into CD4$^+$ and CD8$^+$ subtypes based on surface markers. Obesity is associated with an increase in CD8$^+$ T cells within AT, which promote macrophage differentiation and chemotaxis. CD4$^+$ T cells, recognizing major histocompatibility complex class II on antigen-presenting cells, can be further classified into pro-inflammatory T helper 1 (Th1) and Th17 cells, anti-inflammatory Th2 cells, and regulatory T cells (Tregs). In obesity, the number of CD3$^+$ CD4$^+$ Th1

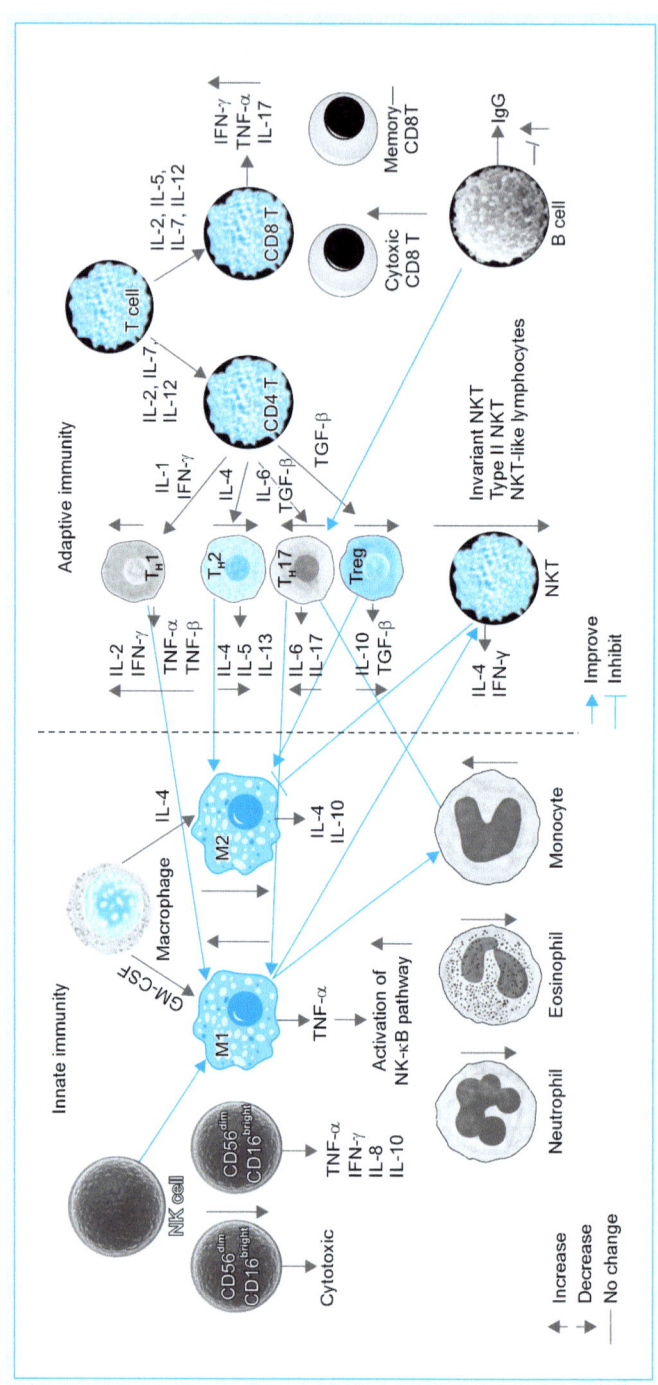

FIG. 6: Change in immune cells during innate and adaptive immunity in the condition of type 2 diabetes mellitus, obesity, or adipose tissue.

(GM-CSF: granulocyte-macrophage colony-stimulating factor; IFN-γ: interferon gamma; IgG: immunoglobulin G; IL-2: interleukin 2; NF-κB: nuclear factor kappa B; NKT: natural killer T; TNF-α: tumor necrosis factor alpha)

Source: With permission from Zhou et al. (2018).[41]

> **BOX 1: Role of immune cells during innate and adaptive immunity in adipose tissue associated with insulin resistance.**
>
> *Macrophages*:
> - Adipocyte death influences macrophage localization and function in adipose tissue and polarization from M2 to M1
> - Pro-inflammatory macrophages in adipose tissue are associated with insulin resistance
> - Cells cluster around necrotic adipose cells in CLSs
>
> *T cells*:
> - Inflammatory T cell profile in adipose tissue is associated with insulin resistance
> - Th2 frequency in visceral adipose tissue inversely correlates with insulin resistance
> - Treg frequency in visceral adipose tissue decreases in obese compared to lean mice
> - Foxp3 expression increases in obese versus lean humans
> - $CD8^+$ T cell frequency increases in visceral adipose tissue compared to subcutaneous adipose tissue
>
> *B cells*:
> - Obesity leads to enhanced infiltration of B cells in visceral adipose tissue
> - B cells undergo class switching to IgG^+ in the context of obesity and insulin resistance
> - Peripheral B cells in type 2 diabetes mellitus exhibit a pro-inflammatory phenotype
> - B cell antigen presentation can promote insulin resistance
>
> *Effects of immune intervention*:
> - Targeted disruption of IKKβ and JNK prevents HFD-induced insulin resistance
> - Transfer of IgG from obese diet-induced obese mice to young mice newly on high-fat/caloric diet accelerates onset of inflammation and insulin resistance
> - B cell depletion via administration of anti-CD20 antibody results in reduced TNF-α-producing M1 cells in visceral adipose tissue and decreased insulin resistance
> - Anti-CD3 antibody therapy results in reversal of insulin resistance
>
> (CLSs: crown-like structures; IgG^+: immunoglobulin G; IKKβ: inhibitor of nuclear factor kappa B kinase subunit beta; JNK: c-Jun N-terminal kinase; Th2: T helper 2; Tregs: regulatory T cells)
>
> *Source*: With permission from McLaughlin et al. (2017).[42]

cells increases and contributes to AT inflammation through IFN-γ secretion, while the number of $CD3^+$ $CD4^+$ Th2 cells decreases. Additionally, the reduction of AT Treg cells during obesity further exacerbates AT inflammation.[31,47]

METABOLIC DYSREGULATION AND HORMONAL IMBALANCES

Metabolic Dysregulation

The 2008 twin cycle hypothesis has explained that when an individual consistently consumes more energy than they expend daily, any excess carbohydrates must be converted to fat in the liver for storage of metabolic energy **(Flowchart 2)**.[48] This process is influenced by endogenous insulin levels, and individuals with insulin resistance tend to accumulate liver fat more easily due to higher plasma insulin levels. If the subcutaneous AT reaches its storage capacity, newly synthesized fat, along with excess dietary fat, accumulates in the liver. This accumulation inhibits the liver's response to insulin, resulting in increased glucose production

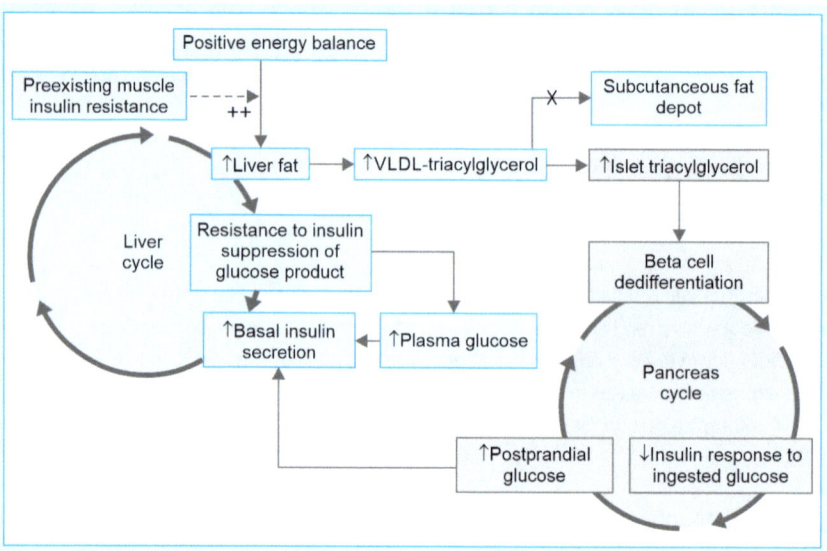

FLOWCHART 2: The 2008 twin cycle hypothesis.

(VLDL: very low-density lipoprotein)

Source: With permission from Taylor R, Barnes AC. Translating aetiological insight into sustainable management of type 2 diabetes. Diabetologia. 2018;61(2):273-83.

and establishing a vicious cycle of hyperinsulinemia and elevated glucose production. Excessive fat in the liver leads to increased export of fat in the form of very low-density lipoprotein (VLDL) triacylglycerol[49] (in **Flowchart 3**, the cyan color indicates the loss of insulin's suppression of liver glucose production). When the storage capacity of subcutaneous fat is exceeded (reaching the personal fat threshold), fat delivery to all tissues, including the pancreatic islets, increases significantly.[50] Postprandial hyperglycemia triggers increased and prolonged insulin secretion, further promoting de novo lipogenesis. This creates a second vicious cycle that enhances de novo lipogenesis and fat delivery to the pancreas. Over many years, the excess fat in the pancreas leads to the loss of specialized function and dedifferentiation of beta cells.[51] Eventually, the inhibitory effects of fatty acids and glucose on the islets reach a critical threshold, resulting in the relatively sudden onset of clinical diabetes. The twin cycle hypothesis suggests that both vicious cycles can be reversed by inducing negative energy balance.

Autophagy: Obesity is associated with various abnormalities in the microenvironment that impair insulin sensitivity. Factors such as lipid accumulation, oxidative stress, inflammation, ER stress, and mitochondrial dysfunction not only affect insulin sensitivity but also have negative consequences for autophagy. Autophagy, the cellular process of self-degradation and recycling, is suppressed in the context of overnutrition. This suppression, coupled with the downregulated secretion of glucagon during nutrient excess, leads to hyperinsulinemia, further inhibiting autophagy. As a result, compromised autophagy compromises insulin signaling, contributing to the development of T2DM **(Flowchart 3)**.[5,52-54] Maintaining metabolic homeostasis relies on the protective role of autophagy in pancreatic beta

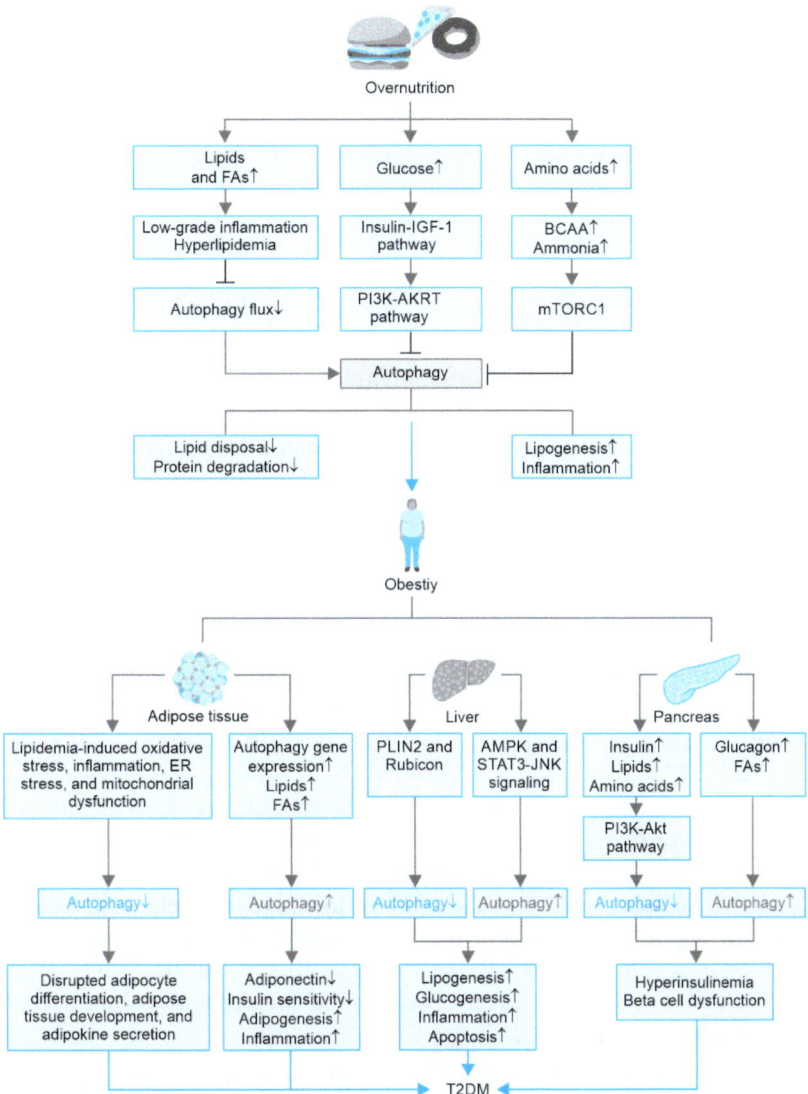

FLOWCHART 3: During the transition from overnutrition and obesity to T2DM, alterations in autophagy occur in various metabolic organs. The excessive intake of nutrients, including lipids, glucose, and amino acids, leads to the suppression of autophagy through different signaling pathways. This suppression of autophagy contributes to the development of obesity by increasing lipid and protein accumulation, promoting low-grade systemic inflammation, and exacerbating insulin signaling dysfunction. In obesity, changes in autophagy can differ among various metabolic sites. In adipose tissue, elevated levels of lipids and FAs and upregulated autophagy genes can enhance autophagy. However, cellular stress can have the opposite effect and suppress autophagy. In the liver, autophagy can either be enhanced or blunted by different signaling pathways. These alterations in hepatic autophagy can contribute to increased lipogenesis, gluconeogenesis, inflammation, and apoptosis. Pancreatic autophagy is influenced by insulin as well as metabolites such as lipids, amino acids, glucagon, and FAs. These factors can have a dual impact on pancreatic autophagy, initially promoting hyperinsulinemia as a protective mechanism against hyperglycemia. However, over time, this dysregulation of pancreatic autophagy contributes to the development of insulin resistance and

Continued

Continued

dysfunction of beta cells, ultimately favoring the onset of T2DM. In obesity, elevated levels of FFAs and glucagon can also enhance pancreatic autophagy. Collectively, these disruptions in autophagy in different metabolic organs contribute to the abnormal accumulation of protein aggregates, lipids, and other detrimental components within the cellular microenvironment. This accumulation fuels cellular stress, leading to insulin resistance and the subsequent transition from obesity to T2DM.

[AMPK: AMP-activated protein kinase; Akt: protein kinase B; BCAA: branched-chain amino acid; DM: diabetes mellitus; ER: endoplasmic reticulum; FAs: fatty acids; FFAs: free fatty acids; IGF-1: insulin-like growth factor 1; JNK: c-Jun N-terminal kinase; mTORC1: mechanistic target of rapamycin (mTOR) complex 1; NAFLD: nonalcoholic fatty liver disease; NASH: nonalcoholic steatohepatitis; PI3K: phosphatidylinositol 3-kinase; PLIN2: perilipin 2; STAT3: signal transducer and activator of transcription 3; T2DM: type 2 diabetes mellitus]

Source: With permission from Ruze et al. (2023).[5]

cells. However, excessive autophagy, particularly under cellular stress, can lead to beta cell loss and worsen the onset of T2DM. Autophagy also plays a significant role in insulin-sensitive tissues such as AT, skeletal muscles, pancreas, liver, and the brain. The ectopic expansion of AT in these locations disrupts autophagy, leading to the accumulation of dysfunctional organelles, tissue-specific insulin resistance, and impaired pancreatic function. Additionally, the reciprocal relationship between autophagy and pathophysiological changes during insulin resistance further disrupts the autophagic process. As autophagy dysfunction worsens, accompanied by increased accumulation of reactive oxygen species (ROS) and mitochondrial damage, insulin resistance becomes progressively aggravated, ultimately contributing to the development and progression of T2DM.[52,53]

During the slow progression of T2DM, beta cells undergo significant stress and apoptosis **(Flowchart 4)**.[5] Simultaneously, the islets of T2DM show a mild increase in the number of macrophages, and the reduction (~40%) in beta cell mass is attributed to various factors such as glucolipotoxicity and amyloid deposition, which induce apoptosis through oxidative and ER stress. The transition from obesity and insulin resistance to T2DM is initiated by beta cell dysfunction, impaired glucose-stimulated insulin secretion (GSIS), and loss of beta cell function, which occurs independently of cell loss in T2DM. This transition is facilitated by the gradual dedifferentiation of beta cells into endocrine progenitor-like cells or their transdifferentiation into other cell types.[55,56]

Overnutrition: Persistent exposure of pancreatic islets to excessive nutrients and sustained elevation of hormone synthesis and secretion contribute to ER stress, exerting detrimental effects on beta cell function and survival in the context of obesity. In order to compensate for insulin resistance in peripheral tissues, the demand for insulin synthesis is amplified, overwhelming the protein folding capacity of the ER due to the excessive influx of nutrients. This triggers the activation of UPR pathways, including PKR-like ER-associated kinase (PERK), resulting in the inhibition of protein translation and eventual insulin deficiency. Additionally, prolonged hyperglycemia and hyperlipidemia within the islets induce glucolipotoxicity, impairing insulin secretion and promoting beta cell apoptosis. ER stress not only disrupts normal insulin synthesis and secretion but also triggers protein degradation pathways and autophagy. The sustained ER stress ultimately leads to the dedifferentiation and apoptosis of beta cells, further exacerbating the dysfunction of the insulin-producing cells.[57-59]

CHAPTER 2: Obesity and Diabetes Pathophysiology

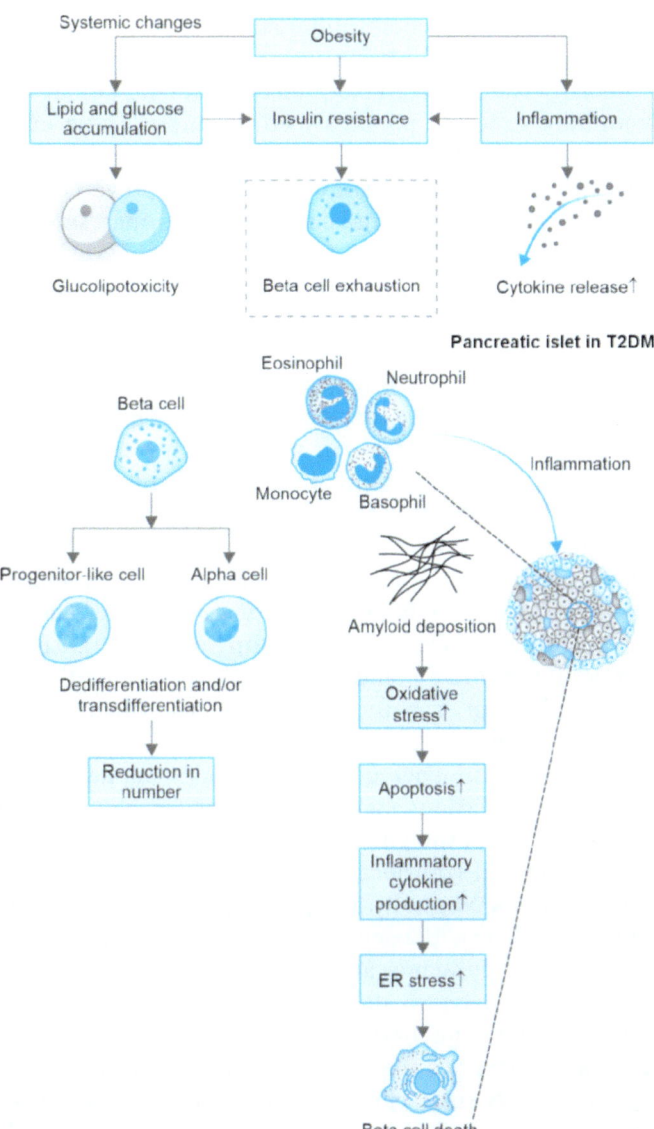

FLOWCHART 4: Obesity contributes to the accelerated loss of beta cells in the pancreatic islets of individuals with type 2 diabetes mellitus (T2DM). The accumulation of lipids and glucose induces a condition known as glucolipotoxicity, which exacerbates insulin resistance and exhausts beta cells. This process is accompanied by enhanced low-grade inflammation due to the increased secretion of pro-inflammatory cytokines into the microenvironment. In the islets of individuals with T2DM, a microenvironment similar to that found in adipose tissue is established, characterized by inflammation. In this inflammatory milieu, the deposition of amyloid compounds worsens oxidative stress, leading to increased apoptosis of beta cells. Additionally, beta cells may undergo dedifferentiation, transforming into progenitor-like cells or even transdifferentiating into other cell types, such as alpha cells. These changes further compromise the beta cell population. Collectively, the constant proapoptotic and pro-inflammatory signals, coupled with the promotion of ER stress, contribute to the loss of beta cells. This process ultimately contributes to the progression of T2DM.

(ER: endoplasmic reticulum)

Source: With permission from Ruze et al. (2023).[5]

Obesity and high-fat feeding elicit similar effects to the prolonged incubation of islets with FFAs in terms of insulin secretion and distribution of calcium channels. These effects are associated with an elevated accumulation of fat within the islets and the surrounding exocrine pancreas. Furthermore, there exists a negative correlation between pancreatic fat content and GSIS in humans. As pancreatic fat decreases, glucose tolerance and insulin secretion improve concomitantly. This suggests that intrapancreatic or intra-islet fat deposits may serve as a local and persistent source of FFAs, exerting detrimental effects on beta cell function.[58,59]

The microbiome–gut–brain axis, regulated by various factors, plays a pivotal role in regulating overall metabolism, adiposity, energy balance as well as central appetite and food reward signaling in humans. When this axis becomes dysregulated, it becomes closely linked to several metabolic diseases, such as obesity and T2DM. A key factor in this dysregulation is microbiome dysfunction, which is primarily responsible for disrupting energy balance, promoting fat deposition, triggering inflammation, inducing insulin resistance, causing glucolipotoxicity, and disrupting endocrine signaling pathways. These effects can occur through direct interactions or indirect influences on the body's systems. The microbiome's impact on the microbiome–gut–brain axis and its subsequent influence on metabolic health highlights the critical role of microbiome homeostasis in maintaining overall well-being and preventing metabolic diseases.[60] **Figure 7** described the role of the microbiome–gut–brain axis dysfunction in obesity and T2DM.[5] The interaction between the gut microbiota, glucose metabolism, and the immune system involves a complex, three-way relationship. Firstly, the gut microbiota plays a role in influencing the host's glucose metabolism and hormone production by producing various metabolites. Elevated blood glucose levels can increase the permeability of the gut, allowing bacterial components to enter the bloodstream. This bacterial translocation triggers a (pro)inflammatory response from the immune system. Normally, the gut microbiota helps train the immune system through interactions with bacterial components and metabolites. Secondly, the immune system actively shapes and regulates the gut microbiota to maintain a symbiotic relationship between the host and the microbiota. It also works to maintain the integrity of the gut barrier, preventing bacterial translocation. When bacterial translocation occurs, inflammation can arise in various tissues, leading to functional impairments such as beta cell dysfunction, insulin resistance, and fatty liver disease. Lastly, glucose metabolism can stimulate a pro-inflammatory response from the immune system through the interplay of metabolic and inflammatory pathways, known as immunometabolism. In this way, all three factors (gut microbiota, glucose metabolism, and the immune system) interact with and influence each other, potentially contributing to the development of metabolic diseases. Overall, the intricate interplay between the gut microbiota, glucose metabolism, and the immune system demonstrates their interconnectedness and highlights their collective impact on metabolic health.[61] Overall, although the field of microbiota research is still in its early stages, the combination of technical advancements and the dedication of researchers worldwide provides a solid foundation for exploring the complexities of the microbiota and unlocking its vast potential to prevent or treat metabolic diseases like obesity and diabetes.

CHAPTER 2: Obesity and Diabetes Pathophysiology

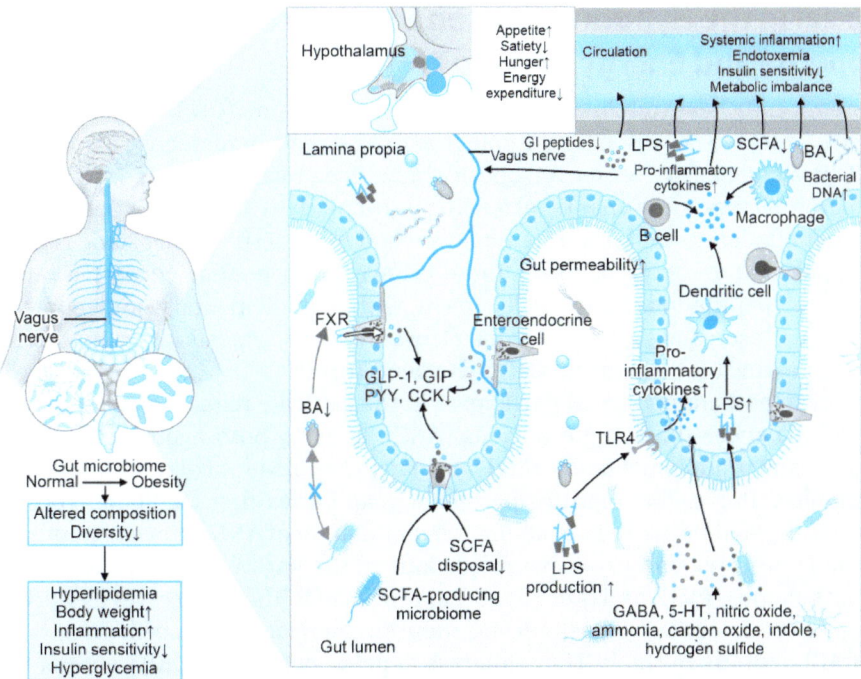

FIG. 7: Dysfunction of the microbiome–gut–brain axis plays a significant role in obesity and type 2 diabetes mellitus (T2DM). In obesity, there are notable changes in the composition and diversity of the gut microbiome. These alterations lead to various metabolic abnormalities and changes in microbial metabolites. For instance, there is a decrease in the production of beneficial compounds like BAs and SCFAs, while there is an increase in LPS levels. These changes compromise the protective function of the gut and contribute to increased gut permeability. Inflammatory stimuli such as nitric oxide, ammonia, carbon oxide, indole, and hydrogen sulfide contribute to this heightened permeability. As a result, there is a significant increase in the flux of LPS, which has multiple effects. LPS can activate TLR4 on enterocytes, leading to the secretion of inflammatory cytokines and the recruitment of inflammatory immune cells like dendritic cells, B cells, and macrophages. Moreover, these immune cells themselves produce inflammatory cytokines upon exposure to LPS. Simultaneously, the reduced production of SCFAs and BAs leads to decreased activation of GPCRs and FXR in enteroendocrine cells. These cells play a crucial role in producing GI hormones essential for energy homeostasis, such as GLP-1, GIP, PYY, and CCK. These hormones have both peripheral and central effects on regulating metabolism and appetite, either directly through the vagus nerve or indirectly via immunoneuroendocrine mechanisms. Centrally, the abnormal hormonal signals transmitted from the gut to the hypothalamus in the brain disrupt eating behavior and metabolic control. Peripherally, the influx of LPS, pro-inflammatory cytokines, and bacterial DNA, coupled with inadequate levels of SCFAs, BAs, and GI peptides in the circulation, further impairs insulin signaling and metabolic balance. These central and peripheral abnormalities in metabolic control ultimately contribute to the development of hyperglycemia in T2DM.

(5-HT: 5-hydroxytryptamine; BA: bile acid; CCK: cholecystokinin; FXR: farnesoid X receptor; GABA: gamma aminobutyric acid; GI: gastrointestinal; GIP: glucose-dependent insulinotropic polypeptide; GLP-1: glucagon-like peptide 1; GPCR: G-protein coupled receptor; LPS: lipopolysaccharide; PYY: peptide YY; SCFA: short-chain fatty acid; TLR4: toll-like receptor 4)

Source: With permission from Ruze et al. (2023).[5]

Nuclei in the Hypothalamus and Brain Stem Regulating Appetite and Energy Balance

More recently, research into the central nervous system's (CNS) metabolic role has opened doors to the discovery of potential drug targets in metabolic disorders such as T2DM and obesity. Moreover, obesity induces enduring alterations in the brain's cytoarchitecture and synaptic plasticity, particularly within the hypothalamus.[5-7] The hypothalamus and brain stem play pivotal roles in the homeostatic regulation of appetite and energy balance. These critical brain regions encompass distinct neuronal populations and nuclei, each with complementary and contrasting functions, exerting significant control over various aspects of energy balance, encompassing both energy intake and expenditure.[62]

Key hypothalamic nuclei participate in the intricate regulation of appetite and energy balance. The arcuate nucleus (ARC), housing both agouti-related protein (AGRP) and proopiomelanocortin (POMC) neurons, resides adjacent to the median eminence. This region features permeable capillaries that facilitate exposure to circulating signals, thereby enabling the modulation of ARC neuronal populations. These neurons extend extensive projections to the paraventricular nucleus of the hypothalamus (PVH) and other hypothalamic nuclei. The PVH serves as a principal hypothalamic satiety center. POMC neurons activate melanocortin-4 receptor (MC4R) neurons in the PVH to suppress appetite, whereas AGRP neurons inhibit PVH-MC4R neurons, promoting appetite. Additionally, AGRP neurons also inhibit POMC neurons by stimulating inhibitory gamma aminobutyric acid (GABA)-ergic input to POMC neurons. Anorexigenic signals like leptin and glucagon-like peptide 1 (GLP-1) enhance satiety by acting on POMC neurons, whereas orexigenic signals like ghrelin can increase appetite by affecting AGRP neurons. Other hypothalamic neuronal populations maintain extensive connections with neighboring nuclei. For instance, the dorsomedial hypothalamus (DMH) primarily exerts inhibitory projections to the PVH and POMC but also features activating inhibitory GABAergic neurons projecting to the ARC's AGRP neurons. The ventromedial hypothalamus (VMH) primarily sends excitatory projections to POMC neurons, while AGRP neurons send inhibitory projections to the VMH. Furthermore, postprandial satiety signals originating from enteroendocrine cells within the gastrointestinal tract can also influence the dorsal vagal complex (DVC) located in the brain stem to suppress appetite (**Fig. 8**).[62]

Divergent Functions of AGRP and POMC Neurons in Maintaining Glucose and Lipid Homeostasis

The CNS, encompassing both hypothalamic and brain stem neuronal populations, plays a pivotal role in maintaining the balance of energy intake and expenditure. These neuronal populations respond to circulating signals, orchestrating the adjustment of autonomic nervous system activity toward various metabolic organs and endocrine glands. This intricate communication between the CNS and the periphery is crucial for preserving glucose and lipid homeostasis.[62]

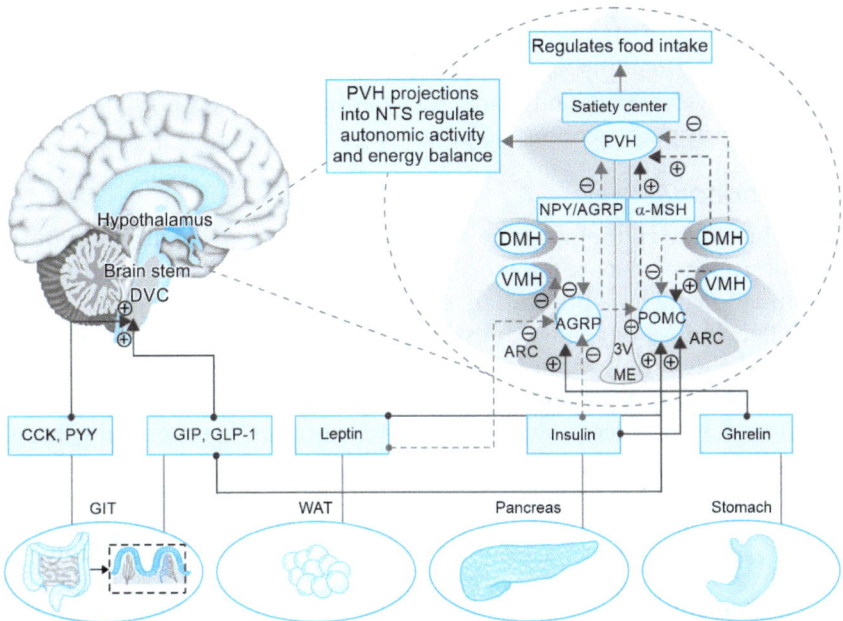

FIG. 8: Key hypothalamic nuclei involved in the regulation of appetite and energy balance.

(AGRP: agouti-related protein; ARC: arcuate nucleus; CCK: cholecystokinin; DMH: dorsomedial hypothalamus; DVC: dorsal vagal complex; GIP: glucose-dependent insulinotropic polypeptide; GLP-1: glucagon-like peptide 1; GIT: gastrointestinal tract; ME: median eminence; α-MSH: alpha melanocyte-stimulating hormone; NPY: neuropeptide Y; NTS: nucleus tractus solitarius; POMC: proopiomelanocortin; PVH: paraventricular nucleus of the hypothalamus; PYY: peptide YY; VMH: ventromedial hypothalamus; WAT: white adipose tissue; 3V: third ventricle)

Numerous brain regions, including specific hypothalamic and brain stem nuclei, harbor intricate neural networks that govern the function of pancreatic islets through autonomic efferent pathways. These neural circuits have been functionally validated, unveiling the significant roles of several hypothalamic nuclei in regulating pancreatic insulin release. Within these hypothalamic nuclei, a bidirectional control over insulin secretion is evident. Activation of a specific subset of oxytocin neurons in the PVH leads to the suppression of insulin secretion, whereas increased glucokinase activity in the ARC enhances GSIS and improves glucose tolerance. Additionally, neurons projecting to the pancreas within the dorsal motor nucleus of the vagus (DMV) have been observed to be stimulated by GLP-1, suggesting a potential vagal efferent pathway for enhancing insulin release. IRs are widely distributed throughout the brain, enabling circulating insulin to modulate neuronal populations crucial for metabolic regulation. Notably, the hypothalamus stands as a pivotal insulin-responsive brain region dedicated to the maintenance of euglycemia. Intriguingly, the divergent effects of central insulin signaling on glucose and lipid homeostasis may be attributed to the distinct outcomes of IR activation in AGRP neurons versus POMC neurons. Insulin's impact on AGRP neurons contributes to enhanced glucose homeostasis, while its influence on POMC neurons brings about alterations in lipid metabolism.[62]

Hormonal Imbalances

Type 2 diabetes mellitus is a multifaceted, genetically influenced condition characterized by dysregulation or insufficiency in various key hormonal pathways, contributing to its pathogenesis and progression.

Incretin Hormones

The gastrointestinal epithelium secretes incretin hormones, which play a vital role in maintaining normal glucose tolerance. These hormones stimulate insulin secretion in response to glucose, preventing excessive postprandial glucose levels. The incretin effect is dose-dependent, ensuring consistent postprandial glucose control regardless of the carbohydrate content of the meal.[63] The two primary incretin hormones, GLP-1 and glucose-dependent insulinotropic polypeptide (GIP), are crucial in regulating glucose metabolism. Upon nutrient ingestion, these hormones are secreted by the gastrointestinal tract, and they play a role in modulating the release of insulin and glucagon from pancreatic islet cells. However, their activity is short-lived as they are rapidly degraded into inactive metabolites by dipeptidyl peptidase 4 (DPP-4).[64]

Glucose-dependent insulinotropic polypeptide: This is the first discovered incretin hormone, which contributes to approximately 60% of the total incretin effect. It is released by duodenal K cells in the proximal small intestine in response to the absorption of fats and carbohydrates after a meal. In the pathogenesis of T2DM, there is a genetic component with reduced expression of beta cell GIP receptors, which may be an early event in the development of the disease. This is supported by observations of reduced insulinotropic response to exogenous GIP in patients with T2DM and the decreased GIP effect seen in about 50% of their nondiabetic first-degree relatives. However, other data indicate that rapid desensitization of signaling through GIP receptors occurs in T2DM, which may be associated with GIP hypersecretion, chronic hyperglycemia, or other metabolic abnormalities **(Figs. 9A and B)**.[63,64]

Glucagon-like peptide 1: In patients with T2DM, the loss of the insulinotropic effect of GIP may be either a primary cause of the disease or a consequence of ongoing hyperglycemia, limiting the potential of GIP analogs or mimetics. On the other hand, GLP-1, discovered in 1985, is secreted by L cells in the distal small intestine and colon, alpha cells of the pancreas, and neurons in the hypothalamus. It induces satiety and regulates feeding behavior. Similar to GIP, GLP-1 levels increase after food ingestion, with plasma concentrations rising six- to eightfold following a carbohydrate meal. GLP-1 not only stimulates insulin secretion but also inhibits glucagon secretion, HGP, gastric emptying, and appetite. Additionally, GLP-1 has stimulative and regenerative effects on beta cells. In individuals with T2DM, there appears to be a deficit of GLP-1. Reduced postprandial GLP-1 response has been observed in patients with T2DM, and the degree of reduction correlates with the subject's obesity level **(Fig. 8)**.[62,63] The diminished incretin effect observed in T2DM is primarily attributed to the significant decline in beta cell function and reduced insulinotropic response to GIP. While GLP-1 secretion and activity may remain intact, they are unable to fully compensate for the impaired GIP activity at

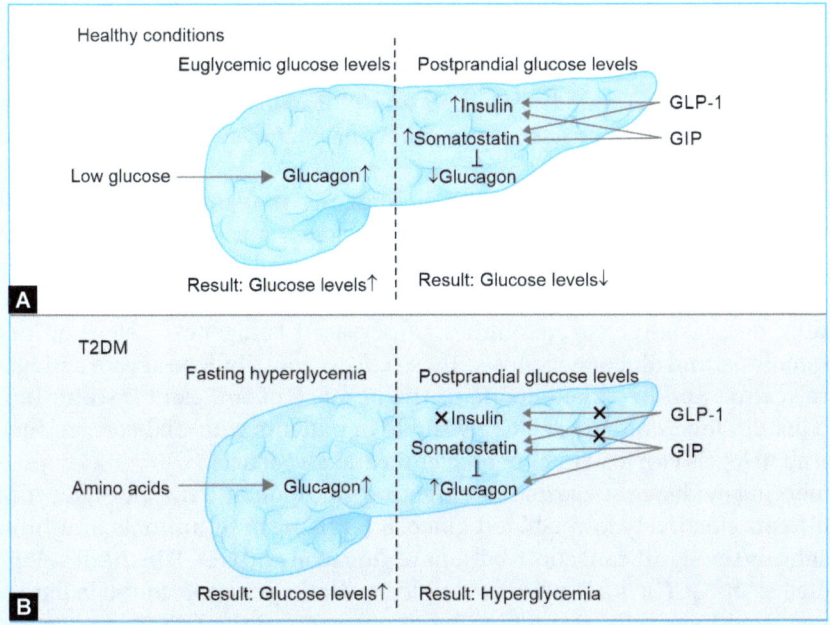

FIGS. 9A AND B: Actions of glucagon-like peptide 1 (GLP-1) and glucose-dependent insulinotropic polypeptide (GIP) in the pancreas. The diagrams show the actions of the incretins under fasting and postprandial glucose levels in (A) healthy individuals and (B) patients with type 2 diabetes mellitus (T2DM).

Source: With permission from Boer et al. (2020).[63]

physiological levels. Recent studies, such as the comprehensive review by Meier et al., have provided detailed insights into the role of reduced insulinotropic response to GIP in T2DM, highlighting its association with decreased beta cell mass and impaired maximum insulin secretory capacity.[65]

Recent research has shed light on the contribution of impaired alpha cell function in the pathophysiology of T2DM. This dysfunction leads to the inadequate suppression of glucagon secretion and HGP, even in the presence of a meal. In the context of insufficient insulin levels and increased insulin resistance, this dysregulated glucagon secretion contributes to the development of hyperglycemia in individuals with T2DM. The incretins, including GLP-1, play a crucial role in mediating insulin release and suppressing glucagon secretion. While GIP activity is impaired in individuals with T2DM, the insulinotropic effects of GLP-1 remain preserved. Therefore, GLP-1 represents a promising therapeutic option for the management of T2DM due to its ability to enhance insulin secretion and suppress glucagon levels.[64]

Glucagon: A Hormone by the Alpha Cells

Glucagon, a peptide hormone consisting of 29 amino acids, is primarily secreted from the pancreatic alpha cells. Its main role is to stimulate HGP, thereby increasing plasma glucose levels. Glucagon is recognized as the counterregulatory hormone to insulin, and the balance between insulin and glucagon secretion is crucial for maintaining normal glucose homeostasis. Interestingly, in the pathophysiology of T2DM, dysfunction of the pancreatic alpha cells is observed. Individuals with T2DM often exhibit elevated fasting plasma glucagon levels, and their glucagon concentrations fail to decrease appropriately or may even increase paradoxically following meal ingestion.[66]

The theory of bihormonal regulation suggests that diabetes is the result of abnormal secretion of both insulin and glucagon. Insulin deficiency leads to metabolic disorders such as elevated lipolysis, increased proteolysis, and decreased glucose utilization. On the other hand, excess glucagon has various effects including decreased glycogen synthesis, increased ketogenesis, elevated hepatic glycogenolysis, and gluconeogenesis. These effects contribute to severe endogenous hyperglycemia and hyperketonemia in the absence of sufficient insulin. In cases where insulin levels remain relatively stable in patients with diabetes, an increase in glucagon levels can lead to hyperglycemia and glycosuria.[67]

Emerging evidence suggests that targeting glucagon and the glucagon receptor (GCGR) can effectively lower blood glucose levels in both animals and humans, highlighting the significant contributions of glucagon and GCGR in the development of diabetes. The GCGR is a G-protein-coupled receptor primarily found in pancreatic beta cells and liver cells. Upon binding of glucagon to the GCGR, it triggers liver glycogen breakdown and elevates blood glucose levels, which stimulates insulin release. GLP-1, predominantly expressed in intestinal L cells, activates the GLP-1 receptor to regulate metabolism. Both glucagon and GLP-1 are derived from the same precursor molecule, proglucagon, and they play crucial roles in the regulation of lipid and bile acid metabolism, exerting significant influences on glucose metabolism and the development of diabetes.[67]

Adipocytokines: The Adipose Tissue Hormones

Adipose tissue has many important functions other than energy storage that are mediated through hormones or substances synthesized and released by adipocytes. These substances, termed "adipocytokines", act on distant targets in an endocrine fashion or locally in paracrine and autocrine fashions. The adipocyte-derived hormones, such as adiponectin and leptin, have been shown to improve insulin sensitivity, a key factor in the pathogenesis of T2DM. Indeed, obesity induced by eating a high-energy diet is a risk factor for the development of insulin resistance and subsequently, T2DM. AT, in addition to being a fat storage organ, can also secrete several hormones and some proteins (called adipokines), which may act as markers of deteriorating pancreatic islet function. Some of these adipocytokines can increase insulin sensitivity by increasing fatty acid oxidation and reducing the triglyceride levels in skeletal muscle.[68,69]

- *Leptin*: Serum concentrations of leptin increase in proportion to increasing adiposity. In patients with obesity, high leptin levels are associated with low circulating soluble leptin receptors (SLRs) consistent with a state of leptin resistance. Leptin must cross the blood–brain barrier (BBB) to reach the hypothalamus and exert its anorexigenic functions. Decreased transport across the BBB and a decreased ability of leptin to activate hypothalamic signaling in diet-induced obesity may be crucial in the pathogenesis of leptin resistance. Leptin receptors are also present in peripheral organs, such as the liver, skeletal muscles, pancreatic beta cells, and even adipose cells, indicating endocrine, autocrine, and paracrine roles of leptin in energy regulation. Leptin signaling in these organs is thought to mediate important metabolic effects. For example, leptin has been implicated in glucose and lipid metabolism as an insulin sensitizer.[68,69]

- *Adiponectin*: This is an insulin-sensitizing adipocytokine whose plasma levels were found to be decreased in T2DM, insulin resistance and obesity. It is well known that AMPK is an energy sensor and that it regulates cellular metabolism. AMPK stimulates glucose uptake and lipid oxidation to produce energy during deficient nutrient status. It turns off energy utilization mechanisms through the synthesis of lipid and glucose molecules to reinstate the energy balance.[69]

  Accumulation of excess visceral fat was found to modify the liberation of adipocytokines molecules like resistin, leading to central nervous system-mediated skeletal muscle and hepatic insulin resistance.

- *Resistin*: It is known that resistin increases blood glucose and insulin concentrations in mice and impairs the hypoglycemic response to insulin infusion. Earlier studies reported lower resistin mRNA in AT in various mouse models of obesity, such as diet-induced obesity. Resistin also suppresses insulin-stimulated glucose uptake in cultured 3T3-L1 adipocytes, and antiresistin antibodies reverse this effect. These observations from the above studies clearly suggest that resistin induces insulin resistance and hyperresistinemia that contribute to impaired insulin sensitivity in the obese models studied.[69]

Beyond serving as sites for energy storage, adipocytokines play a pivotal role in governing cellular metabolic pathways in response to the nutritional status. The upregulation of adipocytokines, such as resistin, vaspin, apelin, and TNF-α, has been linked to the development of insulin resistance associated with obesity and T2DM. The evolving understanding of adipocytokines' impact on glucose homeostasis and insulin sensitivity offers valuable insights for shaping therapeutic interventions aimed at mitigating vascular diseases.

Role of Gut Peptide in Obesity

Obesity occurs when energy intake chronically exceeds energy expenditure. By consistently overriding homeostatic signals of energy availability, eating becomes disjointed from energy requirements, resulting in dysregulation of the metabolic mechanisms controlling energy homeostasis, including impaired gut hormone secretion. Abnormal gut hormone responses have been demonstrated in adults and children with obesity. Individuals with obesity have blunted ghrelin reductions post-meal, together with reduced circulating baseline and meal-stimulated levels of the anorectic peptides, peptide YY (PYY), GLP-1, and neurotensin (NT), compared to individuals with normal weight. However, a recent study in rats with diet-induced obesity, akin to a western diet, showed reduced circulating PYY and GLP-1 concentrations and a loss of circadian secretion profiles of PYY, GLP-1, and amylin. In addition, sustained exposure to a high-fat diet in mice has been shown to lead to an increase in ghrelin-producing cells. These findings suggest that high-energy intake per se may chronically impair gut hormone responsiveness to ingested nutrients. Studies investigating the role of ghrelin in obesity have shown blunted post-meal ghrelin suppression, loss of premeal peaks, along with reduced diurnal variability; these changes are thought to contribute to the lack of regular meals and the frequent snacking behavior often observed in individuals with obesity.[70]

MECHANISM OF ACTION OF GUT MICROBIOTA IN OBESITY

The gut microbiota can achieve this through various means. First, gut microbiota influences host energy balance through sensors of microbial products. Short-chain fatty acids are a subgroup of fatty acids composed of acetate, propionate, and butyrate, which are end products of bacterial fermentation. These metabolites may act as signaling molecules that regulate various transcription factors involved in energy balance. The short-chain fatty acids and conjugated fatty acids can modulate the brain via direct or indirect mechanisms and affect its ability to regulate appetite and food intake.[71] On the other hand, pro-obesity microbiomes have been reported to be involved in various activities that promote body weight gain. Some microbes, such as those belonging to the phylum Firmicutes are involved in promoting adiposity or could enhance host-mediated adaptive response mechanisms that limit energy uptake, such as reducing the capacity to ferment polysaccharides.[72] Firmicutes have been described to possess many carbohydrate metabolism enzymes, which can contribute to the metabolization of carbohydrates allowing a greater energy absorption and contributing to obesity.[73] Furthermore, the pro-obesity gut microbiota is involved in inducing low-grade inflammation by promoting metabolic expression of inflammatory markers in AT and pro-inflammatory cytokines associated with increased risks of weight gain. It was discovered that gut microbiota-associated inflammation is controlled by microbiota lipopolysaccharide (LPS). The LPS from intestinal bacteria may increase the risk of developing obesity and cause insulin resistance via means including inducing obesity–inflammatory markers in AT.[74-76]

ENDOCRINE CAUSE OF OBESITY AND DIABETES

Endocrine Cause of Obesity

Endocrine disorders, such as hypothyroidism and hypercortisolism, are recognized causes of secondary obesity. However, individuals with primary (simple) obesity can also exhibit various hormonal abnormalities. Some of these issues stem from dysfunction in AT, which secretes adipokines influencing endocrine organ function and can often be reversed with weight loss. However, there are cases where these abnormalities indicate a genuine endocrine disorder requiring specific treatment.

The secretion of thyroid hormones (TH) is regulated by the hypothalamic–pituitary–thyroid (HPT) axis. Thyroid-stimulating hormone (TSH or thyrotropin) is released by the anterior pituitary lobe in response to thyrotropin-releasing hormone (TRH) from the hypothalamus. TH, including triiodothyronine (T3) and thyroxine (T4), then regulate both TRH and TSH release in a feedback loop to maintain overall bodily homeostasis. TH exerts diverse effects, including control of energy expenditure, basal metabolic rate (BMR), adaptive thermogenesis, and appetite regulation. Clinical research has indicated that thyroid status correlates with changes in body weight and adiposity. Even among euthyroid individuals, those with higher TSH levels tend to have a higher BMI than those with TSH levels closer to the lower end of the normal range. Variations in TH levels, even within the normal range, can influence weight gain or impact the effectiveness of weight loss treatments.[77,78]

The secretion of sex hormones is regulated by the hypothalamic–pituitary–gonadal (HPG) axis. In brief, gonadotropin-releasing hormone (GnRH) is produced by the hypothalamus and stimulates the anterior pituitary lobe to release gonadotropins: luteinizing hormone (LH) and follicle-stimulating hormone (FSH). These gonadotropins, in turn, stimulate the gonads (ovaries and testes) to secrete estrogen and testosterone and regulate reproductive processes. While testosterone, through negative feedback, inhibits GnRH and gonadotropin secretion, the regulation of female sex steroids is more complex.[79]

Hypogonadism can both cause and result from obesity in both men and women. A recent meta-analysis found that the prevalence of hypogonadism in obese men was 43.8% when measuring total testosterone (TT), but this figure rose to 75.0% in severely obese individuals undergoing bariatric surgery. Several mechanisms contribute to the development of obesity-related hypogonadism in men. Obesity increases aromatase cytochrome P450 activity in AT, leading to enhanced conversion of testosterone to estradiol. Elevated estradiol levels, in turn, downregulate GLUT4 via estrogen receptor beta stimulation, resulting in insulin resistance. This insulin resistance reduces sex hormone-binding globulin (SHBG) synthesis in the liver, increasing the amount of TT available for conversion to estradiol in AT. Elevated estrogen levels then inhibit gonadotropin secretion from the pituitary gland, further contributing to hypogonadism. Consequently, obesity can adversely affect sperm concentration, motility, and morphology in men.[80-82]

ENDOCRINE CAUSE OF DIABETES

The co-occurrence of T2DM alongside various hormonal disorders, such as pituitary, adrenal, and thyroid diseases, is a common observation. For instance, impaired glucose tolerance (IGT) and full-blown diabetes mellitus often accompany conditions like acromegaly and hypercortisolism (Cushing syndrome). The heightened cardiovascular risks and increased mortality associated with acromegaly and Cushing syndrome may, in part, result from the enhanced insulin resistance that typically accompanies excess hormone production.[83]

In acromegalic patients, insulin resistance is apparent both in the liver and the peripheral tissues, leading to elevated insulin levels and increased glucose turnover, especially during the fasting state. The prevalence of diabetes and IGT in acromegaly varies between 16 and 56%. This variation seems to be correlated with circulating growth hormone (GH) levels, patient age, and the duration of the disease. GH has physiological effects on glucose metabolism, including the promotion of gluconeogenesis and lipolysis, resulting in elevated blood glucose and FFA levels. Conversely, insulin-like growth factor 1 (IGF-1) enhances insulin sensitivity primarily in skeletal muscles. However, in acromegaly, increased IGF-1 levels cannot fully counteract the insulin resistance caused by excess GH.[83]

Hyperproduction of cortisol in hypercortisolism leads to visceral obesity, insulin resistance, and dyslipidemia. These metabolic abnormalities, along with other factors like hypertension, hypercoagulability, and structural and functional changes in the heart ventricles, collectively heighten cardiovascular risk. Even after the resolution of hypercortisolism, these metabolic effects can persist for up to 5 years. Hypercortisolism induces hyperglycemia, reduces glucose tolerance, promotes insulin resistance, and stimulates hepatic gluconeogenesis and glycogenolysis.[83]

In patients with neuroendocrine tumors (NETs), disruptions in glucose tolerance can arise due to decreased insulin secretion, as seen in individuals who have undergone pancreatic surgery or those with pheochromocytoma. Additionally, an imbalance between hormones can contribute to altered glucose metabolism in conditions such as glucagonoma and somatostatinoma. The use of somatostatin analogs (SSAs) for the symptomatic treatment of NETs can also impact glucose metabolism.[83]

In thyroid disorders, abnormal glucose tolerance is primarily encountered in hyperthyroidism. The underlying causes are complex, and there is limited data available on the prevalence and severity of glucose-related issues. Nonetheless, it is crucial to provide appropriate treatment for glucose imbalances in these specific patient populations, aligning with the guidelines set forth by the American Diabetes Association and the European Association for the Study of Diabetes.[83]

REFERENCES

1. Lloyd-Jones DM, Liu K, Colangelo LA, Yan LL, Klein L, Loria CM, et al. Consistently stable or decreased body mass index in young adulthood and longitudinal changes in metabolic syndrome components: the Coronary Artery Risk Development in Young Adults Study. Circulation. 2007;115(8):1004-11.
2. Colditz GA, Willett WC, Rotnitzky A, Manson JE. Weight gain as a risk factor for clinical diabetes mellitus in women. Ann Intern Med. 1995;122(7):481-6.
3. Chan JM, Rimm EB, Colditz GA, Stampfer MJ, Willett WC. Obesity, fat distribution, and weight gain as risk factors for clinical diabetes in men. Diabetes Care. 1994;17(9):961-9.
4. Schienkiewitz A, Schulze MB, Hoffmann K, Kroke A, Boeing H. Body mass index history and risk of type 2 diabetes: results from the European Prospective Investigation into Cancer and Nutrition (EPIC)-Potsdam Study. Am J Clin Nutr. 2006;84(2):427-33.
5. Ruze R, Liu T, Zou X, Song J, Chen Y, Xu R, et al. Obesity and type 2 diabetes mellitus: connections in epidemiology, pathogenesis, and treatments. Front Endocrinol (Lausanne). 2023;14:1161521.
6. Youngren JF. Regulation of insulin receptor function. Cell Mol Life Sci. 2007;64(7-8):873-91.
7. Khalid M, Alkaabi J, Khan MAB, Adem A. Insulin Signal Transduction Perturbations in Insulin Resistance. Int J Mol Sci. 2021;22(16):8590.
8. Leto D, Saltiel AR. Regulation of glucose transport by insulin: traffic control of GLUT4. Nat Rev Mol Cell Biol. 2012;13(6):383-96.
9. Agius L. Role of glycogen phosphorylase in liver glycogen metabolism. Mol Aspects Med. 2015;46:34-45.
10. Dong XC, Copps KD, Guo S, Li Y, Kollipara R, DePinho RA, et al. Inactivation of hepatic Foxo1 by insulin signaling is required for adaptive nutrient homeostasis and endocrine growth regulation. Cell Metab. 2008;8(1):65-76.
11. Tzivion G, Dobson M, Ramakrishnan G. FoxO transcription factors; Regulation by AKT and 14-3-3 proteins. Biochim Biophys Acta. 2011;1813(11):1938-45.
12. Perry RJ, Camporez JG, Kursawe R, Titchenell PM, Zhang D, Perry CJ, et al. Hepatic acetyl CoA links adipose tissue inflammation to hepatic insulin resistance and type 2 diabetes. Cell. 2015;160(4):745-58.

13. Ros S, García-Rocha M, Domínguez J, Ferrer JC, Guinovart JJ. Control of liver glycogen synthase activity and intracellular distribution by phosphorylation. J Biol Chem. 2009;284(10):6370-8.
14. Cignarelli A, Genchi VA, Perrini S, Natalicchio A, Laviola L, Giorgino F. Insulin and Insulin Receptors in Adipose Tissue Development. Int J Mol Sci. 2019;20(3):759.
15. Petersen MC, Shulman GI. Mechanisms of Insulin Action and Insulin Resistance. Physiol Rev. 2018;98(4):2133-223.
16. Kersten S. Mechanisms of nutritional and hormonal regulation of lipogenesis. EMBO Rep. 2001;2(4):282-6.
17. Spiegelman D, Israel RG, Bouchard C, Willett WC. Absolute fat mass, percent body fat, and body-fat distribution: which is the real determinant of blood pressure and serum glucose? Am J Clin Nutr. 1992;55(6):1033-44.
18. Rexrode KM, Manson JE, Hennekens CH. Obesity and cardiovascular disease. Curr Opin Cardiol. 1996;11(5):490-5.
19. Després JP, Moorjani S, Lupien PJ, Tremblay A, Nadeau A, Bouchard C. Regional distribution of body fat, plasma lipoproteins, and cardiovascular disease. Arteriosclerosis. 1990;10(4):497-511.
20. Harrison LC, Martin FI, Melick RA. Correlation between insulin receptor binding in isolated fat cells and insulin sensitivity in obese human subjects. J Clin Invest. 1976;58(6):1435-41.
21. Bonadonna RC, Groop L, Kraemer N, Ferrannini E, Del Prato S, DeFronzo RA. Obesity and insulin resistance in humans: a dose–response study. Metabolism. 1990;39(5):452-9.
22. Wilcox G. Insulin and insulin resistance. Clin Biochem Rev. 2005;26(2):19-39.
23. Pearson T, Wattis JA, King JR, MacDonald IA, Mazzatti DJ. The Effects of Insulin Resistance on Individual Tissues: An Application of a Mathematical Model of Metabolism in Humans. Bull Math Biol. 2016;78(6):1189-217.
24. DeFronzo RA, Tripathy D. Skeletal muscle insulin resistance is the primary defect in type 2 diabetes. Diabetes Care. 2009;32 Suppl 2(Suppl 2):S157-63.
25. Coelho M, Oliveira T, Fernandes R. Biochemistry of adipose tissue: an endocrine organ. Arch Med Sci. 2013;9(2):191-200.
26. Rosen ED, Spiegelman BM. Adipocytes as regulators of energy balance and glucose homeostasis. Nature. 2006;444(7121):847-53.
27. Czech MP. Insulin action and resistance in obesity and type 2 diabetes. Nat Med. 2017;23(7):804-14.
28. Lewis GF, Carpentier AC, Pereira S, Hahn M, Giacca A. Direct and indirect control of hepatic glucose production by insulin. Cell Metab. 2021;33(4):709-20.
29. Basu R, Chandramouli V, Dicke B, Landau B, Rizza R. Obesity and type 2 diabetes impair insulin-induced suppression of glycogenolysis as well as gluconeogenesis. Diabetes. 2005;54(7):1942-8.
30. Magnusson I, Rothman DL, Katz LD, Shulman RG, Shulman GI. Increased rate of gluconeogenesis in type II diabetes mellitus. A 13C nuclear magnetic resonance study. J Clin Invest. 1992;90(4):1323-7.
31. Zatterale F, Longo M, Naderi J, Raciti GA, Desiderio A, Miele C, et al. Chronic Adipose Tissue Inflammation Linking Obesity to Insulin Resistance and Type 2 Diabetes. Front Physiol. 2020;10:1607.
32. Rohm TV, Meier DT, Olefsky JM, Donath MY. Inflammation in obesity, diabetes, and related disorders. Immunity. 2022;55(1):31-55.
33. Burhans MS, Hagman DK, Kuzma JN, Schmidt KA, Kratz M. Contribution of Adipose Tissue Inflammation to the Development of Type 2 Diabetes Mellitus. Compr Physiol. 2018;9(1):1-58.
34. Yung JHM, Giacca A. Role of c-Jun N-terminal Kinase (JNK) in Obesity and Type 2 Diabetes. Cells. 2020;9(3):706.
35. Baker RG, Hayden MS, Ghosh S. NF-κB, inflammation, and metabolic disease. Cell Metab. 2011;13(1):11-22.
36. Russo L, Lumeng CN. Properties and functions of adipose tissue macrophages in obesity. Immunology. 2018;155(4):407-17.
37. Goldberg RB. Cytokine and cytokine-like inflammation markers, endothelial dysfunction, and imbalanced coagulation in development of diabetes and its complications. J Clin Endocrinol Metab. 2009;94(9):3171-82.
38. Richardson VR, Smith KA, Carter AM. Adipose tissue inflammation: feeding the development of type 2 diabetes mellitus. Immunobiology. 2013;218(12):1497-504.
39. Lee CH, Lam KS. Obesity-induced insulin resistance and macrophage infiltration of the adipose tissue: a vicious cycle. J Diabetes Investig. 2018;9(6):1239-48.
40. Berrou J, Fougeray S, Venot M, Chardiny V, Gautier JF, Dulphy N, et al. Natural killer cell function, an important target for infection and tumor protection, is impaired in type 2 diabetes. PLoS One. 2013;8(4):e62418.
41. Zhou T, Hu Z, Yang S, Sun L, Yu Z, Wang G. Role of Adaptive and Innate Immunity in Type 2 Diabetes Mellitus. J Diabetes Res. 2018;2018:7457269.

42. McLaughlin T, Ackerman SE, Shen L, Engleman E. Role of innate and adaptive immunity in obesity-associated metabolic disease. J Clin Invest. 2017;127(1):5-13
43. Fernández-Real JM, Pickup JC. Innate immunity, insulin resistance and type 2 diabetes. Diabetologia. 2012;55(2):273-8.
44. Chmelar J, Chung KJ, Chavakis T. The role of innate immune cells in obese adipose tissue inflammation and development of insulin resistance. Thromb Haemost. 2013;109(3):399-406.
45. Blaszczak AM, Jalilvand A, Hsueh WA. Adipocytes, Innate Immunity and Obesity: A Mini-Review. Front Immunol. 2021;12:650768.
46. Shu CJ, Benoist C, Mathis D. The immune system's involvement in obesity-driven type 2 diabetes. Semin Immunol. 2012;24(6):436-42.
47. Sell H, Habich C, Eckel J. Adaptive immunity in obesity and insulin resistance. Nat Rev Endocrinol. 2012;8(12):709-16.
48. Schwarz JM, Linfoot P, Dare D, Aghajanian K. Hepatic de novo lipogenesis in normoinsulinemic and hyperinsulinemic subjects consuming high-fat, low-carbohydrate and low-fat, high-carbohydrate isoenergetic diets. Am J Clin Nutr. 2003;77(1):43-50.
49. Adiels M, Taskinen MR, Packard C, Caslake MJ, Soro-Paavonen A, Westerbacka J, et al. Overproduction of large VLDL particles is driven by increased liver fat content in man. Diabetologia. 2006;49(4):755-65.
50. Lalloyer F, Vandewalle B, Percevault F, Torpier G, Kerr-Conte J, Oosterveer M, et al. Peroxisome proliferator-activated receptor alpha improves pancreatic adaptation to insulin resistance in obese mice and reduces lipotoxicity in human islets. Diabetes. 2006;55(5):1605-13.
51. White MG, Shaw JAM, Taylor R. Type 2 diabetes: the pathologic basis of reversible β-cell dysfunction. Diabetes Care. 2016;39(11):2080-8.
52. Stienstra R, Haim Y, Riahi Y, Netea M, Rudich A, Leibowitz G. Autophagy in adipose tissue and the beta cell: implications for obesity and diabetes. Diabetologia. 2014;57(8):1505-16.
53. Tao T, Xu H. Autophagy and obesity and diabetes. In: Le W (Ed). Autophagy: Biology and Diseases. Clinical Science. Singapore: Springer; 2020. pp. 425-45.
54. Barlow AD, Thomas DC. Autophagy in diabetes: β-cell dysfunction, insulin resistance, and complications. DNA Cell Biol. 2015;34(4):252-60.
55. Costes S, Bertrand G, Ravier MA. Mechanisms of Beta-Cell Apoptosis in Type 2 Diabetes-Prone Situations and Potential Protection by GLP-1-Based Therapies. Int J Mol Sci. 2021;22(10):5303.
56. Kahn SE. Clinical review 135: The importance of beta-cell failure in the development and progression of type 2 diabetes. J Clin Endocrinol Metab. 2001;86(9):4047-58.
57. Campbell JE, Newgard CB. Mechanisms controlling pancreatic islet cell function in insulin secretion. Nat Rev Mol Cell Biol. 2021;22(2):142-58.
58. Oh YS, Bae GD, Baek DJ, Park EY, Jun HS. Fatty Acid-Induced Lipotoxicity in Pancreatic Beta-Cells During Development of Type 2 Diabetes. Front Endocrinol (Lausanne). 2018;9:384.
59. Cerf ME. Beta cell dysfunction and insulin resistance. Front Endocrinol (Lausanne). 2013;4:37.
60. Richards P, Thornberry NA, Pinto S. The gut-brain axis: Identifying new therapeutic approaches for type 2 diabetes, obesity, and related disorders. Mol Metab. 2021;46:101175.
61. Scheithauer TPM, Rampanelli E, Nieuwdorp M, Vallance BA, Verchere CB, van Raalte DH, et al. Gut Microbiota as a Trigger for Metabolic Inflammation in Obesity and Type 2 Diabetes. Front Immunol. 2020;11:571731.
62. Haspula D, Cui Z. Neurochemical Basis of Inter-Organ Crosstalk in Health and Obesity: Focus on the Hypothalamus and the Brainstem. Cells. 2023;12(13):1801.
63. Boer GA, Holst JJ. Incretin Hormones and Type 2 Diabetes-Mechanistic Insights and Therapeutic Approaches. Biology (Basel). 2020;9(12):473.
64. Fujioka K. Pathophysiology of type 2 diabetes and the role of incretin hormones and beta-cell dysfunction. JAAPA. 2007;Suppl:3-8.
65. Nauck MA. Incretin-based therapies for type 2 diabetes mellitus: properties, functions, and clinical implications. Am J Med. 2011;124(1 Suppl):S3-18.
66. Lund A, Bagger JI, Christensen M, Knop FK, Vilsbøll T. Glucagon and type 2 diabetes: the return of the alpha cell. Curr Diab Rep. 2014;14(12):555.
67. Jia Y, Liu Y, Feng L, Sun S, Sun G. Role of Glucagon and Its Receptor in the Pathogenesis of Diabetes. Front Endocrinol (Lausanne). 2022;13:928016.

68. Ylli D, Sidhu S, Parikh T, Burman KD. Endocrine Changes in Obesity. In: Feingold KR, Anawalt B, Blackman MR, et al. (Eds). Endotext [Internet]. South Dartmouth (MA): MDText.com, Inc.; 2000.
69. Jaganathan R, Ravindran R, Dhanasekaran S. Emerging Role of Adipocytokines in Type 2 Diabetes as Mediators of Insulin Resistance and Cardiovascular Disease. Can J Diabetes. 2018;42(4):446-456.e1.
70. Mok JK, Makaronidis JM, Batterham RL. The Role of Gut Hormones in Obesity. Curr Opin Endocr Metab Res. 2019;4:4-13.
71. Torres-Fuentes C, Schellekens H, Dinan TG, Cryan JF. The microbiota-gut-brain axis in obesity. Lancet Gastroenterol Hepatol. 2017;2(10):747-56.
72. Ley RE, Bäckhed F, Turnbaugh P, Lozupone CA, Knight RD, Gordon JI. Obesity alters gut microbial ecology. Proc Natl Acad Sci U S A. 2005;102(31):11070-5.
73. Crovesy L, Masterson D, Rosado EL. Profile of the gut microbiota of adults with obesity: a systematic review. Eur J Clin Nutr. 2020;74(9):1251-62.
74. Caesar R, Reigstad CS, Bäckhed HK, Reinhardt C, Ketonen M, Lundén GÖ, et al. Gut-derived lipopolysaccharide augments adipose macrophage accumulation but is not essential for impaired glucose or insulin tolerance in mice. Gut. 2012;61(12):1701-7.
75. Muccioli GG, Naslain D, Bäckhed F, Reigstad CS, Lambert DM, Delzenne NM, et al. The endocannabinoid system links gut microbiota to adipogenesis. Mol Syst Biol. 2010;6:392.
76. Saad MJ, Santos A, Prada PO. Linking Gut Microbiota and Inflammation to Obesity and Insulin Resistance. Physiology (Bethesda). 2016;31(4):283-93.
77. Mullur R, Liu YY, Brent GA. Thyroid hormone regulation of metabolism. Physiol Rev. 2014;94:355-82.
78. Pasquali R, Casanueva F, Haluzik M, van Hulsteijn L, Ledoux S, Monteiro MP, et al. European Society of Endocrinology Clinical Practice Guideline: Endocrine work-up in obesity. Eur J Endocrinol. 2020;182:G1-G32.
79. Klein CE. The hypothalamic-pituitary-gonadal axis. In: Kufe DW, Pollock RE, Weichselbaum RR, Bast RC Jr, Gansler TS, Holland JF, et al. (Eds). Holland-Frei Cancer Medicine, 6th edition. Hamilton (ON): BC Decker; 2003.
80. van Hulsteijn LT, Pasquali R, Casanueva F, Haluzik M, Ledoux S, Monteiro MP, et al. Prevalence of endocrine disorders in obese patients: systematic review and meta-analysis. Eur J Endocrinol. 2020;182:11-21.
81. Cohen PG. Obesity in men: the hypogonadal-estrogen receptor relationship and its effect on glucose homeostasis. Med Hypotheses. 2008;70:358-60.
82. Liu Y, Ding Z. Obesity, a serious etiologic factor for male subfertility in modern society. Reproduction. 2017;154:R123-R131.
83. Resmini E, Minuto F, Colao A, Ferone D. Secondary diabetes associated with principal endocrinopathies: the impact of new treatment modalities. Acta Diabetol. 2009;46(2):85-95.

CHAPTER 3

Genetics of Human Obesity

> **Key Highlights**
> - Genetic factors play a significant role in the development of human obesity. Twin and family studies have consistently shown a strong familial clustering of obesity, indicating a genetic component.
> - The heritability of obesity is estimated to be around 40–70%, indicating that a substantial proportion of the variance in body weight and adiposity can be attributed to genetic factors.
> - Rare genetic syndromes and monogenic forms of obesity have provided valuable insights into the specific genes and pathways involved in body weight regulation. Mutations in genes such as *MC4R*, *LEPR*, and *POMC* have been associated with severe early-onset obesity.
> - Polygenic obesity refers to the influence of multiple genetic variants, each with a small effect size, on an individual's risk of developing obesity. Genome-wide association studies (GWAS) have identified numerous common genetic variants that contribute to polygenic obesity.
> - Gene-environment interactions play a crucial role in the development of obesity. Environmental factors, such as diet and physical activity, can modify the expression of obesity-related genes and influence individual susceptibility to weight gain.

INTRODUCTION

Obesity is a grave public health concern and is strongly associated with increased mortality rates. It contributes significantly to the burden of noncommunicable diseases worldwide, including type 2 diabetes mellitus (T2DM), cardiovascular disease, hypertension, and certain forms of cancer.[1] Defined clinically as a body mass index (BMI) above 30 kg/m², obesity imposes an ever-growing burden on global public health. Individuals with obesity face an elevated risk of various health conditions, such as T2DM, hypertension, cardiovascular disease, osteoarthritis, and several types of cancer.[2]

The pathogenesis of obesity is undeniably complex, involving intricate interactions among behavioral, environmental, and genetic factors. The rising prevalence of obesity can be partially attributed to the consumption of highly calorific foods and the sedentary lifestyle prevalent in modern times. Interestingly, obesity may have had advantages in primitive times when food availability was limited, and high energy expenditure through physical activity was a way of life. In such circumstances, individuals with a "thrifty phenotype" had a survival advantage due to their more efficient calorie utilization.[3] However, there exists a wide range of variability in obesity susceptibility among individuals or communities exposed to the same environmental risk factors. This observation suggests that genetic differences play a significant role in the variation of body weight and susceptibility to obesity. Notably, there is a strong genetic component underlying the substantial interindividual variation in body weight, as supported by twin and family studies. These studies consistently estimate the heritability of corpulence and adiposity in humans to be between 40 and 70%.[1,4]

Nevertheless, the heritability of obesity is also influenced by environmental factors. For instance, Finnish twin studies have reported a heritability of fat mass of up to 90% among twins with low physical activity. However, this percentage decreases to approximately 20% among the most active pairs of twins of the same ethnicity. This finding suggests that genetic influences on obesity are amplified in an obesogenic environment, while intense and sustained physical activity can mitigate some of the detrimental effects of obesity susceptibility variants.[4]

The origins of the "thrifty gene" hypothesis can be traced back to the influential paper by JV Neel. According to this theory, genes that predispose individuals to obesity may have provided a selective advantage in populations that frequently experienced periods of food scarcity and starvation. In today's obesogenic environment, individuals carrying these genes may exhibit an exaggerated response to the abundance of calorie-rich foods, resulting in not just mild overweight but extreme obesity. This phenomenon is particularly evident in certain high-risk populations, such as Pima Indians and Pacific Islanders, where the prevalence of obesity is notably higher. Moreover, recent studies conducted in the United States have revealed a disproportionate level of obesity among African-Americans and Hispanic-Americans compared to Caucasians, suggesting a significant role of genetics that cannot be solely attributed to lifestyle, economic, or environmental factors. These findings highlight the importance of genetics in shaping an individual's susceptibility to obesity. While lifestyle and environmental factors certainly contribute to the obesity epidemic, the presence of specific genes can lead to an overreaction in today's obesogenic environment, resulting in severe obesity. Understanding the genetic factors involved is crucial for developing targeted interventions and addressing the disparities observed in various populations. It emphasizes the complex interplay between genetic predisposition and the modern environment in shaping obesity levels.[5-7]

There is mounting evidence suggesting a significant genetic component in the risk of developing obesity. Twin studies have been instrumental in assessing the genetic contribution to this trait. Monozygotic (MZ) twins, who share identical genetic material, exhibit a concordance for fat mass ranging from 70 to 90%, whereas nonidentical dizygotic (DZ) twins, who share only 50% of their genetic material, have a lower concordance of 35–45%. Although twin studies provide strong evidence for the genetic influence on obesity, the variability in heritability estimates can be attributed to the methodology employed. For example, a study conducted by Stunkard reported a heritability of 77% for BMI, which increased to 84% in a 25-year follow-up of a sample of 1,974 MZ and 2,097 DZ male twin pairs. Adoption and family studies have further supported the role of genetics, showing a strong correlation between the BMI of adoptees and their biological parents, but not with adoptive parents. Additionally, studies on twins separated at birth have demonstrated a significant association in BMI for identical twins raised apart, while no such association was found for nonidentical twins.[3]

These findings strongly support the notion that genes play a central role in determining BMI and, consequently, in the development of obesity. However, identifying the specific genetic factors underlying obesity has proven challenging due to the complex interactions involved in the regulation of adiposity.

HERITABILITY AND FAMILIAL CLUSTERING OF OBESITY

Heritability Reported in Twin Studies

Epidemiological studies examining common obesity have consistently demonstrated a genetic component in the susceptibility to obesity. The concordance rates, which measure the similarity in obesity status, decrease as the degree of relatedness decreases. For example, the concordance rate between MZ twin pairs is more than twice that of DZ twin pairs, with values of approximately 0.68 compared to 0.28, respectively.[8-11]

Poulsen et al. conducted a study to investigate the relative contributions of genetic and environmental factors to the development of different components of the obesity syndrome in male and female twins. They enrolled 303 elderly twin pairs and utilized classic twin analysis to estimate concordance and heritability for these components. The findings revealed significantly higher concordance rates for glucose intolerance and overall obesity among MZ twins compared to DZ twins (0.64 vs. 0.43 and 0.71 vs. 0.56, respectively), indicating a stronger genetic influence on the development of these phenotypes. Heritability estimates for glucose concentration and BMI among MZ twins further supported these results. When analyzing the data separately for men and women, the researchers observed the difference in concordance rates between male MZ and DZ twin pairs (0.70 vs. 0.41), suggesting a genetic influence specifically among male twins. However, for glucose intolerance, the concordance rates were similar between female MZ and DZ twins. The study also revealed significant differences in interclass correlation, a measure of similarity, between MZ and DZ twins for postoral glucose tolerance test plasma glucose at 120 minutes and BMI (0.52 vs. 0.26 and 0.68 vs. 0.28, respectively).[8]

The National Academy of Sciences-National Research Council (NAS-NRC) Twin Registry conducted a study involving the assessment of height, weight, and BMI in a sample of 1,974 MZ (identical) and 2,097 DZ (fraternal) male twin pairs. The findings from this study were consistent with concordance rates reported in the Danish registry, indicating that the rates of overweight were twice as high for MZ twins compared to DZ twins. Using classic twin methods, the study estimated the heritability of height, weight, and BMI at two different time points—at age 20 years and at a 25-year follow-up. The heritability estimates were found to be high for all three measures. At age 20, the heritability estimates were 0.80 for height, 0.78 for weight, and 0.77 for BMI. At the 25-year follow-up, the heritability estimates increased slightly to 0.80 for height, 0.81 for weight, and 0.84 for BMI. These results suggest that approximately 80% of the variance in BMI can be attributed to genetic factors. These findings align with the results of other twin studies investigating the heritability of height, weight, and BMI. The data consistently point toward a substantial genetic influence on obesity, indicating that genetic factors play a significant role in determining an individual's susceptibility to obesity.[9]

The Finnish Twin Cohort, a European twin study, aimed to assess the genetic and environmental contributions to the variance in BMI. The study involved 7,245 nonpregnant MZ and DZ twin pairs of the same sex. The results of the study indicated that genetic effects played a substantial role in the variation of BMI. Among men, genetic factors contributed to 72% of the total variance, indicating a strong genetic influence on BMI. Among nonpregnant women, genetic effects accounted for 66.4% of the total variance in BMI. In addition to genetic factors, the study also identified nonshared environmental effects that contributed to the variance in BMI. These nonshared environmental factors accounted for 27.8% of the variance among men and 33.6% among women. These findings suggest that both genetic and nonshared environmental factors play significant roles in the development of BMI. The study highlights the complex interplay between genetic predisposition and environmental influences in determining an individual's BMI.[10]

The prevalence of abdominal obesity has been on the rise, particularly in pediatric populations, surpassing the increase in overall BMI. This upward trend is concerning as visceral fat, which accumulates in the abdomen, is considered a major contributor to obesity-related health risks. Twin studies provide valuable insights into the heritability of abdominal fatness and help determine whether genetic influences are shared or unique to BMI. Previous research has demonstrated high heritability for various adiposity measures in adults, including truncal skinfold thickness, percentage body fat, and waist circumference (WC). Associations with BMI have implicated both common and distinct genetic factors. To explore the genetic and environmental influences on BMI and central adiposity in children during the peak of the pediatric obesity epidemic, Wardle et al. conducted a study using data from United Kingdom registries. The study included 5,092 twin pairs aged 8-11 years. The findings revealed that DZ twins had significantly higher BMIs and WCs compared to MZ twins. By doubling the difference between the correlations of MZ and DZ twins, the researchers estimated the heritability of BMI scores and WC. The results indicated substantial genetic influences, with heritability estimates of 74% for BMI and 74% for WC. When the estimates were combined across sexes, the heritability estimates reached 77% for BMI and 76% for WC. In conclusion, this study highlighted the significant genetic influences on BMI and abdominal adiposity among children born since the onset of the pediatric obesity epidemic. The majority of the genetic effect on abdominal adiposity is shared with BMI, indicating common genetic determinants. However, around 40% of the genetic influence on abdominal adiposity is attributable to independent genetic factors. These findings contribute to our understanding of the complex genetic underpinnings of obesity and emphasize the need for comprehensive strategies to address the rising prevalence of abdominal obesity in children.[11]

The "Linosa Study" was conducted in a unique and isolated population of 293 Caucasian individuals, including 123 parents and 170 offspring. The purpose of this study was to investigate the potential for genetic analysis of complex diseases, specifically focusing on the metabolic syndrome (MetS). The researchers aimed to leverage the distinct characteristics of this islander population to provide epidemiological insights and estimate heritability for MetS and its related traits based on the National Cholesterol Education Program/Adult Treatment Panel III (NCEP/ATP III) criteria. In the Linosa group, the overall prevalence of MetS was found to be relatively high, reaching 29.9%. This prevalence appeared notably higher compared to data reported from NHANES III, a population study conducted in the United States, as well as other Caucasian populations in Europe. These findings highlight the unique nature of the Linosa population and the potential influence of genetic factors on the development of MetS. Significantly, the study yielded remarkable heritability estimates for MetS, central obesity, and WC, amounting to 27%, 27%, and 38%, respectively. These estimates suggest a substantial genetic contribution to the observed variability in these traits. Similarly, when investigating insulin resistance (IR) as a discrete trait, appreciable heritability of 32% was observed ($p < 0.001$). Additionally, when assessing IR using HOMA-IR (homeostatic model assessment for IR) quantitative values, a heritability estimate of 38% was obtained ($p < 0.001$). These findings from the Linosa Study emphasize the potential role of genetic factors in the development of MetS and its related traits, including central obesity and IR. The high heritability estimates underscore the importance of genetic influences in these complex diseases. The unique characteristics of the Linosa population provide valuable insights for further genetic analysis of complex diseases, paving the way for future research in this field.[12]

The high prevalence of diabetes among South Asians is closely associated with a significant propensity for abdominal obesity. In a study conducted by Davey et al., the researchers aimed to develop a measure of central obesity that accounts for total adiposity and environmental factors, and to assess the genetic contribution to familial aggregation in Indian families. The study involved a community-based cross-sectional investigation in Chennai, India, with a total of 1,295 individuals from 300 families participating. The researchers focused on the adjusted sagittal abdominal diameter as a measure of central obesity. The intrasibship correlation for this adjusted parameter was found to be 0.46, suggesting a high degree of similarity within siblings. This correlation indicates a sibship heritability estimate of approximately 0.9, suggesting that around 90% of the observed variation in abdominal fat accumulation adjusted for total adiposity, sex, and age could be attributed to genetic factors within the studied population. Interestingly, when individuals with diabetes were excluded from the analysis, the intrasibship correlation slightly increased to 0.48. This finding implies that the genetic contribution to familial aggregation in central obesity remains strong even in the absence of diabetes. Furthermore, the researchers accounted for possible assortative mating, a process where individuals with similar phenotypes are more likely to form partnerships, and found that the results still support a heritability estimate exceeding 90% for the defined trait of adjusted abdominal fat accumulation. These findings suggest that conducting linkage studies focused on abdominal obesity could potentially identify one or more genes associated with this highly heritable trait. Identifying such genes may offer valuable insights into the genetic factors underlying T2DM among South Asians, given the strong association between abdominal obesity and the increased risk of developing this disease in this population.[13]

In a study conducted by the Twins UK Registry, a cohort of 430 MZ (215 pairs) and 1,750 DZ (875 pairs) British female twins was examined to investigate the potential impact of obesity on the genetic susceptibility to T2DM. The primary outcome measure used in the study was insulin sensitivity, which was assessed using the quantitative insulin-sensitivity check index (QUICKI). The study findings revealed that the influence of unique environmental factors on QUICKI decreased as BMI increased. This indicates that genetic factors play a more significant role in determining insulin sensitivity at higher levels of BMI. At the average BMI level of 25 kg/m^2, the heritability of QUICKI was estimated to be 0.61, indicating that 61% of the variation in insulin sensitivity could be attributed to genetic factors. Furthermore, the study observed a notable gene-obesity interaction. Among twins who were concordant for overweight, the heritability of QUICKI was found to be 31 percentage points higher [h^2 = 0.81; 95% confidence interval (CI) 0.65–0.90] compared to twins who were concordant for normal weight (h^2 = 0.50; 95% CI 0.37–0.60). This indicates that the genetic influence on insulin sensitivity is even more pronounced in individuals who are overweight. In conclusion, this twin study provides further evidence supporting the existence of a gene-obesity interaction concerning insulin sensitivity at an aggregate level.[14]

HERITABILITY REPORTED IN ADOPTEE STUDIES

In adoptee studies, such as the Danish registry and the Muscatine Ponderosity Family Study, the influence of genetic factors on BMI becomes evident. These studies have shown that the BMI of adopted individuals is more closely correlated with the BMI of their biological parents rather than their adoptive parents, emphasizing the importance of genetic factors over the shared familial environment. In the Danish adoptee study, a sample of 540 adult Danish adoptees, selected from a population of 3,580, was categorized into four weight classes—(1) thin, (2) median weight, (3) overweight, and (4) obese. The study aimed to assess the contributions of genetic factors and family environment to human fatness. The findings indicated that the BMI of the adopted individuals was most strongly associated with the BMI of their biological parents, providing further evidence for the role of genetic factors in determining fatness. Similarly, the Muscatine Ponderosity Family Study investigated the role of genetic and environmental factors in determining the variability in BMI among 1,302 relatives identified through 284 schoolchildren from Muscatine. The study aimed to understand the contributions of genetics and environmental factors to BMI variation. The results supported the significance of genetic factors in determining BMI, further highlighting the influence of genetics overshared environmental factors. The Adoptee studies consistently demonstrate that genetic factors play a substantial role in determining BMI and fatness.[15,16]

Overall, these twin studies and adoptee studies consistently demonstrate that genetic factors play a substantial role in determining BMI and WC. The correlation between the BMI of adopted individuals and their biological parents' BMI suggests a strong genetic influence on weight and body composition. They also highlight the significant role of genetic factors in influencing insulin sensitivity, particularly in individuals with higher BMI levels. Understanding the interplay between genes, obesity, and insulin sensitivity can contribute to a better comprehension of the mechanisms underlying T2DM and may have implications for personalized approaches to prevention and treatment.

Familial Clustering of Obesity

Familial clustering of a disease refers to its occurrence within specific families at a higher rate than what would be expected in the general population. This phenomenon has been observed in various diseases, such as kidney disease, Ménière's disease, cardiovascular diseases, and different types of cancer. Numerous studies have focused on examining the familial clustering of obesity in diverse countries across the globe.[17-23] Parental obesity is a significant factor associated with obesity during childhood and adolescence, with both genetic and environmental influences playing a role. The presence of parental obesity contributes to familial patterns of adiposity through gene-environment interactions. Extensive research has consistently demonstrated that parental obesity is a notable risk factor for childhood obesity. Studies consistently show a direct correlation between parental and childhood fatness, indicating that as parental fatness increases, so does childhood fatness. Children with two obese parents are particularly vulnerable to obesity compared to those with one or neither parent being obese. While some studies suggest potential variations in the impact of maternal and paternal obesity, this finding is not consistently observed. Understanding the etiology of obesity during childhood and adolescence is crucial for developing effective prevention programs. By identifying the underlying causes and risk factors, targeted prevention strategies can be implemented to encourage healthier lifestyles and reduce the prevalence of obesity in this age group.[22] Overall, familial clustering of obesity is a complex phenomenon influenced by a combination of genetic, environmental, early life, and shared lifestyle factors. Understanding the factors contributing to familial clustering can help in the development of effective strategies for obesity prevention and management, with a focus on both individual and family-based interventions.

In a cross-sectional study conducted by Li et al. in Northern China, the prevalence of overweight and obesity was found to be alarmingly high, particularly among boys and their fathers. The study aimed to investigate the existence of familial clustering of overweight and obesity among schoolchildren and their family members in this region. A large sample of 95,292 schoolchildren was included in the study, and a subgroup of 450 overweight and obese children was selected for further analysis. Detailed questionnaires were administered to collect data on nutrition and behaviors of the children and their families, which were then subjected to statistical analysis. The results revealed a significant prevalence of familial clustering, with 75.3% of families showing clustering of overweight and 20.3% showing clustering of obesity. Both parents (first-generation relatives) and grandparents (second-generation relatives) exhibited high rates of overweight, with prevalence rates of 54.6% and 53.1% respectively. Interestingly, the study also identified a significant association between familial clustering of obesity and family income, indicating that socioeconomic factors may play a role in the development of obesity within families. Importantly, the study also found a significant association between familial clustering of obesity and family income. This suggests that socioeconomic factors may contribute to the development of obesity within families. Overall, the results of this study confirmed the presence of familial aggregation of high adiposity, indicating that the tendency toward overweight and obesity runs in families in this population.[24]

The Resilience for Eating and Activity Despite Inequality (READI) study conducted in Australia shed light on the familial clustering of behaviors, specifically focusing on the concordance of clusters between children and their mothers. The study findings suggest that parents, particularly mothers, play a crucial role in modeling sedentary behavior and shaping the eating environment for their children. The analysis of concordance in clustering between mothers and children revealed strong relationships in clusters where sedentary behavior or consumption of energy-dense food and drinks were predominant traits. This indicates that parental influence, specifically in terms of modeling sedentary behavior and creating an environment conducive to consuming high-calorie foods, may be particularly important in shaping these behaviors in children. Furthermore, the Cluster Analysis of Behaviors demonstrated significant correlations between BMI and both sedentary time and physical activity. Specifically, higher sedentary time was positively associated with BMI, while physical activity showed a negative association. These findings highlight the importance of these behaviors in relation to weight status, with sedentary behavior being linked to higher BMI ($r = 0.04$; $p < 0.05$) and physical activity potentially playing a role in its reduction ($r = -0.08$; $p < 0.05$).[25]

In a population-based family study conducted in Eastern Finland, the findings supported the relationship of familial aggregation of BMI between mothers and their children. Mother-offspring pairs showed a correlation coefficient of 0.31 ($p < 0.001$), father-offspring pairs had a correlation coefficient of 0.23 ($p = 0.017$), mother-daughter pairs had a correlation coefficient of 0.26 ($p = 0.044$), and mother-son pairs had the highest correlation coefficient of 0.36 ($p = 0.001$). The presence of maternal obesity was associated with three times higher proportion of children being in the highest quartile of BMI. Similarly, when one or both parents were obese, there was a 2.8 times increased likelihood of children being in the highest quartile of BMI, and it increased to 4.6 times when both parents were obese. These findings confirm the aggregation of BMI within families, indicating a familial predisposition to obesity. The consistent relationship between maternal obesity and offspring obesity suggests that mothers may play a key role in primary prevention efforts against obesity.[26]

A cross-sectional study conducted on a Japanese population focused on analyzing family cluster patterns between families and preschool children. The study included 2,114 preschool children aged 3-6 years who attended childcare facilities, including nursery schools and kindergartens. The findings of the study highlighted the importance of certain factors in preventing overweight and obesity in children. The results indicated that reducing screen time and increasing nighttime sleep duration are key factors in preventing children's overweight and obesity. The study identified clusters of children based on various factors such as screen time, sleep duration, dinner timing, and outside playtime. The cluster with the highest prevalence of overweight and obesity (15.1%) was characterized by excessive screen time, shorter nighttime sleep duration, average dinner timing, and average outside playtime. On the other hand, the cluster with the lowest prevalence of overweight and obesity (4.0%) exhibited the least screen time, longest sleep duration, earliest dinner timing, and average outside playtime. Additionally, the study found that family environments, specifically mealtime regularity and parents' screen time, varied significantly across clusters. The cluster with the highest prevalence of overweight and obesity had a higher proportion of irregular mealtimes and the highest screen time for both parents. These findings emphasize the importance of creating healthy family environments and routines to prevent childhood overweight and obesity. By promoting consistent mealtimes, reducing screen time for both children and parents, and ensuring adequate nighttime sleep, the risk of overweight and obesity in preschool children can be mitigated.[27]

Overall, parental obesity has been identified as an important independent risk factor for adiposity in children. The association between parental obesity and childhood adiposity can be influenced by factors such as gender and age. It is crucial to recognize that parents play a significant role in shaping the lifestyle patterns of their children, and this influence extends to their risk of developing obesity. When addressing the issue of childhood obesity, it is essential to consider the familial environmental factors that contribute to its development. The home environment, including dietary habits, physical activity levels, and sedentary behaviors, can greatly influence a child's risk of obesity. Parents serve as role models and gatekeepers in promoting healthy behaviors and creating a supportive environment for their children.

MONOGENIC AND POLYGENIC FORMS OF OBESITY

The classification of obesity into monogenic and polygenic categories has been traditionally used to differentiate between rare, severe, and early-onset forms of obesity (monogenic) and more common forms influenced by multiple genetic factors (polygenic). Monogenic obesity is associated with specific genetic mutations or chromosomal abnormalities that have a significant impact on body weight regulation. On the other hand, polygenic obesity results from the cumulative effect of numerous genetic variants, each contributing a small effect to overall obesity risk. While monogenic and polygenic obesity have been considered distinct forms, recent research has revealed common underlying biological mechanisms. Both forms of obesity involve the central nervous system (CNS) and neuronal pathways that control the hedonic aspects of food intake. These pathways play a crucial role in regulating body weight, appetite, and energy balance. Furthermore, there is evidence suggesting that the expression and effects of monogenic obesity-causing mutations may be influenced, at least to some extent, by an individual's polygenic susceptibility to obesity.[1] In the past, the search for genes associated with obesity was guided by specific hypotheses and focused on a limited number of candidate genes believed to be involved in regulating body weight. However, recent advancements in high-throughput genome-wide genotyping and sequencing technologies, along with a deeper understanding of human genetic architecture, have revolutionized the field. These advances now allow researchers to explore the entire genome and investigate the role of genetic variants in body weight regulation without preconceived hypotheses. This hypothesis-generating approach has opened up new possibilities for uncovering genetic factors contributing to obesity and has significantly advanced our understanding of the complex genetic basis of this condition.

Monogenic Forms of Obesity

Monogenic obesity refers to a group of rare and severe forms of obesity caused by mutations with significant effects in a single gene or chromosomal region. While these monogenic forms of obesity are uncommon, studying their genetic basis has greatly contributed to our understanding of obesity's development and shed light on various pathways and mechanisms involved. The discovery of the ob/ob mutant mouse strain in the 1950s was an early milestone in obesity research. These mice exhibited excessive adipose tissue, reproductive issues, and a mature weight approximately three times higher than normal mice. However, identifying the specific mutation responsible for the ob phenotype took several years. In 1994, positional cloning techniques were employed to locate and characterize the gene involved. It was found that the gene encoded a 16-kDa secreted protein, which was named leptin, derived from the Greek word "leptos" meaning thin. Interestingly, another strain of severely obese mice, db/db, was later discovered to have a mutation in the leptin receptor gene. The discovery of the leptin gene and its receptor mutation provided crucial insights into the regulation of body weight and appetite. These findings emphasized the importance of the leptin signaling pathway in the control of energy balance and highlighted the role of defective leptin signaling in the development of obesity. Studying monogenic forms of obesity, such as the ob/ob and db/db mouse models, has been instrumental in uncovering key genetic factors and unraveling the biological mechanisms involved in obesity.[1,3,4] **Table 1** provides a concise summary of the various underlying causes of monogenic obesity. It presents an overview of the specific genetic mutations and associated genes that contribute to this rare form of severe obesity.[28]

The genetics of obesity can be categorized into two main groups—(1) syndromic and (2) nonsyndromic obesity, each with distinct characteristics. Syndromic obesity refers to severe obesity that is accompanied by additional phenotypes, such as mental retardation, dysmorphic features, and specific developmental abnormalities. Examples of syndromic obesity include conditions such as Prader-Willi syndrome, fragile X syndrome, Bardet-Biedl syndrome, Cohen syndrome, and Albright hereditary osteodystrophy (AHO), all of which are associated with developmental delay and the early onset of obesity **(Table 2)**. On the other hand, nonsyndromic obesity can have various genetic origins. It can be monogenic, meaning caused by mutations in a single gene, polygenic, involving multiple genes,

TABLE 1: The genetic architecture of monogenic obesity.

Name	Gene	Mode of inheritance	Chromosomal position	Associated phenotype
Leptin	LEP	Autosomal recessive	7q32.1	• Severe early-onset obesity • Extreme hyperphagia • Hyperinsulinemia • Hypothalamic hypothyroidism • Hypogonadotropic hypogonadism
Leptin receptor	LEPR	Autosomal recessive	1p31.2	• Severe obesity with hyperphagia • Delayed or absent puberty • Reduced IGF-1 (insulin-like growth factor 1) levels • Growth abnormalities
Proopio-melanocortin	POMC	Autosomal recessive	2p23.2	• Severe pediatric-onset obesity • Hyperphagia • Red hair pigmentation • Pale skin
Melanocortin 4 receptor	MC4R	Autosomal dominant/ Autosomal recessive	18q21.32	• Severe early-onset obesity • Hyperphagia • Highly elevated plasma insulin concentrations • Increased bone mineral density (BMD)
Single-minded drosophila homolog-1	SIM1	Autosomal dominant	6q16.3	• Early-onset obesity • Hypotonia • Developmental delay • Short extremities
Neurotrophic tyrosine kinase receptor type 2	NTRK2	Autosomal dominant	9q21.33	• Severe early onset obesity • Deregulation of food intake
Kinase suppressor of Ras 2	KSR2	Autosomal dominant	12q24.22-q24.23	• Hyperphagia in childhood • Low heart rate • Reduced metabolic rate • Severe insulin resistance
Carboxy-peptidase	CPE	Autosomal dominant	4q32.3	• Intellectual disability • Type 2 diabetes mellitus • Hypogonadotropic • Hypogonadism
Proconvertase 1	PCSK1	Autosomal recessive	5q15	• Severe childhood obesity • Abnormal glucose homeostasis • Reduced plasma insulin with elevated proinsulin levels • Hypogonadotropic hypogonadism hypocortisolemia

Continued

Continued

Name	Gene	Mode of inheritance	Chromosomal position	Associated phenotype
Brain-derived neurotropic factor (PWS)	BDNF	Autosomal dominant	11p14.1	• Early-onset obesity • Deregulation of food intake
SH2B adaptor protein	SH2B1	Autosomal dominant	16p11.2	• Severe early-onset obesity • Hyperphagic • Hyperinsulinemia without diabetes • Delayed speech and language • Aggressive behavior
Tubby, homolog of mouse	TUB	Autosomal recessive	11p15.4	• Obesity • Decreased visual acuity • Night blindness • Rod-cone dystrophy

TABLE 2: Syndromic forms of human obesity.

Syndrome	Gene	Mode of inheritance	Phenotype
Prader–Willi syndrome (PWS)	Contiguous gene disorder	Imprinting defect with loss of paternally expressed genes on 15q11–13	Neonatal hypotonia, poor feeding, evolving into extreme hyperphagia, central obesity, decreased lean body mass, short stature, hypothalamic hypogonadism, mild mental retardation, and obsessive-compulsive behavior
Bardet–Biedl syndrome	At least 12 loci (BBS1–BBS12) 12 genes identified	Oligogenic: Either autosomal recessive or tri-tetra allelic	Progressive rod-cone dystrophy, post axial polydactyly, renal cysts, progressive renal disease, dyslexia, learning disabilities, hypogonadism, occasional congenital heart disease, and progressive late childhood obesity
Alstrom syndrome	ALMS1	Autosomal recessive	Mild truncal obesity, short stature, type 2 diabetes mellitus, retinopathy, sensorineural hearing loss, nephropathy, and dilated cardiomyopathy
WAGR syndrome	BNDF	Autosomal dominant	Obesity, Wilms' tumor, aniridia, genitourinary anomalies, and mental retardation
16p11.2 deletion		Autosomal dominant	Progressive obesity, autism/mental retardation
Fragile X syndrome (FXS)	FMR1 gene at chromosome Xq27.3	Autosomal dominant	Intellectual disability, large ears, a narrow head, long face, and prognathism. Joint laxity, mitral valve prolapse, and macroorchidism

Continued

Continued

Syndrome	Gene	Mode of inheritance	Phenotype
Down syndrome	Extracopy of chromosome 21	Chromosomal disorders	Developmental disabilities specifically targeting children with physical disabilities, coordination disorder, and intellectual disability
Albright hereditary osteodystrophy	GNAS1	Autosomal dominant	Short stature, brachydactyly, developmental delay, pseudo-hypoparathyroidism, a round face, and early-onset obesity
Cohen syndrome	Vacuolar protein sorting 13 homolog B (VPS13B) gene on chromosome 8q22.2		Progressive retinochoroidal dystrophy and myopia, acquired microcephaly, developmental delay, hypotonia, joint laxity, characteristic facial features with prominent central incisors, truncal obesity, cheerful disposition, and neutropenia
Smith–Magenis syndrome	Interstitial deletion of chromosome 17p11.2	Autosomal dominant	Mental retardation, developmental delay, renal anomalies, sleep disturbances, dysmorphic features, and behavioral problems including maladaptive/self-injurious, aggressive, and food seeking behaviors like patients with PWS
Kallmann syndrome	KAL1, FGFR1, FGF8, PROKR2, and PROK2 genes	Autosomal recessive or dominant pattern	Gonadotropin-releasing hormone deficiency, anosmia, abnormal eye movements, ptosis, hearing loss, unilateral renal agenesis, cleft lip or palate, and obesity

or chromosomal, resulting from abnormalities in chromosomes. This classification reflects the complexity of nonsyndromic obesity, where multiple genetic factors may contribute to an individual's susceptibility to obesity.[29,30]

Leptin, a hormone primarily produced and secreted by white adipose tissue, is also present in smaller amounts in other tissues such as brown adipocytes, the stomach, placenta, skeletal muscle, and ovaries. In the db/db mouse strain, a mutation in the leptin receptor gene has been identified as the underlying cause, resulting in severe diabetes mellitus, obesity, and dyslipidemia.[3,4]

To better comprehend the impact of genetic mutations, it is helpful to have a basic understanding of the central regulatory pathway involved in appetite regulation **(Fig. 1)**. The CNS, specifically the hypothalamic leptin-melanocortin pathway, plays a crucial role in maintaining energy balance by regulating food intake through the brain-gut axis.[31] Signals originating from various tissues and organs, such as the gut (hormones such as ghrelin, peptide YY, cholecystokinin, and glucagon-like peptide-1) and the pancreas (insulin), as well as adipokine hormones such as leptin and adiponectin, are received by the hypothalamus. These signals are integrated, and downstream pathways are activated to maintain energy balance.

CHAPTER 3: Genetics of Human Obesity

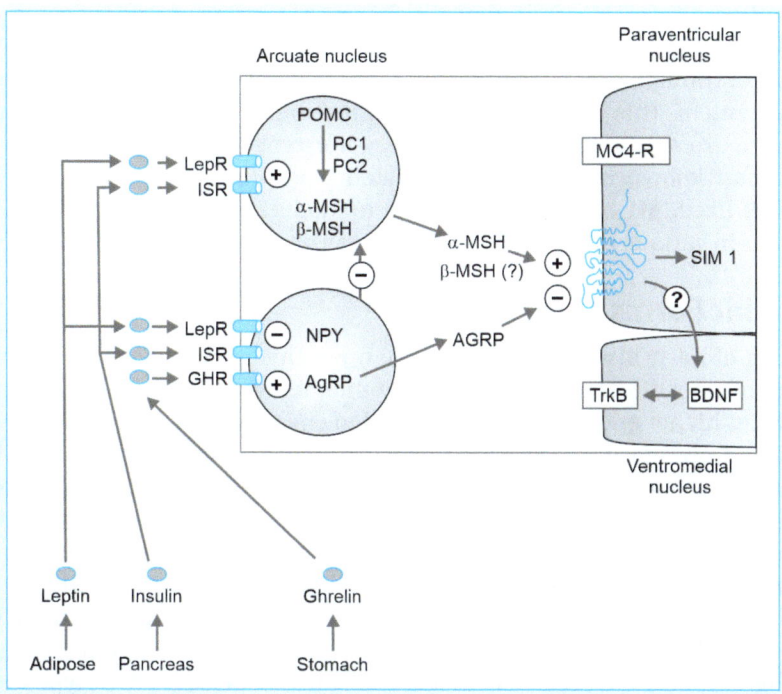

FIG. 1: The leptin/melanocortin pathway. The integration of signals within the hypothalamus plays a critical role in maintaining energy balance and regulating food intake. Various molecules from peripheral tissues communicate with distinct neuronal populations, contributing to the control of satiety and hunger. For example, POMC neurons in the arcuate nucleus are stimulated by leptin and insulin, leading to the production of α-MSH. This molecule activates the *MC4R* receptor in the paraventricular nucleus, triggering a signal of satiety. Ongoing research is investigating the downstream functions of *SIM1*, *BDNF*, and *TKRB* in this pathway. In contrast, another group of neurons that express *NPY* and *AgRP* produces molecules that strongly inhibit MC4R signaling. Any malfunction in these pathways can disrupt energy homeostasis, leading to imbalances in appetite regulation and metabolism.

[AgRP: agouti-related protein; α-MSH: alpha-melanocyte stimulating hormone; BDNF: brain-derived neurotrophic factor; GHR: ghrelin receptor; ISR: insulin receptor; LepR: leptin receptor; NPY: neuropeptide Y; PC1 and 2: proprotein convertase 1 and 2; POMC: proopiomelanocortin; SIM1: single-minded homolog 1 (Drosophila); TrkB: tyrosine kinase receptor]

The leptin/melanocortin pathway is activated by the binding of leptin to leptin receptors (LepR) and insulin-to-insulin receptors (INSR) present on the surface of arcuate nucleus neurons. This process is regulated by two sets of neurons in a feedback loop. The proopiomelanocortin and cocaine- and amphetamine-regulated transcript neurons (POMC/CART) regulate the production of the anorexigenic peptide POMC. Simultaneously, another set of neurons regulates the production of the orexigenic peptides agouti-related peptide (AgRP) and neuropeptide-Y (NPY).[32] POMC undergoes post-translational processing by proprotein convertase 1 (PC1) and proprotein convertase 2 (PC2), resulting in the production of various peptides, including α-, β-, and γ-melanocyte stimulating hormone (MSH) and β-endorphins.[31,33] The melanocortin-4 receptor (MC4R), highly expressed in the paraventricular nucleus (PVN) of the hypothalamus, is the target for binding by both AgRP and α-MSH. Binding of α-MSH to MC4R triggers anorexigenic signals, while binding of AgRP elicits orexigenic signals.[34] Signals from MC4R influence food intake through secondary effector neurons that transmit the signals to higher cortical centers. This process involves brain-derived neurotrophic factor (BDNF) and the neurotrophic tyrosine kinase receptor type 2 (NTRK2), which codes for the receptor known as tropomyosin-related kinase B (TrkB). Additionally, other regulators like SIM1 have been identified to modulate the effects of this pathway. Mutations in various genes within this pathway have been linked to obesity.[35-37]

Polygenic Forms of Obesity

Polygenic obesity, also known as common obesity, occurs when an individual's genetic composition increases their vulnerability to an environment that encourages higher energy intake compared to energy expenditure. The prevalence of common obesity has escalated into a significant epidemic in many Western societies due to factors such as abundant food availability and sedentary lifestyles, posing a substantial challenge to these populations.[38] Polygenic obesity, also known as "common obesity", is a form of obesity that is thought to result from the combined effect of variants in multiple genes acting in concert with environmental risk factors. Early studies investigating the genetic basis of common obesity relied on linkage analyses and candidate gene approaches. Linkage analysis identifies chromosomal regions cosegregating with a disease phenotype in related individuals by leveraging the relationship between recombination frequency and physical distance. Genetic markers coinherited with the phenotype indicate proximity of the markers and the disease locus, analyzed using polymorphic markers on a genome-wide or targeted scale. Candidate gene studies aim to identify associations between genetic markers in specific genes of interest and a particular phenotype. These studies focus on functional or positional candidates based on biological evidence or genomic mapping, and rely on existing knowledge in the field.[4] The candidate gene approach, initiated in the mid-1990s, aimed to confirm the involvement of genes identified in extreme obesity models, both in humans and animals, in the development of common obesity. This approach involved testing common variants within candidate genes for associations with obesity risk, BMI, or other body composition traits. Despite studying hundreds of candidate genes over the following 15 years, only six genes (*ADRB3, BDNF, CNR1, MC4R, PCSK1,* and *PPARG*) demonstrated consistent associations with obesity outcomes.[1] The advent of high-density single nucleotide polymorphism (SNP) genotyping arrays has revolutionized the study of common genetic variants in relation to obesity. Genome-wide association studies (GWAS) now allow for the analysis of millions of SNPs across thousands of individuals, leading to the identification of multiple genomic loci associated with BMI and obesity. These associations have been replicated in numerous studies, providing robust evidence. GWAS employ unbiased approaches, testing the frequency of alleles or genotypes at each SNP for their association with the phenotype of interest. These studies require large sample sizes to detect associations, particularly for complex diseases with small effect sizes of common variants. In obesity-related research, GWAS focus on BMI as a quantitative trait and examine extreme obesity phenotypes through case-control studies.[4]

GENETIC MARKERS AND VARIANTS ASSOCIATED WITH OBESITY

Monogenic Genes Associated with Obesity

The genetic architecture of monogenic obesity is characterized by specific gene variants that have a large effect on body weight regulation. These variants disrupt various biological pathways involved in appetite control, energy balance, and metabolism. Examples of genes associated with monogenic obesity include *MC4R*, *LEPR*, *POMC*, and *PCSK1*, among others. Individuals with monogenic obesity often exhibit early-onset and severe forms of obesity, and the identification of specific gene mutations can aid in the diagnosis and management of this condition (**Table 1**).[28]

Polygenic Genes Associated with Obesity

In the late 1990s, the genome-wide linkage approach emerged in the field of obesity research. This approach utilizes the relatedness of individuals to investigate whether specific chromosomal regions cosegregate with obesity traits across generations. Although over 80 genome-wide linkage studies identified >300 chromosomal loci potentially linked to obesity, only a few loci were replicated, and none were successfully fine-mapped to identify the causal genes involved.[1]

Genome-wide association studies of BMI have previously identified 10 loci with genome-wide significant ($p < 5 \times 10^{-8}$) associations in or near (1) *FTO*, (2) *MC4R*, (3) *TMEM18*, (4) *GNPDA2*, (5) *BDNF*, (6) *NEGR1*, (7) *SH2B1*, (8) *ETV5*, (9) *MTCH2*, and (10) *KCTD15*. Many of these genes are expressed or known to act in the CNS, highlighting a likely neuronal component in the predisposition to obesity. The 10 previously identified loci account for only a small fraction of the variation in BMI. Furthermore, power calculations based on the effect sizes of established variants have suggested that increasing the sample size would likely lead to the discovery of additional variants. A summary of genetic variants associated with BMI and obesity identified through GWAS is presented in **Figure 2**.[39-44] The initial significant finding in GWAS of adiposity was the identification of a robust association between BMI, obesity, and a region on chromosome *16q12* containing the *FTO* gene. Multiple studies published in 2007 reported the association of SNPs within the *FTO* gene with BMI and obesity. Expression analyses have demonstrated high levels of *FTO* expression in various tissues, including the hypothalamus, suggesting its potential involvement in body weight regulation.[39-45]

To enhance the statistical power in investigating gene variants linked to BMI, the Genetic Investigation of ANthropometric Traits (GIANT) consortium, a multinational collaboration, was established. In their initial meta-analysis, utilizing a discovery sample of 16,876 individuals, the consortium identified a significant association between common *MC4R* variants and BMI.[41] Concurrently, Chambers et al. reported an association between *MC4R* SNPs and WC as well as IR in individuals of east-Asian descent. Previous associations of rare pathogenic *MC4R* variants with monogenic obesity suggest that genes carrying deleterious mutations leading to extreme obesity may also contain variants associated with

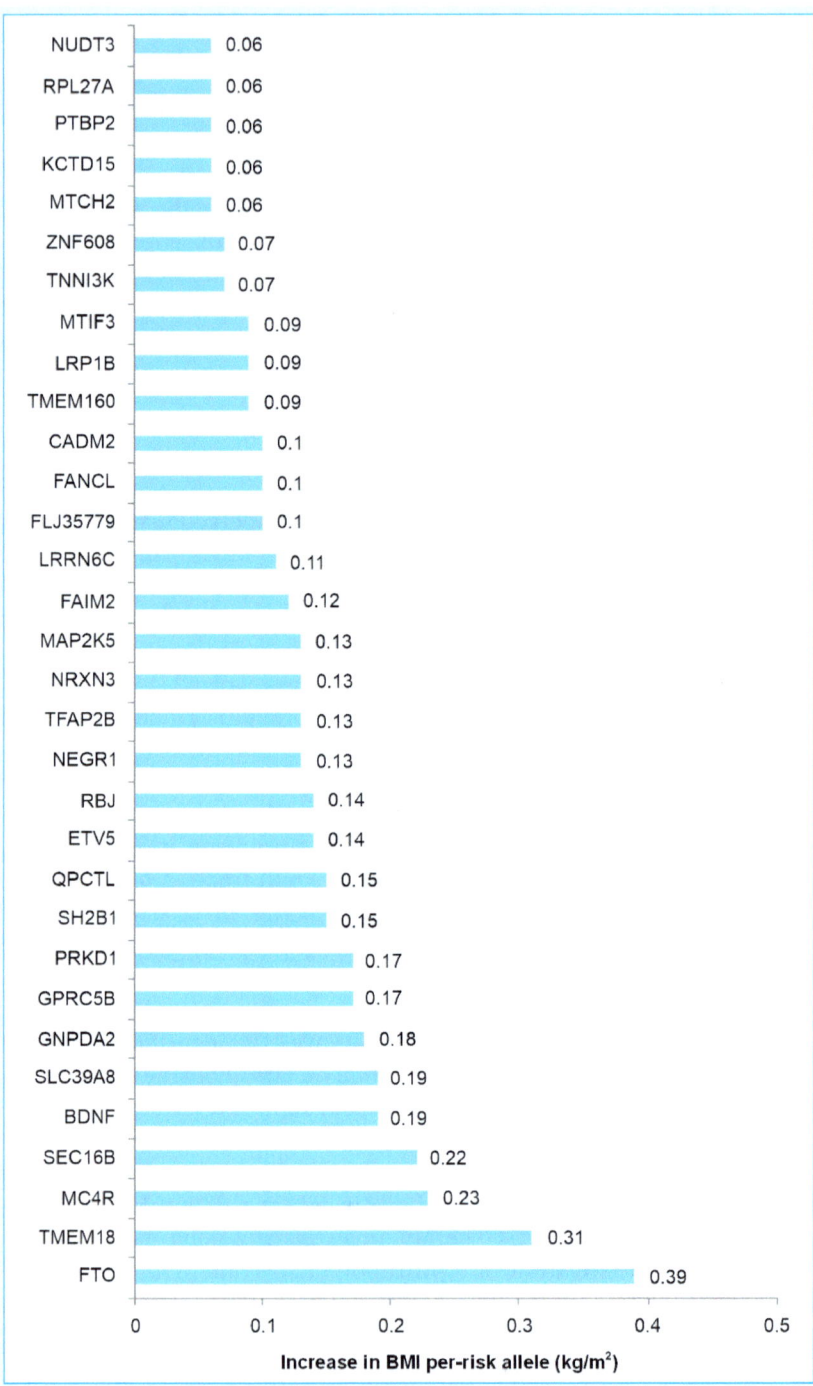

FIG. 2: The BMI increment per risk allele is reported for the SNP marker demonstrating the highest level of association with BMI at each locus.[44]

(BMI: Body mass index; SNP: single nucleotide polymorphism)

common phenotypic variations in BMI.[46] In a larger meta-analysis involving a discovery sample of 32,387 individuals, the GIANT consortium expanded their findings and identified variants within or near six additional genes associated with BMI. These genes include transmembrane protein 18 (*TMEM18*), potassium channel tetramerization domain containing 15 (*KCTD15*), glucosamine-6-phosphate deaminase 2 (*GNPDA2*), SH2B adaptor protein 1 (*SH2B1*), mitochondrial carrier homolog 2 (*MTCH2*), and neuronal growth regulator 1 (*NEGR1*) **(Fig. 2)**.[42]

A study conducted by investigators from deCODE genetics in a population sample of 31,392 individuals, including Icelandic (*n* = 25,344), Dutch (*n* = 2,998), European-American (*n* = 1,890), and African-American (*n* = 1,160) descent, validated the association of four previously mentioned loci (*TMEM18*, *NEGR1*, *KCTD15*, and *SH2B1*) with BMI and identified significant associations with BMI at three additional loci (*SEC16B*, *BDNF*, and near *ETV5*) **(Fig. 2)**.[42,43] In the most extensive meta-analysis of GWAS on BMI conducted to date, involving a discovery sample of over 123,865 individuals and an additional 125,931 individuals in the replication stage, the GIANT consortium confirmed the association of several previously identified adiposity loci with obesity and obesity-related traits. Additionally, they reported significant associations between SNPs at 18 additional loci and BMI.[44]

In addition to confirming the association of known loci with BMI, case-control studies have identified specific variants associated with susceptibility to obesity **(Fig. 3)**. Meyre et al. (2009) confirmed the association of *FTO* and *MC4R* with obesity and discovered variants within the *MAF*, *PTER*, and *NPC1* genes that were associated with extreme obesity. A meta-analysis of child obesity case-control

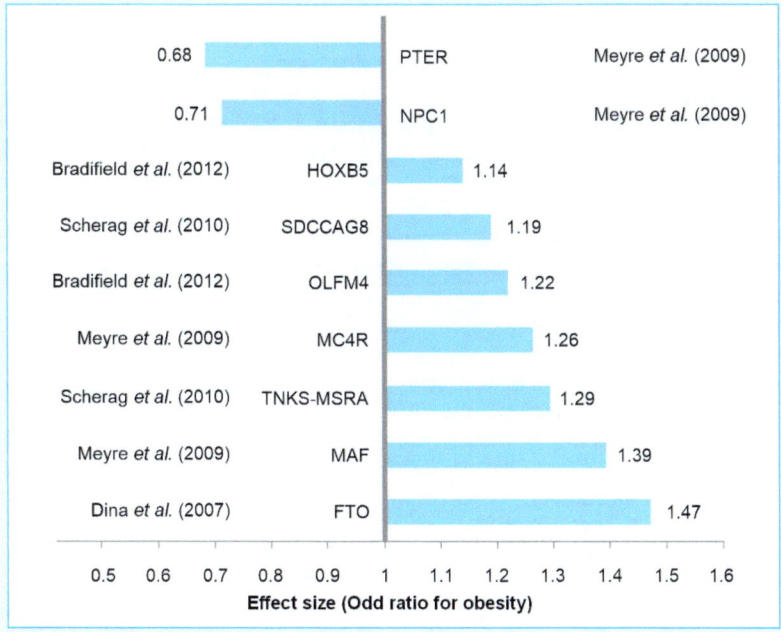

FIG. 3: Effect sizes have been reported for genetic variants associated with BMI in genome-wide association studies (GWAS).

studies from Germany and France revealed an association between SNPs in the *SDCCAG8*, *TNKS*, and *MSRA* genes and early-onset obesity. Furthermore, the Early Growth Genetics consortium conducted a meta-analysis of child obesity case-control studies and identified variants in nine loci associated with childhood obesity, including two novel loci (*OLFM4* and *HOXB5*).[47-49]

REFERENCES

1. Loos RJF, Yeo GSH. The genetics of obesity: From discovery to biology. Nat Rev Genet. 2022;23(2):120-33.
2. Haslam DW, James WP. Obesity. Lancet. 2005;366(9492):1197-209.
3. Xia Q, Grant SF. The genetics of human obesity. Ann N Y Acad Sci. 2013;1281(1):178-90.
4. El-Sayed Moustafa JS, Froguel P. From obesity genetics to the future of personalized obesity therapy. Nat Rev Endocrinol. 2013;9(7):402-13.
5. Friedman JM. A war on obesity, not the obese. Science. 2003;299(5608):856-8.
6. Fee M. Racializing narratives: Obesity, diabetes and the "Aboriginal" thrifty genotype. Soc Sci Med. 2006;62(12):2988-97.
7. Cossrow N, Falkner B. Race/ethnic issues in obesity and obesity-related comorbidities. J Clin Endocrinol Metab. 2004;89(6):2590-4.
8. Poulsen P, Vaag A, Kyvik K, Beck-Nielsen H. Genetic versus environmental aetiology of the metabolic syndrome among male and female twins. Diabetologia. 2001;44(5):537-43.
9. Stunkard AJ, Foch TT, Hrubec Z. A twin study of human obesity. JAMA. 1986;256(1):51-4.
10. Turula M, Kaprio J, Rissanen A, Koskenvuo M. Body weight in the Finnish Twin Cohort. Diabetes Res Clin Pract. 1990;10 Suppl 1:S33-6.
11. Wardle J, Carnell S, Haworth CM, Plomin R. Evidence for a strong genetic influence on childhood adiposity despite the force of the obesogenic environment. Am J Clin Nutr. 2008;87(2):398-404.
12. Bellia A, Giardina E, Lauro D, Tesauro M, Di Fede G, Cusumano G, et al. "The Linosa Study": epidemiological and heritability data of the metabolic syndrome in a Caucasian genetic isolate. Nutr Metab Cardiovasc Dis. 2009;19(7):455-61.
13. Davey G, Ramachandran A, Snehalatha C, Hitman GA, McKeigue PM. Familial aggregation of central obesity in Southern Indians. Int J Obes Relat Metab Disord. 2000;24(11):1523-7.
14. Wang X, Ding X, Su S, Spector TD, Mangino M, Iliadou A, et al. Heritability of insulin sensitivity and lipid profile depend on BMI: evidence for gene-obesity interaction. Diabetologia. 2009;52(12):2578-84.
15. Stunkard AJ, Sørensen TI, Hanis C, Teasdale TW, Chakraborty R, Schull WJ, et al. An adoption study of human obesity. N Engl J Med. 1986;314(4):193-8.
16. Moll PP, Burns TL, Lauer RM. The genetic and environmental sources of body mass index variability: the Muscatine Ponderosity Family Study. Am J Hum Genet. 1991;49(6):1243-55.
17. Borch-Johnsen K, Olsen JH, Sørensen TI. Genes and family environment in familial clustering of cancer. Theor Med. 1994;15(4):377-86.
18. Satko SG, Sedor JR, Iyengar SK, Freedman BI. Familial clustering of chronic kidney disease. Semin Dial. 2007;20(3):229-36.
19. Requena T, Espinosa-Sanchez JM, Cabrera S, Trinidad G, Soto-Varela A, Santos-Perez S, et al. Familial clustering and genetic heterogeneity in Ménière's disease. Clin Genet. 2014;85(3):245-52.
20. Nielsen M, Andersson C, Gerds TA, Andersen PK, Jensen TB, Køber L, et al. Familial clustering of myocardial infarction in first-degree relatives: a nationwide study. Eur Heart J. 2013;34(16):1198-203.
21. Seger HM, Soisson AP, Dodson MK, Rowe KG, Cannon-Albright LA. Familial clustering of endometrial cancer in a well-defined population. Gynecol Oncol. 2011;122(1):75-8.
22. Parent ME, Ghadirian P, Lacroix A. Familial clustering of obesity and breast cancer. Genet Epidemiol. 1996;13(1):61-78.
23. Xi B, Mi J, Duan JL, Yan SJ, Cheng H, Hou DQ, et al. Familial clustering of obesity and the role of lifestyle factors among children in Beijing. Zhonghua Yu Fang Yi Xue Za Zhi. 2009;43(2):122-7.
24. Li Z, Luo B, Du L, Hu H, Xie Y. Familial clustering of overweight and obesity among schoolchildren in northern China. Int J Clin Exp Med. 2014;7(12):5778-83.

25. Cameron AJ, Crawford DA, Salmon J, Campbell K, McNaughton SA, Mishra GD, et al. Clustering of obesity-related risk behaviors in children and their mothers. Ann Epidemiol. 2011;21(2):95-102.
26. Fuentes RM, Notkola IL, Shemeikka S, Tuomilehto J, Nissinen A. Familial aggregation of body mass index: a population-based family study in eastern Finland. Horm Metab Res. 2002;34(7):406-10.
27. Watanabe E, Lee JS, Mori K, Kawakubo K. Clustering patterns of obesity-related multiple lifestyle behaviours and their associations with overweight and family environments: A cross-sectional study in Japanese preschool children. BMJ Open. 2016;6(11):e012773.
28. Thaker VV. Genetic and epigenetic causes of obesity. Adolesc Med State Art Rev. 2017;28(2):379-405.
29. Chung WK. An overview of monogenic and syndromic obesities in humans. Pediatr Blood Cancer. 2012;58(1):122-8.
30. Mahmoud R, Kimonis V, Butler MG. Genetics of obesity in humans: A clinical review. Int J Mol Sci. 2022;23(19):11005.
31. Morton GJ, Cummings DE, Baskin DG, Barsh GS, Schwartz MW. Central nervous system control of food intake and body weight. Nature. 2006; 443(7109):289-95.
32. Cowley MA, Smart JL, Rubinstein M, Cerdán MG, Diano S, Horvath TL, et al. Leptin activates anorexigenic POMC neurons through a neural network in the arcuate nucleus. Nature. 2001;411(6836):480-4.
33. Millington GWM, Tung YCL, Hewson AK, O'Rahilly S, Dickson SL. Differential effects of α-, β-, and γ2-melanocyte-stimulating hormones on hypothalamic neuronal activation and feeding in the fasted rat. Neuroscience. 2001;108(3):437-45.
34. Harrold JA, Williams G. Melanocortin-4 receptors, beta-MSH and leptin: Key elements in the satiety pathway. Peptides. 2006;27(2):365-71.
35. Mountjoy KG, Wong J. Obesity, diabetes and functions for proopiomelanocortin-derived peptides. Mol Cell Endocrinol. 1997;128(1–2):171-7.
36. Michaud JL, Rosenquist T, May NR, Fan CM. Development of neuroendocrine lineages requires the bHLH-PAS transcription factor SIM1. Genes Dev. 1998;12(20):3264-75.
37. Han JC, Liu QR, Jones M, Levinn RL, Menzie CM, Jefferson-George KS, et al. Brain-derived neurotrophic factor and obesity in the WAGR syndrome. N Engl J Med. 2008;359(9):918-27.
38. Mutch DM, Clément K. Unraveling the genetics of human obesity. PLoS Genet. 2006;2(12):e188.
39. Frayling TM, Timpson NJ, Weedon MN, Zeggini E, Freathy RM, Lindgren CM, et al. A common variant in the FTO gene is associated with body mass index and predisposes to childhood and adult obesity. Science. 2007;316(5826):889-94.
40. Scuteri A, Sanna S, Chen WM, Uda M, Albai G, Strait J, et al. Genome-wide association scan shows genetic variants in the FTO gene are associated with obesity-related traits. PLoS Genet. 2007;3(7):e115.
41. Loos RJF, Lindgren CM, Li S, Wheeler E, Zhao JH, Prokopenko I, et al. Common variants near MC4R are associated with fat mass, weight and risk of obesity. Nat Genet. 2008;40(6):768-75.
42. Willer CJ, Speliotes EK, Loos RJF, Li S, Lindgren CM, Heid IM, et al. Six new loci associated with body mass index highlight a neuronal influence on body weight regulation. Nat Genet. 2009;41(1):25-34.
43. Thorleifsson G, Walters GB, Gudbjartsson DF, Steinthorsdottir V, Sulem P, Helgadottir A, et al. Genome-wide association yields new sequence variants at seven loci that associate with measures of obesity. Nat Genet. 2009;41(1):18-24.
44. Speliotes EK, Willer CJ, Berndt SI, Monda KL, Thorleifsson G, Jackson AU, et al. Association analyses of 249,796 individuals reveal 18 new loci associated with body mass index. Nat Genet. 2010;42(11):937-48.
45. Dina C, Meyre D, Gallina S, Durand E, Körner A, Jacobson P, et al. Variation in FTO contributes to childhood obesity and severe adult obesity. Nat Genet. 2007;39:724-6.
46. Chambers JC, Elliott P, Zabaneh D, Zhang W, Li Y, Froguel P, et al. Common genetic variation near MC4R is associated with waist circumference and insulin resistance. Nat Genet. 2008;40:716-8.
47. Meyre D, Delplanque J, Chèvre JC, Lecoeur C, Lobbens S, Gallina S, et al. Genome-wide association study for early-onset and morbid adult obesity identifies three new risk loci in European populations. Nat Genet. 2009;41:157-9.
48. Scherag A, Dina C, Hinney A, Vatin V, Scherag S, Vogel CI, et al. Two new loci for body-weight regulation identified in a joint analysis of genome-wide association studies for early-onset extreme obesity in French and German study groups. PLoS Genet. 2010;6:e1000916.
49. Bradfield JP, Taal HR, Timpson NJ, Scherag A, Lecoeur C, Warrington NM, et al. A genome-wide association meta-analysis identifies new childhood obesity loci. Nat Genet. 2012;44:526-31.

CHAPTER 4

Clinical Manifestations and Diagnosis

Key Highlights

- Obesity is characterized by excessive body weight due to an accumulation of adipose tissue. It can present with physical signs such as increased body mass index (BMI), enlarged waist circumference (WC), and presence of excess body fat in various areas of the body.
- Diagnosis of obesity is primarily based on BMI, which is calculated by dividing weight in kilograms by the square of height in meters (kg/m^2). A BMI of 30 or higher is indicative of obesity.
- Recent and updated guidelines recommend to use the cutoff mark for overweight (BMI 25.0–29.9 kg/m^2) and obesity (BMI ≥ 30 kg/m^2) to identify the population on risk of cardiovascular disease (CVD) and mortality.
- Diabetes mellitus (DM) is a metabolic disorder characterized by high blood sugar levels. Common clinical manifestations include increased thirst, frequent urination, unexplained weight loss, fatigue, blurred vision, slow wound healing, and recurrent infections.
- The diagnosis of diabetes involves assessing fasting plasma glucose (FPG) levels, oral glucose tolerance test (OGTT), or glycated hemoglobin (HbA1c) levels. The American Diabetes Association (ADA) defines diabetes as FPG ≥ 126 mg/dL, 2-hour plasma glucose ≥ 200 mg/dL during OGTT, or HbA1c ≥ 6.5%.

INTRODUCTION

Obesity is widely recognized as a disease by various government institutions, health organizations, and medical societies, including the American Academy of Family Physicians, American Heart Association, American Society of Bariatric Physicians, Federal Trade Commission, Maternal and Child Health Bureau, National Academy of Sciences Institute of Medicine, National Institutes of

Health, and the World Health Organization (WHO). According to the definition provided by Dorland's Illustrated Medical Dictionary, a disease is characterized by any deviation or interruption of the normal structure or function of a body part, organ, or system, accompanied by specific symptoms and signs, with a known or unknown cause, pathology, and prognosis. Obesity fulfills all these criteria, as it has a known etiology, recognizable signs and symptoms, and leads to structural and functional changes that result in pathological consequences. The diagnosis of obesity is commonly established by determining a patient's body mass index (BMI), calculated by dividing weight in kilograms by height in meters squared (kg/m^2). The WHO defines overweight as a BMI of approximately 25 kg/m^2, and obesity as a BMI of approximately 30 kg/m^2. However, it is important to note that while BMI provides a general measure of overall body fat, individuals with similar BMIs can have varying body compositions. Overall, recognizing obesity as a disease acknowledges its complex nature and the significant impact it has on the structure and function of the body. By considering obesity as a disease, appropriate attention can be given to its prevention, diagnosis, and management, leading to improved health outcomes for individuals affected by this condition.[1]

Diabetes mellitus (DM) is a global health concern, characterized by disruptions in lipid and carbohydrate metabolism and persistent hyperglycemia. It can result from impaired insulin secretion, insulin receptor resistance, or a combination of both. DM affects individuals of all ages and is escalating at an alarming rate worldwide, approaching epidemic proportions.[2] Mismanagement or uncontrolled hyperglycemia can lead to acute complications, while untreated or undetected symptoms can progress to chronic complications. Timely diagnosis and effective management have been shown to prevent or delay the onset of chronic complications and even mortality. Failure to control hyperglycemia in individuals with DM increases the risk of developing conditions like cardiovascular diseases (CVDs).[3] Despite available treatments, DM remains a leading cause of death globally. A comprehensive understanding of the pathophysiology of symptoms is crucial for the diagnosis, management, and prevention of the disorder. However, many people underestimate the significance of early signs and symptoms due to the chronic nature of the disease. Unlike some acute conditions, the consequences of hyperglycemia may not immediately manifest. Unfortunately, damage can occur years before noticeable symptoms emerge. Raising awareness about the early symptoms is vital as it enables prompt disease control and helps prevent vascular complications.[4,5]

This chapter puts together information on the clinical manifestation (sign and symptoms with its pathophysiology) and diagnosis (early detection with updated diagnostic criteria and assessment) of obesity and diabetes.

SYMPTOMS AND SIGNS OF OBESITY AND DIABETES

The primary manifestation of obesity is the excessive accumulation of adipose tissue, or body fat. While BMI serves as a general indicator of overall body fat, it is important to recognize that individuals with similar BMI values can exhibit significant differences in body composition. Research has shown that abdominal obesity, particularly the accumulation of visceral fat, is a stronger predictor of cardiometabolic risk and associated conditions such as CVD and insulin resistance, compared to overall body fat.[6] A reliable method for assessing abdominal obesity is measuring waist circumference (WC), which correlates well with the amount of visceral fat present. The measurement of WC can serve as a valuable tool for clinicians in identifying patients who should undergo further evaluation for cardiometabolic risk factors, including dyslipidemia and hyperglycemia. Additionally, WC measurement can be instrumental in monitoring the effectiveness of diet and exercise interventions. It has been observed that regular aerobic exercise can lead to a reduction in both WC and cardiometabolic risk, even in the absence of significant changes in BMI. Therefore, WC measurement offers additional information beyond BMI and can aid in assessing an individual's response to lifestyle modifications aimed at improving their overall health and reducing cardiometabolic risk factors.[7] Consequently, WC measurement was recommended by a panel of experts as a valuable tool in identifying obesity and determining individuals at a higher risk of developing type 2 diabetes mellitus (T2DM) or CVD.[8] Apart from abdominal obesity, other indications of obesity include insulin resistance, elevated blood glucose levels, hypertension (HTN), raised cholesterol and triglyceride levels, decreased levels of high-density lipoprotein cholesterol (HDL-c), respiratory difficulties, and back pain **(Figs. 1A and B)**.[9,10]

Obesity is a condition marked by the accumulation of excess fat in the body, and it is a progressive systemic disease with a range of specific effects on various organs and systems. This condition leads to a multitude of debilitating symptoms encompassing physical, psychological, social, and medical consequences as outlined below in **Table 1**, along with secondary metabolic effects. Many of these factors collectively contribute to the development of ischemic heart disease (IHD). Over time, obesity can have life-threatening implications, primarily by increasing the risk of conditions such as diabetes, coronary heart disease (CHD), various cancers, and in some cases, directly through complications like Pickwickian syndrome, sleep apnea, venous thrombosis embolus, or cellulitis. Many of these pathological consequences are linked to the "metabolic syndrome", characterized by both central fat distribution and an overall excess of body fat. It is important to note that these two components have distinct genetic influences, but both can be exacerbated by a sedentary lifestyle and a diet rich in high-fat foods.[11]

The signs and symptoms of DM can be categorized into three main groups. The first category includes physical symptoms such as polydipsia (increased thirst and subsequent increased fluid intake), polyuria (frequent urination), glycosuria (glucose in urine), polyphagia (extreme hunger or increased appetite), unexplained weight loss despite normal or increased eating, decreased skin turgor (very dry skin), unexplained tiredness or fatigue, significant decrease in the level of consciousness or dizziness, acetonic breath, nocturia, tachycardia (fast heart rate), dehydration, and dry mouth or hyposalivation. It is important to note that most individuals experience the classical triad of DM symptoms, known as the "3Ps": polyuria, polydipsia, and polyphagia. The second category encompasses specific long-term complications associated with DM, such as microangiopathy. Retinopathy, which leads to sudden changes in vision, nephropathy affecting the kidneys, and neuropathy, characterized by a tingling sensation or numbness in the

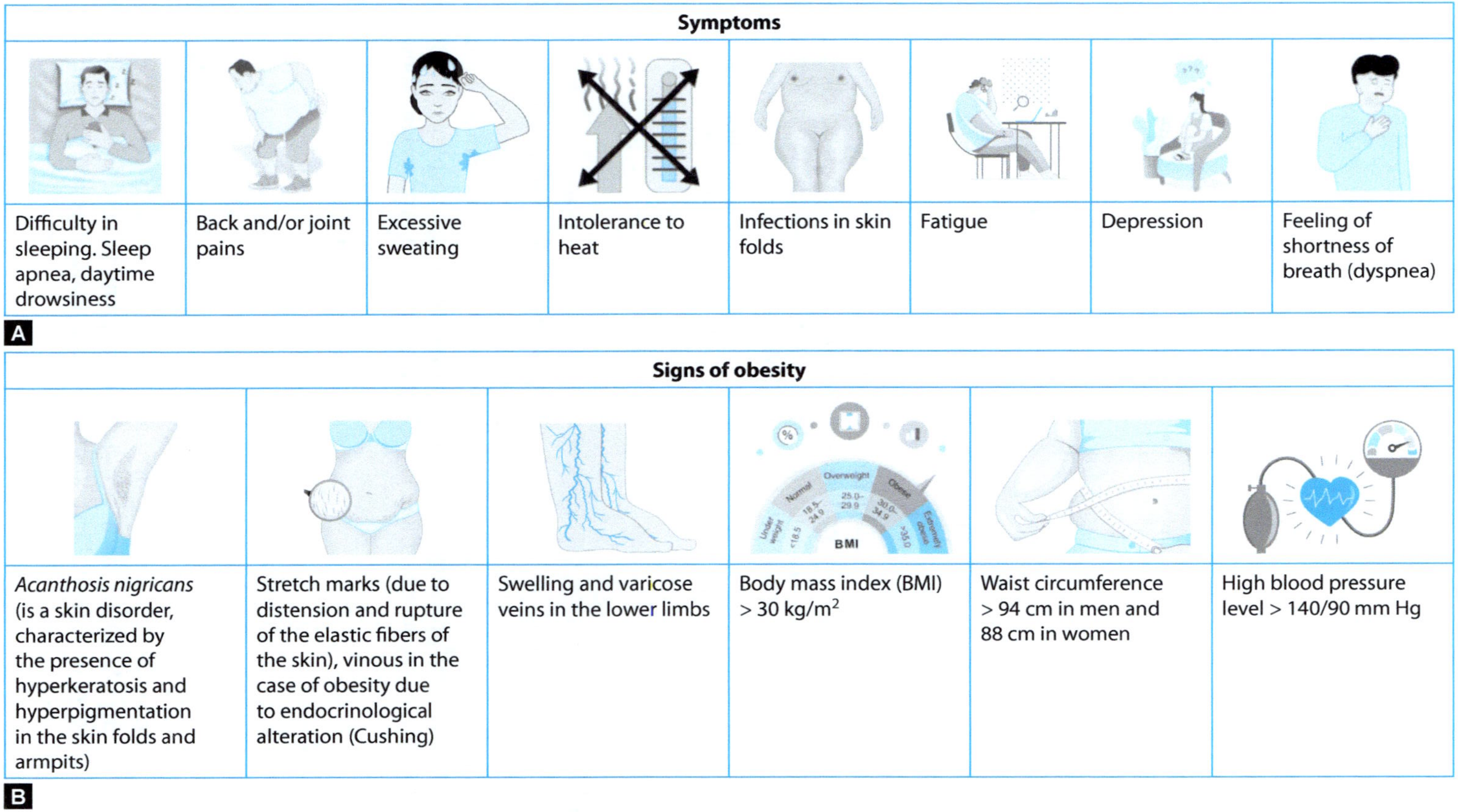

CHAPTER 4: Clinical Manifestations and Diagnosis

Symptoms

Back and/or joint pains	Excessive sweating	Intolerance to heat	Infections in skin folds	Fatigue	Depression	Feeling of shortness of breath (dyspnea)
Difficulty in sleeping. Sleep apnea, daytime drowsiness						

A

Signs of obesity

	Stretch marks (due to distension and rupture of the elastic fibers of the skin), vinous in the case of obesity due to endocrinological alteration (Cushing)	Swelling and varicose veins in the lower limbs	Body mass index (BMI) > 30 kg/m²	Waist circumference > 94 cm in men and 88 cm in women	High blood pressure level > 140/90 mm Hg
Acanthosis nigricans (is a skin disorder, characterized by the presence of hyperkeratosis and hyperpigmentation in the skin folds and armpits)					

B

FIGS. 1A AND B: (A) Symptoms and (B) signs of obesity.

TABLE 1: Debilitating symptoms due to obesity.

Physical symptoms	Metabolic problems	Social	Psychological	Endocrine	Anesthetic and surgical hazards
• Breathlessness • Varicose veins • Back pain • Arthritis • Edema, cellulitis • Sweating • Stress incontinence	• Hypertension • NIDDM • Hyperlipidemia • Hypercoagulation, IHD and stroke	• Isolation • Agoraphobia • Unemployment • Family, marital stress	• Tiredness • Low self-esteem • Self-deception • Distortion of thought	• Hirsutism • Oligomenorrhea, infertility • Menorrhagia • Estrogen-dependent cancers (breast, endometrium, prostate)	• Sleep apnea • Wound dehiscence • Hernia • Chest infections

(IHD: ischemic heart disease; NIDDM: non-insulin-dependent diabetes mellitus)

hands or feet, are examples of these complications. The third category involves an increased predisposition to other diseases and conditions. DM can accelerate the progression of diseases such as atherosclerosis and can lead to more frequent or recurrent skin and urinary tract infections. Overall, recognizing and understanding these signs and symptoms is essential for the early detection, management, and prevention of complications associated with DM. The pathophysiology for the occurrence of symptoms associated with diabetes is explained in the following text **(Fig. 2)**:[12]

Polyuria

Persistent hyperglycemia or uncontrolled DM results in incomplete reabsorption of glucose in the proximal renal tubule of the kidney. This leads to the presence of glucose in the urine, a condition known as glycosuria. The presence of glucose increases the osmotic pressure of the urine, inhibiting the reabsorption of water by the kidney. As a consequence, there is an increase in urine production, known as polyuria.[12]

Polydipsia

Polyuria often occurs at night, causing frequent urination, which disrupts sleep cycles and contributes to daytime fatigue. The excretion of glucose in the urine leads to the simultaneous loss of water and electrolytes necessary for maintaining normal urine osmolarity. This polyuria–glycosuria condition results in a decrease in blood volume, which is compensated for by water from body cells, leading to dehydration in individuals with DM and subsequent weight loss. The loss of water also triggers increased thirst, known as polydipsia. **Figure 2** illustrates the relationship between these symptoms.[12]

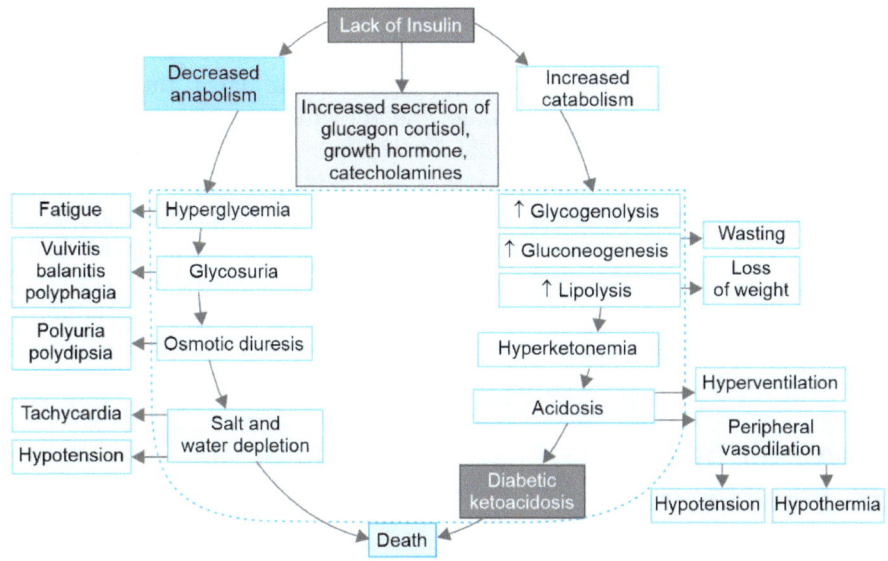

FIG. 2: The interrelationship between impaired glucose, protein, and lipid metabolism and signs and symptoms experienced in poorly controlled diabetes mellitus.

Polyphagia (Fatigue)

The negative caloric balance caused by glycosuria and tissue catabolism triggers an increase in appetite and food intake, a condition known as polyphagia. In uncontrolled DM, glucose from the blood is unable to enter cells, leading to intracellular glucose starvation. As a result, the body is unable to efficiently convert the food consumed into adenosine triphosphate (ATP), the energy currency of cells. This contributes to feelings of weakness and fatigue, even after consuming a substantial meal.[12]

Sudden Weight Loss

The inability of the body to transport glucose for energy production in individuals with DM leads to the utilization of muscle protein through a process called gluconeogenesis. This utilization of muscle protein contributes to weight loss in these individuals. Furthermore, the absence of insulin, which normally inhibits the breakdown of fat in adipose tissue, leads to increased lipolysis or the breakdown of triglycerides into fatty acids. This can result in sudden weight loss in obese individuals who develop DM and are unaware of their condition.[12]

Shortness of Breath

The combination of insulin deficiency and hyperglycemia leads to a decrease in fructose 2,6-bisphosphate levels in the liver, which affects the activity of enzymes such as phosphofructokinase and fructose 1,6-bisphosphatase. The increased levels of hormones like glucagon, cortisol, growth hormone, and catecholamines due to low or absent insulin levels promote processes such as glycogenolysis, gluconeogenesis, and lipolysis. However, in diabetic ketoacidosis (DKA), the elevated glucagon levels alter hepatic metabolism to favor the formation of ketone bodies. This is achieved through the activation of the enzyme carnitine palmitoyltransferase I, which is crucial for regulating the transport of fatty acids into the mitochondria where they undergo beta oxidation and are converted into ketone bodies. The accumulation of ketone bodies in the blood leads to increased acidity and depletion of bicarbonate alkali reserves, resulting in metabolic acidosis. Initially, the body attempts to buffer this acidosis using bicarbonate, but eventually, other compensatory mechanisms come into play, such as hyperventilation. This hyperventilation, known as Kussmaul respiration, is an extreme form of increased breathing rate aimed at eliminating carbon dioxide and reducing blood acidity.[12]

Tachycardia (Rapid Heart Rate) and Hypotension (Low Blood Pressure)

Ketone bodies also contribute to osmotic diuresis, leading to additional losses of electrolytes. Consequently, individuals experiencing DKA may have a deficit in total body water of approximately 6.0 L, along with significant deficiencies in sodium, potassium, chloride, phosphate, magnesium, and calcium. Dehydration is a characteristic feature of DKA, often accompanied by symptoms such as a dry mouth or hyposalivation and decreased skin turgor. In severe cases of dehydration, tachycardia (rapid heart rate) and hypotension (low blood pressure) may occur.[12]

Hyposalivation and Increase in Infection Rate

Hyposalivation, or reduced salivary flow, is a common symptom associated with polyuria in individuals with DKA. It is suggested that the replacement of functional tissue with adipose tissue alters both the quantity and quality of saliva production, contributing to the occurrence of hyposalivation. When saliva production is decreased, there may be an increased risk of fungal infections, such as *Candida albicans*, as well as the potential development of other species. Other factors that can contribute to increased infections in individuals with DM include insulin hyposecretion, impaired glucose utilization, and increased glucose production. Infections in diabetic patients are caused by a hyperglycemic environment that impairs immune function and leads to complications such as angiopathies, neuropathy, and dysmotility, along with increased medical interventions.[12,13]

Acetonic Breath

Another sign and symptom exhibited by individuals with DM is the production of acetonic breath, a condition known as DKA. This can be characterized by a distinctive "fruity" odor. DKA occurs when there are inadequate levels of insulin, resulting in high blood glucose levels and the accumulation of organic acids and ketones in the blood.[12]

DIAGNOSTIC CRITERIA FOR DIABETES AND PREDIABETES

Evolution of Diagnostic Criteria

The diagnostic criteria for diabetes have evolved over time. In 1979, the US National Diabetes Data Group (NDDG) established diagnostic blood glucose targets based on correlations with diabetes-related complications. The criteria set the diagnostic blood glucose level at 140 mg/dL (7.78 mmol/L), with an oral glucose tolerance test (OGTT) required if glycemia was between 110 and 140 mg/dL.[14,15] The WHO also adopted these criteria with slight modifications. In 1997, the American Diabetes Association (ADA) expert committee revised the diagnosis criteria, lowering the fasting plasma glucose (FPG) cutoff to ≥126 mg/dL (≥7.0 mmol/L) based on studies showing increased incidence of retinopathy even at blood glucose values >120 mg/dL.[16] This change aimed to reduce discrepancies between FPG and OGTT values, as the latter had technical challenges, lower reproducibility, and higher costs. However, the DECODE study demonstrated that post-OGTT blood glucose levels were more predictive of CVD. While there is no definitive guidance on the best diagnostic test for diabetes, FPG remains widely used in clinical practice, while OGTT is more suitable for research studies or situations requiring a clear differentiation between diabetes and other glucose metabolism disorders.[17] The ADA introduced new diagnostic criteria for impaired fasting glucose (IFG) and impaired glucose tolerance (IGT), defining IFG as fasting blood glucose between 110 and 125 mg/dL, and IGT as blood sugar between 140 and 199 mg/dL 2 hours post-OGTT.[18]

Current Diagnostic Criteria

The diagnostic criteria of diabetes have been constantly evolving. Both type 1 diabetes mellitus (T1DM) and T2DM are diagnosed based on the plasma glucose criteria, either the FPG levels or the 2-hour postprandial plasma glucose (2-hour PPG) levels during a 75-g OGTT, or the newer glycated hemoglobin (HbA1c) criteria which reflects the average plasma glucose concentration over the previous 8–12 weeks.[19] The International Expert Committee Report recommends a cut point of ≥6.5% for HbA1c for diagnosing diabetes as an alternative to FPG (FPG ≥ 7.0 mmol/L). HbA1c testing has some substantial advantages over FPG and OGTT, such as convenience, preanalytical stability, and less day-to-day fluctuations due to stress and illness.[20] Additionally, HbA1c has been recognized as a marker to assess secondary vascular complications due to metabolic derailments in susceptible individuals.[21,22] However, given ethnic differences in sensitivity and specificity of HbA1c, population-specific cutoffs might be necessary.[23,24] Moreover, measuring HbA1c is expensive as compared to FPG assessments and standardization of measurement techniques and laboratories are poorly practiced across the country.[25] Also, in several countries including India, HbA1c demonstrated inadequate predictive accuracy in the diagnosis of diabetes, and there is no consensus on a suitable cutoff point of HbA1c for the diagnosis of diabetes in this high-risk population.[26] Thus, there is concern raised on using HbA1c as the sole criteria for the diagnosis of diabetes, particularly in resource-constrained settings. Therefore, a combination of HbA1c and FPG would improve the identification of individuals with DM and prediabetes in limited resource settings like India **(Flowchart 1)**.

A recent study conducted in Singapore residents of Chinese, Malay, and Indian race aimed to assess the performance of HbA1c as a screening test in Asian populations. The study suggested that HbA1c is an appropriate alternative to FPG as a first-step screening test. It was found that a combination of HbA1c with a cutoff of ≥6.1% and FPG level ≥100 mg/dL would improve detection in patients with diabetes.[23] In resource-constrained settings and countries, the applicability of diagnostic markers such as antibodies, C-peptide levels, serum or plasma insulin, and genetic testing for maturity-onset diabetes of the young (MODY) is limited due to their restricted availability and affordability.[27]

Prediabetes refers to the condition of individuals whose glucose levels do not meet the criteria for diabetes but display abnormal carbohydrate metabolism. Prediabetes is characterized by the presence of IFG, IGT, and/or A1C levels between 5.7 and 6.4% (39–47 mmol/mol) **(Box 1)**. Rather than being considered a distinct

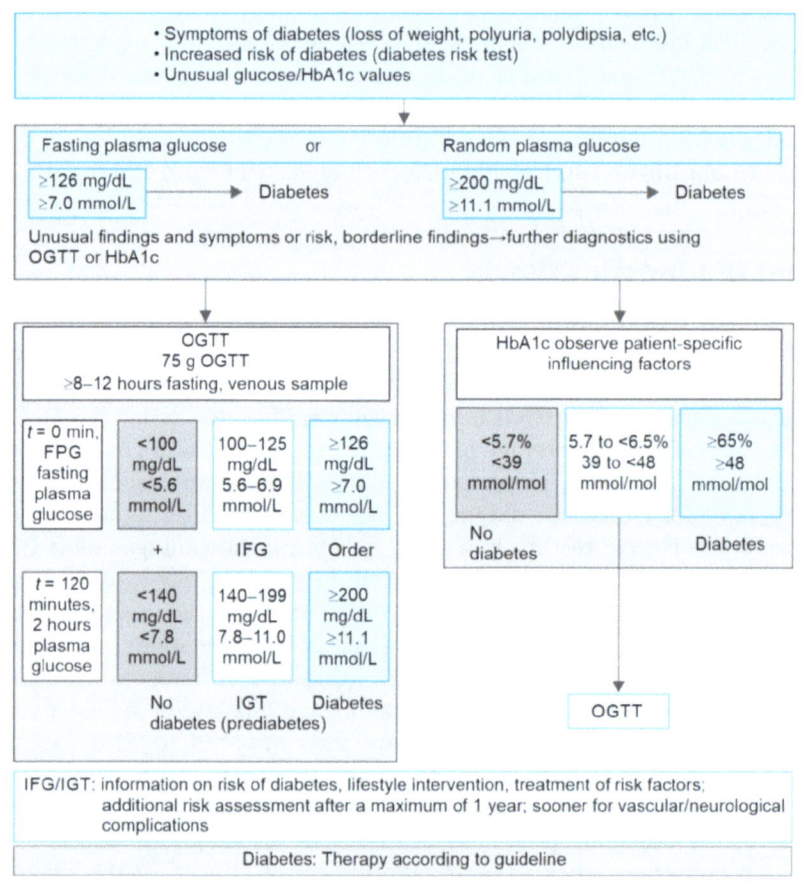

FLOWCHART 1: Diagnostic approach for diagnosing diabetes.

(IFG: impaired fasting glucose; IGT: impaired glucose tolerance; OGTT: oral glucose tolerance test; HbA1c: glycated hemoglobin)

> **BOX 1: Criteria defining prediabetes.***
> - FPG 100 mg/dL (5.6 mmol/L) to 125 mg/dL (6.9 mmol/L) (IFG)
> - 2-hour PG during 75-g OGTT 140 mg/dL (7.8 mmol/L) to 199 mg/dL (11.0 mmol/L) (IGT)
> - A1c 5.7–6.4% (39–47 mmol/mol)
>
> *For all three tests, risk is continuous, extending below the lower limit of the range and becoming disproportionately greater at the higher end of the range.
>
> (FPG: fasting plasma glucose; IFG: impaired fasting glucose; IGT: impaired glucose tolerance; OGTT: oral glucose tolerance testing; PG: plasma glucose)

> **BOX 2: Criteria for the diagnosis of diabetes.**
> - FPG ≥ 126 mg/dL (7.0 mmol/L) after an overnight fast; fasting is defined as no caloric intake for at least 8 hours*
> - 2-hour PG ≥ 200 mg/dL (11.1 mmol/L) during OGTT; the test should be performed as described by WHO, using a glucose load containing the equivalent of 75-g anhydrous glucose dissolved in water*
> - A1c ≥ 6.5% (48 mmol/mol); the test should be performed in a laboratory using a method that is NGSP certified and standardized to the DCCT assay*
> - In a patient with classic symptoms of hyperglycemia or hyperglycemic crisis, a random plasma glucose ≥ 200 mg/dL (11.1 mmol/L)
>
> *In the absence of unequivocal hyperglycemia, diagnosis requires two abnormal test results from the same sample or in two separate test samples.
>
> (DCCT: Diabetes Control and Complications Trial; FPG: fasting plasma glucose; NGSP: National Glycohemoglobin Standardization Program; OGTT: oral glucose tolerance test; PG: plasma glucose; WHO: World Health Organization)

clinical entity, prediabetes should be seen as a risk factor for the development of diabetes and CVD. Screening criteria for diabetes or prediabetes in asymptomatic adults are provided in **Box 1**. Prediabetes is commonly associated with obesity, particularly abdominal or visceral obesity, dyslipidemia characterized by high triglycerides and/or low HDL-c, and HTN. The presence of prediabetes should prompt a comprehensive screening for cardiovascular risk factors.[28] **Boxes 1 to 3** provide the current diagnostic criteria for diabetes, prediabetes, and gestational diabetes as per the ADA.[27]

ASSESSMENT OF OBESITY AND COMORBIDITIES

Assessment of Obesity

According to various clinical guidelines, such as the National Heart, Lung, and Blood Institute's (NHLBI) "Clinical Guidelines on the Identification, Evaluation, and Treatment of Overweight and Obesity in Adults", the "Practical Guide on the Identification, Evaluation, and Treatment of Overweight and Obesity in Adults", and the WHO, the assessment of risk status related to overweight or obesity takes into account several factors, including BMI, WC, and the presence of comorbid conditions. A desirable or healthy BMI falls within the range of 18.5–24.9 kg/m^2, while individuals with a BMI between 25 and 29.9 kg/m^2 are classified as overweight. Obesity is defined as a BMI of 30 kg/m^2 or higher. Obesity is further

> **BOX 3: Screening for and diagnosis of gestational diabetes mellitus (GDM).**
>
> *One-step strategy*:
> - Perform a 75-g OGTT, with plasma glucose measurement when patient is fasting and at 1 and 2 hours, at 24–28 weeks gestation in women not previously diagnosed with diabetes
> - The OGTT should be performed in the morning after an overnight fast of at least 8 hours. The diagnosis of GDM is made when any of the following three plasma glucose values are met or exceeded:
>   1. *Fasting*: 92 mg/dL (5.1 mmol/L)
>   2. *1 hour*: 180 mg/dL (10.0 mmol/L)
>   3. *2 hour*: 153 mg/dL (8.5 mmol/L)
>
> *Two-step strategy*:
> - *Step 1*: Perform a 50-g GLT (nonfasting), with plasma glucose measurement at 1 hour, at 24–28 weeks of gestation in women not previously diagnosed with diabetes
>
>   If the plasma glucose level measured 1 hour after the load is ≥130, 135, or 140 mg/dL (7.2, 7.5, or 7.8 mmol/L, respectively), proceed to 100-g OGTT
> - *Step 2*: The 100-g OGTT should be performed when the patient is fasting
>
>   The diagnosis of GDM is made when at least two* of the following four plasma glucose levels (measured fasting and at 1, 2, and 3 hours during OGTT) are met or exceeded (Carpenter–Coustan criteria):
>   1. *Fasting*: 95 mg/dL (5.3 mmol/L)
>   2. *1 hours*: 180 mg/dL (10.0 mmol/L)
>   3. *2 hours*: 155 mg/dL (8.6 mmol/L)
>   4. *3 hours*: 140 mg/dL (7.8 mmol/L)
>
> *American College of Obstetricians and Gynecologists notes that one elevated value can be used for diagnosis.
>
> (GLT: glucose load test; OGTT: oral glucose tolerance test)

categorized into class I (30.0–34.9 kg/m^2), class II (35.0–39.9 kg/m^2), and class III (≥40 kg/m^2) **(Fig. 3)**. It should be noted that lower cutoff points have been suggested for the Asian population, considering their specific characteristics. In addition to BMI, the risk associated with overweight and obesity is influenced by excess abdominal fat and fitness level. Studies have shown that individuals with larger WCs have a higher risk of obesity-related health complications compared to those with normal WCs, even within similar BMI categories. Therefore, considering WC along with BMI provides additional information for assessing the risk associated with overweight and obesity.[29]

A comprehensive review of international evidence-based guidelines on the topic of diagnosing and classifying overweight and obesity in adults revealed that 12 guidelines provided recommendations. These guidelines unanimously recommended using BMI as the primary diagnostic criterion for overweight and obesity in adults. According to these guidelines, a BMI of 25–29.9 kg/m^2 was defined as the cutoff point for overweight, while a BMI ≥ 30 kg/m^2 was considered indicative of obesity. This classification was consistent across all guidelines. Furthermore, it was noted that a BMI ≥ 25 to < 30 kg/m^2 was associated with an increased risk of CVD, while a BMI ≥ 30 kg/m^2 was associated with an increased risk of both CVD and mortality. These findings were supported by the American Heart Association guideline [grade of recommendation (GoR) A]. While WC was not recommended

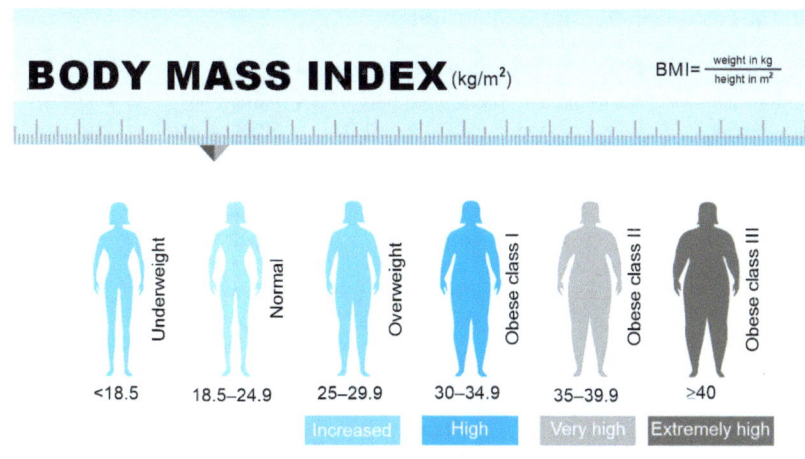

FIG. 3: Classification of overweight in adults according to body mass index.
Courtesy: National Institutes of Health and North American Association for the Study of Obesity.

as a routine measure for diagnosing overweight and obesity [NICE-1 (National Institute for Health and Care Excellence 1): GoR A], it was acknowledged that it provides additional information regarding the risk of developing obesity-related long-term health problems. Several guidelines, including American Association of Clinical Endocrinologists 3, Institute for Clinical Systems Improvement, NICE-1, NICE-2 (GoR A), and Department of Veterans Affairs (GoR B), emphasized the value of WC as a supplementary measure for assessing obesity-related health risks. Overall, the consensus among these guidelines is that BMI remains the primary diagnostic tool for identifying overweight and obesity in adults, with specific cutoff points defined for each category. WC, while not routinely used for diagnosis, offers valuable additional information regarding long-term health risks associated with obesity.[30]

The assessment of obesity has undergone a transformation, shifting away from mere reliance on numerical criteria and cut-off values, particularly recognizing the variations seen among different ethnic groups. Instead, a holistic approach now prevails, which takes into account all associated comorbidities. One exemplary framework that embodies this comprehensive approach is the Edmonton Obesity Staging System (EOSS), a five-stage system for classifying obesity **(Table 2)**. EOSS considers various parameters to determine the most appropriate approach for obesity treatment, making it a valuable tool in clinical practice. Importantly, using the EOSS tool has shown potential to provide more informative insights into obesity compared to relying solely on BMI. This shift in perspective is endorsed by recent clinical practice guidelines from the Canadian Obesity Network. In the Indian context, data from a tertiary care center reveals that a substantial proportion, approximately 68%, of the patient population falls within stage 3 and 4 of this staging system, underscoring the practical utility of adopting such a comprehensive approach in the assessment and management of obesity across diverse populations.[31,32]

TABLE 2: The Edmonton Obesity Staging System.[31]

Stage 0	Stage 1	Stage 2	Stage 3	Stage 4
• NO sign of obesity-related risk factors • NO physical symptoms • NO psychological symptoms • NO functional limitations	• Patient has obesity-related SUBCLINICAL risk factors [borderline hypertension (HTN)], impaired fasting glucose, elevated liver enzymes, etc.] • MILD physical symptoms—patient currently not requiring medical treatment for comorbidities (dyspnea on moderate exertion, occasional aches/pains, fatigue, etc.) • MILD obesity-related psychological symptoms and/or mild impairment of well-being (quality of life not impacted)	• Patient has ESTABLISHED obesity-related comorbidities requiring medical intervention (HTN, T2DM, sleep apnea, polycystic ovary syndrome (PCOS), osteoarthritis, reflux disease) • MODERATE obesity-related psychological symptoms (depression, eating disorders, anxiety disorder) • MODERATE functional limitations in daily activities (quality of life is beginning to be impacted)	• Patient has SIGNIFICANT obesity-related end organ damage (myocardial infarction, heart failure, diabetic complications, incapacitating osteoarthritis) • SIGNIFICANT obesity-related psychological symptoms (major depression, suicide ideation) • SIGNIFICANT functional limitations (e.g., unable to work or complete routine activities, reduced mobility) • SIGNIFICANT impairment of well-being (quality of life is significantly impacted)	• SEVERE (potential end stage) disabilities from obesity-related comorbidities • SEVERELY disabling psychological symptoms • SEVERE functional limitations
(T2DM: type 2 diabetes mellitus)				

In 1998, the NHLBI and the National Institute of Diabetes and Digestive and Kidney Diseases collaborated to release the inaugural federal guidelines for managing overweight and obese adults. These guidelines were developed by a panel comprising 24 members who employed an evidence-based methodology to address 35 clinical questions. The focus was on investigating the impact of various treatment strategies on weight loss and understanding how weight control influences the risk factors associated with major chronic diseases. The NHLBI panel, in formulating their recommendations, operated on the assumption that, for the majority of adults, the benefits of weight loss on overall health outweigh any potential harmful effects. They also believed that many individuals have the capacity to sustain weight loss, leading to long-term health advantages. According to the NHLBI panel, the treatment of obesity should involve a two-step process: assessment and management. The initial step, assessment, entails evaluating the extent of overweight and determining the patient's overall risk status. This process aids in understanding the severity of excess body weight by employing measures such as BMI and considering other relevant factors. Assessment is crucial in identifying associated health risks and comorbid conditions, enabling healthcare professionals to tailor appropriate management strategies. By comprehensively assessing the degree of overweight and evaluating the patient's risk profile, healthcare providers can develop effective treatment goals, select suitable interventions, and monitor progress over time **(Flowchart 2)**.[33]

Obesity can be assessed using various methods, each with its own advantages and disadvantages. The choice of assessment method depends on the specific situation and the desired outcome. Different assessment methods measure different aspects of obesity, such as total or regional adiposity. They may also yield different results when estimating morbidity and mortality associated with obesity. When

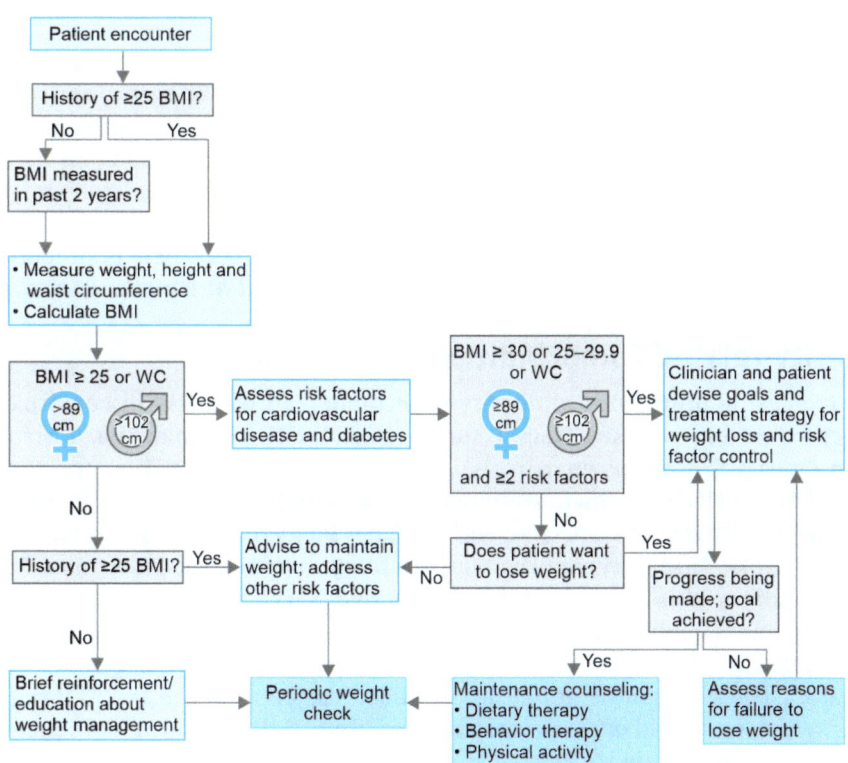

FLOWCHART 2: Treatment algorithm for obesity.

(BMI: body mass index; WC: waist circumference)

Source: Adapted from National Institutes of Health, National Heart, Lung, and Blood Institute Expert Panel on the Identification, Evaluation, and Treatment of Overweight and Obesity in Adults. Clinical guidelines on the identification, evaluation, and treatment of overweight and obesity in adults—The Evidence Report. Obes Res. 1998;6(Suppl 2):51S-209S.

there is an increase in body fat, there are concomitant increases in lean tissues, including fibrous and vascular tissues in adipose tissue, heart muscle, bone mass, and truncal or postural musculature. These nonfat tissues have a higher density (1.0 g/mL) compared to fat (0.7 g/mL). Physical activity can further increase the density of non-fat tissues, which tends to reduce body fat. In general, body weight and body dimension measurements (anthropometry) are commonly used in large-scale epidemiological studies or clinical settings to estimate body fatness and fat distribution. These measurements provide a quick and cost-effective way to assess obesity. On the other hand, densitometry or imaging techniques are typically employed in smaller-scale studies, such as clinical trials, to provide more precise measurements of body composition. The choice of assessment method should be based on the specific research or clinical objectives, considering factors such as sample size, cost, feasibility, and accuracy required for the intended purpose.[34] The most popular methods for measuring body fat from basic body measurements to high-tech body scans along with their strengths and limitations are given in **Table 3**.[35,36]

Updated guidelines of obesity by American College of Cardiology/American Heart Association Task Force on Practice Guidelines and The Obesity Society in 2013 strongly recommend:[37]

- To identify adults who may be at an elevated risk of CVD, the current cut points for overweight (BMI 25.0–29.9 kg/m^2) and obesity (BMI $\geq$ 30 kg/m^2) can be used. Similarly, to identify adults who may be at an elevated risk of mortality from all causes, the current cut point for obesity (BMI $\geq$ 30 kg/m^2) can be employed. These specific BMI thresholds serve as indicators to identify individuals who might be more susceptible to these health risks.
- It is important to advise overweight and obese adults that there is an increased risk of CVD, T2DM, and all-cause mortality associated with higher BMI levels.

Obesity-related Comorbidities

The increasing prevalence of obesity is accompanied by a rise in comorbidities directly linked to excessive weight, such as T2DM, IHD, dyslipidemia, obstructive sleep apnea (OSA), and osteoarthritis. Furthermore, the extended life expectancy of individuals has led to a growing number of patients living with chronic diseases and obesity. Obesity is also associated with a higher incidence of HTN, coronary heart disease, stroke, various types of cancer, disability, and increased mortality.[38,39]

To address this issue, the US Preventive Services Task Force (USPSTF) recommends screening all adults for obesity, recognizing the crucial role of healthcare providers in preventing, identifying, and managing this chronic disease. Once a diagnosis of obesity has been established, the USPSTF suggests that physicians should offer or refer patients with a BMI of 30 kg/m^2 or higher to an intensive, interdisciplinary lifestyle intervention program.[38]

However, it is estimated that <30% of adults with obesity receive this diagnosis during their primary care physician (PCP) visit, indicating a need for improved identification and management of these patients. This population requires access to basic diagnostics and treatment, and in certain cases, specialized bariatric equipment such as beds, chairs, and hoists as well as transportation assistance.

TABLE 3: The most popular methods for measuring body fat from basic body measurements to high-tech body scans along with their strengths and limitations.

Techniques	Description	Strengths	Limitations
Body mass index (BMI)	BMI is the ratio of weight to height, calculated as weight (kg)/height (m^2), or weight (lb)/height (in^2) multiplied by 703	<ul><li>Easy to measure</li><li>Inexpensive</li><li>Cutoff points for overweight 25.0 and 29.9 and obesity 30.0 or higher</li><li>Strongly correlated with body fat levels</li><li>Numerous studies have provided compelling evidence for association of BMI with risk of chronic diseases and mortality</li></ul>	<ul><li>Indirect and imperfect measurement methods</li><li>Less reliable in predicting body fat in older individuals compared to younger adults</li><li>Ethnic and gender differences are unclear</li></ul>
Waist circumference	Waist circumference is the simplest and most common way to measure "abdominal obesity"—the extra fat found around the middle that is an important factor in health, even independent of BMI	<ul><li>Easy to measure</li><li>Inexpensive</li><li>Strongly correlated with body fat in adults as measured by the most accurate methods</li><li>Studies show waist circumference predicts development of disease and death</li></ul>	<ul><li>Measurement procedure has not been standardized</li><li>Lack of good comparison standards (reference data) for waist circumference in children</li><li>May be difficult to measure and less accurate in individuals with a BMI of 35 or higher</li></ul>
Waist-to-hip ratio	It is calculated by measuring the waist and the hip (at the widest diameter of the buttocks), and then dividing the waist measurement by the hip measurement	<ul><li>Good correlation with body fat as measured by the most accurate methods</li><li>Inexpensive</li><li>Studies show waist-to-hip ratio predicts development of disease and death in adults</li></ul>	<ul><li>More prone to measurement error</li><li>More difficult to measure hip than it is to measure waist</li><li>More complex to interpret than waist circumference</li><li>Less accurate in individuals with a BMI of 35 or higher</li></ul>

Continued

Continued

Techniques	Description	Strengths	Limitations
Skinfold thickness	Use a special caliper to measure the thickness of a "pinch" of skin and the fat beneath it in specific areas of the body (the trunk, the thighs, front and back of the upper arm, and under the shoulder blade). Equations are used to predict body fat percentage based on these measurements	• Convenient • Safe • Inexpensive • Portable • Fast and easy (except in individuals with a BMI of 35 or higher)	• Not as accurate or reproducible as other methods • Very hard to measure in individuals with a BMI of 35 or higher
Bioelectric impedance (BIA)	BIA equipment sends a small, imperceptible, safe electric current through the body, measuring the resistance. The current faces more resistance passing through body fat than it does passing through lean body mass and water. Equations are used to estimate body fat percentage and fat-free mass	• Convenient • Safe • Relatively inexpensive • Portable • Fast and easy	• Hard to calibrate • The ratio of body water to fat may be change during illness, dehydration or weight loss, decreasing accuracy • Not as accurate as other methods, especially in individuals with a BMI of 35 or higher
Underwater weighing (densitometry)	Individuals are weighed in air and while submerged in a tank. Researchers use formulas to estimate body volume, body density, and body fat percentage	Accurate	• Time-consuming • Requires individuals to be submerged in water • Generally not a good option for children, older adults, and individuals with a BMI of 40 or higher
Air displacement plethysmography	This method uses a similar principle to underwater weighing but can be done in the air instead of in water. Individuals sit in a small chamber wearing a bathing suit; one commercial example is the "Bod Pod"	• Relatively quick and comfortable • Accurate • Safe • Good choice for children, older adults, pregnant women, individuals with a BMI of 40 or higher	Expensive

Continued

Continued

Techniques	Description	Strengths	Limitations
Dilution method (hydrometry)	Individuals drink isotope-labeled water and give body fluid samples. Researchers analyze these samples for isotope levels, which are then used to calculate total body water, fat-free body mass, and in turn, body fat mass	• Relatively low cost • Accurate • Safe • Can be used in individuals with a BMI of 40 or higher, as well as in children and pregnant women	The ratio of body water to fat-free mass may change during illness, dehydration, or weight loss, decreasing accuracy
Dual-energy X-ray absorptiometry (DEXA)	X-ray beams pass through different body tissues at different rates. So DEXA uses two low-level X-ray beams to develop estimates of fat-free mass, fat mass, and bone mineral density	Accurate	• Equipment is expensive and cannot be moved • Cannot accurately distinguish between different types of fat (fat under the skin, also known as "subcutaneous" fat vs. fat around the internal organs, or "visceral" fat) • Cannot be used with pregnant women, since it requires exposure to a small dose of radiation • Most current systems cannot accommodate individuals with a BMI of 35 or higher
Computerized tomography (CT) and magnetic resonance imaging (MRI)	These two imaging techniques are now considered to be the most accurate methods for measuring tissue, organ, and whole-body fat mass as well as lean muscle mass and bone mass	• Accurate • Allows for measurement of specific body fat compartments, such as abdominal fat and subcutaneous fat	• Equipment is extremely expensive and cannot be moved • CT scans cannot be used with pregnant women or children, due to the high amounts of ionizing radiation used • Some MRI and CT scanners may not be able to accommodate individuals with a BMI of 35 or higher

Providing appropriate long-term care poses logistical challenges and financial burdens for healthcare systems like the National Health Service (NHS), with direct NHS costs for managing obesity amounting to £1 billion in 2002 and projected to rise to £10 billion by 2050.[38,39]

In a cross-sectional survey conducted in three hospital trusts in southern England, the magnitude of the inpatient obesity problem was assessed. The survey included a total of 103 patients, comprising 36 males and 67 females, who had a BMI ≥ 35 kg/m². Among these patients, 37 individuals (10 males and 27 females) had grade III obesity, characterized by a BMI ≥ 40 kg/m², accounting for 36% of the total. The mean BMI of the cohort was 39.1 kg/m², with the highest recorded BMI reaching 52.5 kg/m². Among the surveyed patients, a significant majority of 95 individuals (91%) exhibited at least one comorbidity related to obesity. The most common obesity-related comorbidities observed in the cohort included HTN (20%), T2DM (20%), osteoarthritis (11%), and gastroesophageal reflux disease or IHD (9% each).[39] A cross-sectional analysis was conducted using electronic health record data from a major integrated health system in the USA. The aim was to assess the prevalence of obesity and its associated comorbidities among patients actively receiving care at a US academic medical center. The analysis revealed a higher prevalence of T2DM, prediabetes, HTN, and CVD among the patient population. Among the total number of patients with a BMI ≥ 30 (n = 134,488), only 48% (64,056) had documented evidence of obesity ICD-9 (International Classification of Diseases, Ninth Revision) code. This finding highlights the potential underdiagnosis or underdocumentation of obesity in the medical records of these patients.[38]

A systematic review and meta-analysis were conducted to estimate the incidence of various comorbidities associated with obesity and overweight. A total of 89 relevant studies were included in the analysis. The review identified 18 comorbidities that met the inclusion criteria. The meta-analysis revealed statistically significant associations between overweight and the incidence of several conditions, including T2DM, most cancers (except esophageal in females, pancreatic, and prostate cancer), CVDs (except congestive heart failure), asthma, gallbladder disease, osteoarthritis, and chronic back pain. The strongest association was found between overweight, as defined by BMI, and the incidence of T2DM in females, with a relative risk (RR) of 3.92. Similarly, obesity, as defined by BMI, showed statistically significant associations with the incidence of T2DM, most cancers (except esophageal and prostate cancer), CVDs, asthma, gallbladder disease, osteoarthritis, and chronic back pain. The highest association was observed between obesity and the incidence of T2DM in females, with an RR of 12.41 **(Table 4)**.[40]

The findings of these studies reaffirm that overweight and obesity contribute significantly to the overall health burden. The presence of these conditions is associated with a higher risk of developing various comorbidities, emphasizing the importance of addressing and managing weight-related issues. Furthermore, these findings highlight the substantial impact that overweight and obesity have on healthcare expenditures, underscoring the need for effective interventions and healthcare strategies to address this public health concern.

TABLE 4: Relative comorbidity risks related to being overweight or obese.

Comorbidity	Measure	Overweight		Obesity	
		Male	Female	Male	Female
Type 2 diabetes mellitus*	BMI	2.40 (2.12–2.72)	3.92 (3.10–4.97)	6.74 (5.55–8.19)	12.41 (9.03–17.06)
	WC	2.27 (1.67–3.10)†	3.40 (2.42–4.78)	5.13 (3.81–6.90)†	11.10 (8.23–14.96)
Cancer					
Breast, postmenopausal	BMI	–	1.08 (1.03–1.14)	–	1.13 (1.05–1.22)
Colorectal	BMI	1.51 (1.37–1.67)	1.45 (1.30–1.62)	1.95 (1.59–2.39)	1.66 (1.52–1.81)
Endometrial	BMI	–	1.53 (1.45–1.61)	–	3.22 (2.91–3.56)
Esophageal	BMI	1.13 (1.02–1.26)	1.15 (0.97–1.36)	1.21 (0.97–1.52)	1.20 (0.95–1.53)
Kidney	BMI	1.40 (1.31–1.49)	1.82 (1.68–1.98)	1.82 (1.61–2.05)	2.64 (2.39–2.90)
Ovarian	BMI	–	1.18 (1.12–1.23)	–	1.28 (1.20–1.36)
Pancreatic	BMI	1.28 (0.94–1.75)	1.24 (0.98–1.56)	2.29 (1.65–3.19)	1.60 (1.17–2.20)
Prostate	BMI	1.14 (1.00–1.31)	–	1.05 (0.85–1.30)	–
Cardiovascular diseases					
Hypertension*	BMI	1.28 (1.10–1.50)	1.65 (1.24–2.19)	1.84 (1.51–2.24)	2.42 (1.59–3.67)
	WC	NA	1.38 (1.27–1.51)	NA	1.90 (1.77–2.03)
Coronary artery disease*	BMI	1.29 (1.18–1.41)†	1.80 (1.64–1.98)	1.72 (1.51–1.96)†	3.10 (2.81–3.43)
	WC	1.41 (1.16–1.72)†	1.82 (1.41–2.36)	1.81 (1.45–2.25)†	2.69 (2.05–3.53)
Congestive heart failure*	BMI	1.31 (0.96–1.79)	1.27 (0.68–2.37)†	1.79 (1.24–2.59)	1.78 (1.07–2.95)†

Continued

Continued

Comorbidity	Measure	Overweight		Obesity	
		Male	Female	Male	Female
Pulmonary embolism	BMI	1.91 (1.39–2.64)	1.91 (1.39–2.64)	3.51 (2.61–4.73)	3.51 (2.61–4.73)
Stroke*	BMI	1.23 (1.13–1.34)[†]	1.15 (1.00–1.32)[†]	1.51 (1.33–1.72)[†]	1.49 (1.27–1.74)[†]
Other					
Asthma	BMI	1.20 (1.08–1.33)[†]	1.25 (1.05–1.49)[†]	1.43 (1.14–1.79)[†]	1.78 (1.36–2.32)[†]
Gallbladder disease*	BMI	1.09 (0.87–1.37)[‡]	1.44 (1.05–1.98)[‡]	1.43 (1.04–1.96)[‡]	2.32 (1.17–4.57)[‡]
	WC	1.61 (1.40–1.85)[†]	NA	2.38 (2.06–2.75)[†]	NA
Osteoarthritis	BMI	2.76 (2.05–3.70)	1.80 (1.75–1.85)[†]	4.20 (2.76–6.41)	1.96 (1.88–2.04)[†]
Chronic back pain	BMI	1.59 (1.34–1.89)[†]	1.59 (1.34–1.89)[†]	2.81 (2.27–3.48)[†]	2.81 (2.27–3.48)[†]

*WC measures were considered to be the better risk predictor than BMI measures.
[†]If indicated, the relative risks calculated from the ratios of proportions (RR-Ps) were used; otherwise, the incidence rate ratios (IRRs) were used.
[‡]Both RR-Ps and IRRs were used.

Note: Cancer—cases, not mortality and indicated by physician diagnosis of cancer; coronary artery disease: indicated by myocardial infarction or angina; osteoarthritis: indicated by joint replacement; chronic back pain: indicated by early retirement due to back pain.

(BMI: body mass index; NA: not available; WC: waist circumference; –: not applicable)

REFERENCES

1. Aronne LJ, Nelinson DS, Lillo JL. Obesity as a disease state: a new paradigm for diagnosis and treatment. Clin Cornerstone. 2009;9(4):9-29.
2. Maritim AC, Sanders A, Watkins JB 3rd. Diabetes, oxidative stress, and antioxidants: a review. J Biochem Mol Toxicol. 2003;17(1):24-38.
3. Wild S, Roglic G, Green A, Sicree R, King H. Global prevalence of diabetes: estimates for the year 2000 and projections for 2030. Diabetes Care. 2004;27(5):1047-153.
4. Colagiuri S, Davies D. The value of early detection of type 2 diabetes. Curr Opin Endocrinol Diabetes Obes. 2009;16(2):95-9.
5. Herman WH, Ye W, Griffin SJ, Simmons RK, Davies MJ, Khunti K, et al. Early Detection and Treatment of Type 2 Diabetes Reduce Cardiovascular Morbidity and Mortality: A Simulation of the Results of the Anglo-Danish-Dutch Study of Intensive Treatment in People with Screen-detected Diabetes in Primary Care (ADDITION-Europe). Diabetes Care. 2015;38(8):1449-55.
6. Barnett AH. The importance of treating cardiometabolic risk factors in patients with type 2 diabetes. Diab Vasc Dis Res. 2008;5(1):9-14.
7. Després JP, Lemieux I, Prud'homme D. Treatment of obesity: need to focus on high risk abdominally obese patients. BMJ. 2001;322(7288):716-20.
8. Klein S, Allison DB, Heymsfield SB, Kelley DE, Leibel RL, Nonas C, et al; Association for Weight Management and Obesity Prevention; NAASO; Obesity Society; American Society for Nutrition; American Diabetes Association. Waist circumference and cardiometabolic risk: a consensus statement from shaping America's health: Association for Weight Management and Obesity Prevention; NAASO, the Obesity Society; the American Society for Nutrition; and the American Diabetes Association. Diabetes Care. 2007;30(6):1647-52.
9. Addressing overweight and obesity: Evolving to a medical consensus. J Am Osteopath Assoc. 2008;108(Suppl 1):S2-S15.
10. Garvey WT, Mechanick JI, Brett EM, Garber AJ, Hurley DL, Jastreboff AM, et al; Reviewers of the AACE/ACE Obesity Clinical Practice Guidelines. American Association of Clinical Endocrinologists and American College of Endocrinology Comprehensive Clinical Practice Guidelines for Medical Care of Patients with Obesity. Endocr Pract. 2016;22(Suppl 3):1-203.
11. Lean ME. Pathophysiology of obesity. Proc Nutr Soc. 2000;59(3):331-6.
12. Adinortey MB. Biochemicophysiological Mechanisms Underlying Signs and Symptoms Associated with Diabetes Mellitus. Adv Biol Res. 2017;11(6):382-90.
13. Casqueiro J, Casqueiro J, Alves C. Infections in patients with diabetes mellitus: A review of pathogenesis. Indian J Endocrinol Metab. 2012;16(Suppl1):S27-36.
14. National Diabetes Data Group. Classification and Diagnosis of Diabetes Mellitus and Other Categories of Glucose Intolerance. Diabetes. 1979;28:1039-57.
15. Expert Committee on Diabetes Mellitus. Second Report. Technical Report Series 646. Geneva: World Health Organization; 1980.
16. Report of the Expert Committee on the Diagnosis and Classification of Diabetes Mellitus. Diabetes Care. 1997;20:1183-97.
17. Glucose Tolerance and Mortality: Comparison of WHO and American Diabetes Association Diagnostic Criteria. The DECODE Study Group. European Diabetes Epidemiology Group. Diabetes Epidemiology: Collaborative analysis of Diagnostic criteria in Europe. Lancet. 1999;354:617-21.
18. Rivellese AA, Bozzetto L, Massaro P. Advances in Diabetes Diagnostics. European Endocrine Disease. 2007;(1):20-2.
19. American Diabetes Association. Classification and diagnosis of diabetes: Standards of medical care in diabetes—2019. Diabetes Care. 2019;42(Suppl 1):S13-S28.
20. International Expert Committee. International Expert Committee report on the role of the A1C assay in the diagnosis of diabetes. Diabetes Care. 2009;32(7):1327-34.
21. Hasslacher C, Kulozik F, Platten I. Glycated albumin and HbA1c as predictors of mortality and vascular complications in type 2 diabetes patients with normal and moderately impaired renal function: 5-year results from a 380 patient cohort. J Diabetes Res Clin Metab. 2014;3:9.

22. Lauritzen T, Sandbaek A, Skriver MV, Borch-Johnsen K. HbA1c and cardiovascular risk score identify people who may benefit from preventive interventions: A 7 year follow-up of a high-risk screening programme for diabetes in primary care (ADDITION), Denmark. Diabetologia. 2011;54:1318-26.
23. Lim WY, Ma S, Heng D, Tai ES, Khoo CM, Loh TP. Screening for diabetes with HbA1c: Test performance of HbA1c compared to fasting plasma glucose among Chinese, Malay and Indian community residents in Singapore. Sci Rep. 2018;8:12419.
24. Guo F, Moellering DR, Garvey WT. Use of HbA1c for diagnoses of diabetes and prediabetes: Comparison with diagnoses based on fasting and 2-hr glucose values and effects of gender, race, and age. Metab Syndr Relat Disord. 2014;12:258-68.
25. Radhakrishna P, Vinod KV, Sujiv A, Swaminathan RP. Comparison of hemoglobin A1c with fasting and 2-h plasma glucose tests for diagnosis of diabetes and prediabetes among high-risk South Indians. Indian J Endocrinol Metab. 2018;22:50-6.
26. Prakaschandra R, Naidoo DP. Fasting plasma glucose and the HbA1c are not optimal screening modalities for the diagnosis of new diabetes in previously undiagnosed Asian Indian community participants. Ethn Dis. 2018;28:19-24.
27. Sreenivasamurthy L. Evolution in Diagnosis and Classification of Diabetes. J Diabetes Mellitus. 2021;11:200-7
28. ElSayed NA, Aleppo G, Aroda VR, Bannuru RR, Brown FM, Bruemmer D, et al. 2. Classification and Diagnosis of Diabetes: Standards of Care in Diabetes-2023. Diabetes Care. 2023;46(Suppl 1):S19-S40.
29. Kushner RF. Clinical assessment and management of adult obesity. Circulation. 2012;126(24):2870-7.
30. Semlitsch T, Stigler FL, Jeitler K, Horvath K, Siebenhofer A. Management of overweight and obesity in primary care-A systematic overview of international evidence-based guidelines. Obes Rev. 2019;20(9):1218-30.
31. Sharma AM, Kushner RF. A proposed clinical staging system for obesity. Int J Obes (Lond). 2009;33(3):289-95.
32. S VM, Nitin K, Sambit D, Nishant R, Sanjay K; (on behalf of Endocrine Society of India). ESI Clinical Practice Guidelines for the Evaluation and Management of Obesity in India. Indian J Endocrinol Metab. 2022;26(4):295-318.
33. Lyznicki JM, Young DC, Riggs JA, Davis RM; Council on Scientific Affairs, American Medical Association. Obesity: assessment and management in primary care. Am Fam Physician. 2001;63(11):2185-96.
34. Han TS, Sattar N, Lean M. ABC of obesity. Assessment of obesity and its clinical implications. BMJ. 2006;333(7570):695-8.
35. Harvard TH Chan. Obesity Prevention Source. Measuring obesity. [online] Available from https://www.hsph.harvard.edu/obesity-prevention-source/obesity-definition/how-to-measure-body-fatness/#:~:text=Computerized%20Tomography%20(CT)%20and%20Magnetic,muscle%20mass%20and%20bone%20mass [Last accessed October, 2023].
36. Hu F. Measurements of adiposity and body composition. In: Hu FB (Ed). Obesity Epidemiology. New York City: Oxford University Press; 2008. pp. 53-83.
37. Jensen MD, Ryan DH, Apovian CM, Ard JD, Comuzzie AG, Donato KA, et al; American College of Cardiology/American Heart Association Task Force on Practice Guidelines; Obesity Society. 2013 AHA/ACC/TOS guideline for the management of overweight and obesity in adults: a report of the American College of Cardiology/American Heart Association Task Force on Practice Guidelines and the Obesity Society. Circulation. 2014;129(25 Suppl 2):S102-S38.e
38. Pantalone KM, Hobbs TM, Chagin KM, Kong SX, Wells BJ, Kattan MW, et al. Prevalence and recognition of obesity and its associated comorbidities: cross-sectional analysis of electronic health record data from a large US integrated health system. BMJ Open. 2017;7(11):e017583.
39. Ambrose T, Cullen S, Baker G, Smith M, Elia M, Leach R, et al; Royal College of Physicians Nutrition Committee. Obesity: a window of opportunity to intervene? Characteristics and management of morbidly obese adult inpatients in three trusts in Southern England. Clin Med (Lond). 2013;13(5):472-6.
40. Guh DP, Zhang W, Bansback N, Amarsi Z, Birmingham CL, Anis AH. The incidence of co-morbidities related to obesity and overweight: a systematic review and meta-analysis. BMC Public Health. 2009;9:88.

CHAPTER 5

Prevention and Lifestyle Interventions

> **Key Highlights**
> - A 12-month intensive lifestyle intervention (ILI) with high volumes of exercise in individuals with type 2 diabetes mellitus (T2DM) resulted in >50% of the participants discontinuing glucose-lowering medication compared to standard care.
> - The most effective dietary approach for achieving T2DM remission, with up to 61% of participants experiencing remission at 1 year, was programs that included an induction phase with a "total diet replacement" approach.
> - Regular physical activity and exercise are vital components of diabetes management. Recommendations often include engaging in aerobic exercises such as brisk walking, jogging, or cycling for at least 150 min/week.
> - Physical activity not only helps with weight management but also enhances insulin sensitivity, lowers blood glucose levels, and improves cardiovascular health.
> - Psychosocial support may include counseling, cognitive behavioral therapy, stress management techniques, and peer support groups.

INTRODUCTION

The global prevalence of obesity has experienced a significant surge in recent decades, reaching epidemic proportions. According to the World Health Organization (WHO), the number of obese adults has increased more than seven-fold in the past 40 years.[1] Obesity is closely linked to a high incidence of impaired glucose tolerance (IGT), also known as prediabetes, and serves as an independent risk factor for type 2 diabetes mellitus (T2DM).[2] This relationship has been established through extensive data analysis within the general population.[3] Furthermore, prediabetes has long been recognized as detrimental to cardiovascular health.[4] Additionally, there is mounting evidence indicating a substantial rise in the prevalence of overweight and obesity among adolescents. A recent cohort study focusing on this age group has revealed that an elevated body mass index (BMI) during adolescence is associated with an increased risk of developing T2DM later in life.[5] Considering these findings, it is crucial to prioritize efforts to prevent the progression from obesity to diabetes, while concurrently addressing the comorbidities commonly associated with obesity. These comorbidities primarily include T2DM, metabolic syndrome (MetS), which encompasses a cluster of interrelated disorders such as insulin resistance (IR), elevated triglyceride levels, and hyperglycemia as well as cardiovascular disease (CVD).

The Diabetes Prevention Program (DPP) has proposed prevention strategies aimed at reducing the risk of developing T2DM. These recommendations emphasize the adoption of healthy habits such as maintaining a balanced diet, engaging in regular physical activity, and avoiding smoking, alcohol consumption, and excessive stress. By implementing lifestyle modifications that focus on achieving a modest weight loss (5–10%) and engaging in moderate-intensity physical activity, it is possible to significantly reduce the incidence of T2DM and cardiometabolic risk factors in individuals at high risk.[6-8] In fact, studies conducted under the DPP have demonstrated a remarkable 58% reduction in the development of T2DM through these interventions (DPP). The DPP lifestyle intervention has demonstrated long-lasting benefits in the prevention of T2DM, with its effects shown to persist for up to a decade.[9] Consequently, the prevention of T2DM in the context of obesity plays a critical role in averting metabolic disorders and cardiovascular complications. Evidence-based guidelines strongly endorse the implementation of effective lifestyle interventions as a means of managing weight and preventing disease.[10,11] To successfully implement effective lifestyle interventions in real-world settings, it is essential to adapt them in a way that enhances their generalizability and sustainability without compromising their effectiveness. The Evaluation of Lifestyle Interventions to Treat Elevated Cardiometabolic Risk in Primary Care (E-LITE) study was a randomized trial conducted in primary care settings. The aim of the study was to assess the effectiveness of two adapted lifestyle interventions based on the DPP among overweight or obese adults with prediabetes, MetS, or both. The interventions evaluated were: (1) a coach-led, face-to-face group intervention, and (2) a self-directed DVD intervention. The trial demonstrated that both IT-supported, DPP-based lifestyle interventions resulted in clinically significant reductions in body weight (as measured by changes in BMI). Additionally, improvements in waist circumference and fasting plasma glucose levels were observed when compared to usual care over the 15-month duration of the study. The E-LITE interventions (DPP-based lifestyle interventions) have shown demonstrable benefits and have the potential for significant impact on both clinical outcomes and public health.[12]

Monitoring and evaluation are crucial to assess the effectiveness and impact of the adapted interventions in real-world settings. Collecting data on outcomes and implementation processes can provide insights into areas for improvement and inform future adaptations. Ultimately, the goal of adapting lifestyle interventions is to maximize their reach and impact by making them applicable and sustainable in diverse settings. By considering the unique needs and challenges of different populations and contexts, interventions can be optimized to improve health outcomes and promote long-term behavior change.[13] This chapter puts together information on the effective lifestyle intervention and prevention plan which demonstrates high impact on weight loss and glycemic control in real setting for patients with obesity and diabetes.

DIETARY STRATEGIES FOR WEIGHT LOSS AND GLYCEMIC CONTROL

The process of optimizing and enhancing the efficacy of lifestyle interventions commenced with the inception and execution of the DPP in 1994. Subsequently, the progression and effectiveness of intensive lifestyle interventions (ILIs) over the past 20 years, drawing from four pivotal studies [DPP, Look AHEAD (Action for Health in Diabetes), POUNDS LOST (Preventing Obesity Using Novel Dietary Strategies), CALERIE (Comprehensive Assessment of Long-term Effects of Reducing Intake of Energy)]. These studies aimed to investigate the impact of ILIs on changes in body weight and overall health outcomes. The findings from these studies demonstrated that adopting lifestyle modifications targeting nutrition and physical activity can lead to weight loss and contribute to the prevention or improvement of various obesity-related medical conditions **(Table 1)**. These positive outcomes were observed across different subpopulations, highlighting the broad impact and effectiveness of lifestyle interventions.[8,9,14-24]

TABLE 1: Summary of different lifestyle intervention program outcomes.

Component	DPP[8,9,14-17]	Look AHEAD[18-20]	POUNDS LOST[21,22]	CALERIE[23,24]
Emphasis	Individual	Group	Group	Individual
Group counseling	No	Yes	Yes	Yes
Individual counseling	Yes	Yes	Yes	Yes
Used DPP core	Yes	Yes	Yes	Yes
Diet prescription	CR 1 reduced FI	CR	CR	CR
Exercise goal	150 min/week	175 min/week	90 min/week	NA
Core ILI duration	24 weeks	1 year	2 years	2 years
Follow-up duration	10 years	8 years	2 years	2 years
Weight loss (%)	~7% for 1 years, ~6% in 2 years	~9% after 1 year and 4.7% after 8 years	8.4% after 1 year and 5.3% after 2 years	11.5% after 1 year and 10.4% after 2 years
Waist circumference (%)	1.8% after 1 year and 4.6% after 2.9 years	NA	7.2% after 1 year and 6.1% after 2 years	NA
Cost	$1,826 first year and averaged $305/year	$2,865 first year and $1,120 in years 5–9	NA	NA

(CALERIE: Comprehensive Assessment of Long-term Effects of Reducing Intake of Energy; CR: caloric restriction; DPP: Diabetes Prevention Program; FI: fat intake; Look AHEAD: Action for Health in Diabetes; ILI: intensive lifestyle intervention; NA: not applicable; POUNDS LOST: Preventing Obesity Using Novel Dietary Strategies)

According to the United States Preventive Services Task Force, it is recommended that all adults undergo screening for obesity, and individuals with a BMI of 30 kg/m^2 or higher should be offered "intensive, multicomponent behavioral interventions". This recommendation emphasizes the importance of comprehensive lifestyle interventions for weight loss. The recent Guidelines for the Management of Overweight and Obesity in Adults, published by the American Heart Association/American College of Cardiology/Obesity Society, provide more detailed guidance on the implementation of ILIs. These guidelines suggest that individuals who are overweight (BMI 25.0–29.9 kg/m^2) or obese (BMI ≥ 30 kg/m^2) and would benefit from weight loss should participate in a comprehensive lifestyle intervention program for a minimum of 6 months. These programs typically include instruction in diet, physical activity, and behavior therapy, which are delivered by trained interventionists. The interventionists are often health professionals such as registered dietitians, exercise specialists, psychologists, health counselors, or occasionally trained laypersons. The Obesity Guidelines recommend the provision of face-to-face individual or group counseling sessions as part of the comprehensive lifestyle intervention. It is suggested that individual counseling may lead to greater weight loss compared to group treatment due to the increased opportunity for personalized instruction during individual meetings.[25,26]

Lifestyle changes, including exercise and/or diet modifications, are considered a first-line treatment for T2DM. These lifestyle interventions have shown to improve glycemic control, as measured by HbA1c levels. A recent study reported that a diet-induced weight loss intervention, without an increase in physical activity, resulted in the remission of T2DM. The remission was attributed to the reduction of ectopic fat in the liver and pancreas, along with improvements in beta cell function.[27]

Effective lifestyle interventions often lead to concurrent weight loss, which can independently improve beta cell function. Two studies, namely the DiRECT and DIADEM-I studies, implemented a 12-month ILI with high volumes of exercise in individuals with T2DM.[28-30] These studies resulted in >50% of the participants discontinuing glucose-lowering medication compared to standard care. The DiRECT study, an open-label, cluster-randomized trial conducted in 49 primary care practices, enrolled 306 individuals. At the 12-month mark, the intervention group had 24% participants who achieved a weight loss of 15 kg or more, whereas no participants in the control group achieved this ($p < 0.0001$). The mean body weight decreased by 10.0 kg in the intervention group compared to 1.0 kg in the control group (adjusted difference –8.8 kg, $p < 0.0001$). The study demonstrated that remission of T2DM is an attainable goal in primary care settings. At the 2-year follow-up, 11% participants in the intervention group and 2% participants in the control group achieved a weight loss of at least 15 kg [adjusted odds ratio (aOR) 7.49; $p = 0.0023$]. The DiRECT program maintained sustained remissions at 24 months for over a third of individuals with T2DM, and the extent of sustained weight loss was linked to the maintenance of remission.[28,29]

In another open-label, parallel-group, randomized controlled trial (RCT) called DIADEM-I, conducted in primary care and community settings, the effects of an ILI compared to usual medical care were examined in 158 individuals aged 18–50 years with T2DM. At 12 months, participants in the intervention group experienced a mean body weight reduction of 11.98 kg, whereas the control group had a reduction of 3.98 kg (Δ = –6.08 kg, $p < 0.0001$). Diabetes remission was achieved by 61% of participants in the intervention group, compared with 12% in the control group [odds ratio (OR) 12.03; $p < 0.0001$]. Additionally, 33% of participants in the intervention group achieved normoglycemia, in comparison to 4% of participants in the control group (OR 12.07; $p < 0.0001$). The findings suggest that providing this ILI can lead to significant improvements in key cardiometabolic outcomes in a large proportion of young individuals with early diabetes. These improvements have the potential for long-term benefits in terms of health and well-being.[30] It is well established from above studies that lifestyle interventions, including dietary changes, have a vital role in preventing the progression of impaired fasting glucose or IGT to T2DM.

de la Iglesia et al. conducted a review highlighting various dietary approaches and bioactive compounds employed in the treatment of obesity and diabetes, specifically targeting MetS. The study identified several dietary strategies and their potential positive effects on preventing and treating the different metabolic complications associated with MetS. The review also provided a comprehensive summary of the most relevant dietary approaches and bioactive compounds used in the treatment of obesity and diabetes, with **Flowchart 1** depicting an overview of these approaches. **Tables 2** and **3** presented a summary of the dietary strategies and their potential positive effects on the prevention and treatment of metabolic complications associated with MetS.[31]

An umbrella review of published meta-analyses and systematic reviews, which encompassed 19 meta-analyses of weight loss diets involving 2–23 primary trials (n = 100–1,587) published between 2013 and 2021, revealed several key findings. Firstly, the review indicated that programs incorporating very low energy diets and formula meal replacements were the most effective in managing weight for individuals with T2DM. Secondly, it was found that there were no significant advantages of any specific macronutrient profile or dietary style over others for weight management in this context. Finally, the review highlighted that the most effective dietary approach for achieving T2DM remission, with up to 61% of participants experiencing remission at 1 year, was programs that included an induction phase with a "total diet replacement" approach **(Fig. 1)**.[32]

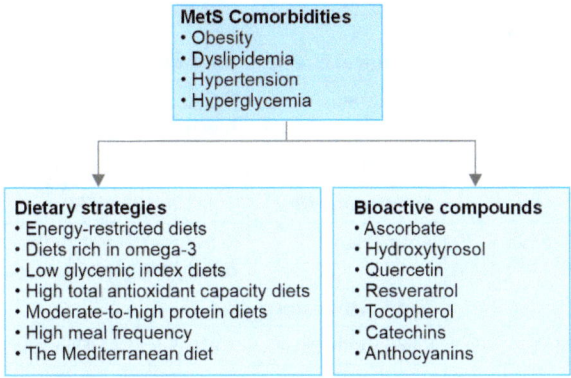

FLOWCHART 1: Diagram of metabolic syndrome (MetS) comorbidities and dietary strategies and bioactive compounds described.

TABLE 2: Potential beneficial effects of different dietary patterns on the treatment of metabolic syndrome (MetS) comorbidities.

Dietary pattern	Metabolic diseases improved	Mechanisms implicated
Energy-restricted diets	Obesity	Lipolysis
	Type 2 diabetes mellitus	Improvements of glycemia and insulin resistance
	Inflammation	↓ Inflammatory markers (e.g., IL-6)
	CV diseases	Improvement of cholesterol profile and ↓ SBP, DBP, and TG
Diets rich in omega-3	Inflammation	↓ Pro-inflammatory cytokines (e.g., IL-6, TNF-α)
	CV diseases	↓ TG, sdLDL particles
Low glycemic index diets	Type 2 diabetes mellitus	↓ HbA1c and fructosamine
High TAC diets	Oxidative stress	Free radicals' scavenger
Moderate-high protein diets	Obesity	↑ Satiety and thermogenesis
High meal frequency	Obesity	↓ Plasma glucose levels oscillations and ↓ insulin secretion
The Mediterranean diet	Type 2 diabetes mellitus	Glycemic control, ↓ HbA1c, ↓ fasting glucose levels
	CV diseases	↓ TC, LDL-c, TG, and ↑ HDL-c
	Obesity	↑ Satiety and ↓ body weight and waist circumference

(CV: cardiovascular; DBP: diastolic blood pressure; HbA1c: glycated hemoglobin; HDL-c: high density lipoprotein cholesterol; IL-6: interleukin-6; LDL-c: low density lipoprotein cholesterol; SBP: systolic blood pressure; sdLDL particles: small dense low density lipoprotein particles; TAC: total antioxidant capacity; TC: total cholesterol; TG: triglycerides; TNF-α: tumor necrosis factor alpha; ↓: reduction; ↑: increment)

TABLE 3: Dietary bioactive compounds with potential positive effects on metabolic syndrome (MetS), biological effects, and molecular mechanisms of action involved.

Bioactive component	Metabolite class	Biological effects	Mechanisms
Anthocyanins	Polyphenol	Antidiabetic	↑ Glucose uptake in an insulin-independent mechanism
		Cardioprotective	↑ BAFMD, HDL-c and ↓ VCAM-1, LDL-c
		Antinflammatory	↓ IL-8, IL-1β, or CRP
Ascorbate	Vitamin	Antioxidant	Scavenger of free radicals and regeneration of oxidized molecules
		Anti-inflammatory	↓ CRP
		Cardioprotective	↑ eNOS and ↓ HDL-c glycation
		Antidiabetic	↑ SVCTs

Continued

Continued

Bioactive component	Metabolite class	Biological effects	Mechanisms
Catechin	Polyphenol	Anti-obesity	↑ ACAD and peroxisomal β-oxidation enzymes, ↓ COMT and PDE
		Cardioprotective	↑ HDL-c and ↓ LDL-c, TC
		Antidiabetic	↓ Fasting glucose levels and insulin sensitivity improvement
Hydroxytyrosol	Polyphenol	Antioxidant	Free radical scavenger, radical chain breaker, and metal chelator
		Anti-inflammatory	↑ eNOS, ↓ COX
		Cardioprotective	↑ HDL-c, ↓ LDL-c oxidation, ICAM-1, VCAM-1, LDL-c and TC
Quercetin	Polyphenol	Antioxidant	↓ Lipid peroxidation, ↑ antioxidant enzymes (e.g., SOD, CAT, GPX)
		Anti-inflammatory	↓ PI3K, GLUT2, NF-κB, TNF-α, MAPK, IL-6, IL-1β, IL-8 or MCP-1
		Anti-obesity	↓ Adipogenesis through ↑ AMPK and ↓ C/EBPα, PPARγ, and SREBP-1
		Antidiabetic	PPARγ, GLUT2, PI3K, and TK
		↓ Blood pressure	↑ eNOS and ↓ platelet aggregation
Resveratrol	Polyphenol	Antioxidant	Scavenger of hydroxyl, superoxide, and metal-induced radicals
		Anti-inflammatory	↓ NF-κB, IL-6, IL-8, TNF-α, MCP-1, eNOS, COX
		Cardioprotective	↑ NO and Nrf2, ↓ ICAM-1, VCAM-1
		Anti-obesity	↑ Lipolysis, ↓ lipogenesis
		Anti-inflammatory	↓ CRP, COX, PKC, IL-8, PAI-1
		Antiatherogenic	↓ Oxidation of LDL-c and PUFAs
Tocopherol	Vitamin	Antioxidant	↓ Lipid peroxyl radicals
		Anti-inflammatory	↓ CRP, COX, PKC, IL-8

(ACAD: acyl-CoA dehydrogenase; AMPK: AMP-activated protein kinase; BAFMD: brachial artery flow-mediated dilation; CAT: catalase; C/EBPα: CCAAT-enhancer-binding protein alpha; COMT: catechol-O-methyltransferase; COX: cyclooxygenase; CRP: C-reactive protein; eNOS: endothelial nitric oxide synthase; GLUT2: glucose transporter 2; GPX: glutathione peroxidase; HDL-c: high-density lipoprotein cholesterol; ICAM-1: intercellular adhesion molecule 1; IL-8: interleukin 8; LDL-c: low-density lipoprotein cholesterol; MAPK: mitogen-activated protein kinases; MCP-1: monocyte chemoattractant protein-1; NF-κB: nuclear factor kappa-light-chain-enhancer of activated B cells; NO: nitric oxide; Nrf2: NF-E2-related factor 2; PAI-1: plasminogen activator inhibitor 1; PDE: phosphodiesterase; PI3K: phosphatidylinositol 3-kinase; PKC: protein kinase C; PPARγ: peroxisome proliferator-activated receptor gamma; PUFAs: polyunsaturated fatty acids; SOD: superoxide dismutase; SREBP-1: sterol regulatory element-binding protein 1; SVCTs: sodium-dependent vitamin C transporters; TC: total cholesterol; TK: tyrosine kinase; TNF-α: tumor necrosis factor alpha; VCAM-1: vascular cell adhesion protein 1; ↓: reduction; ↑: increment)

In a recent clinical study conducted by Ben-Yacov et al. in 2021, it was demonstrated that a personalized portion-controlled (PPT) diet led to significant improvements in glycemic control compared to a Mediterranean (MED) diet. The study assessed the daily time of glucose levels exceeding 140 mg/dL (7.8 mmol/L)

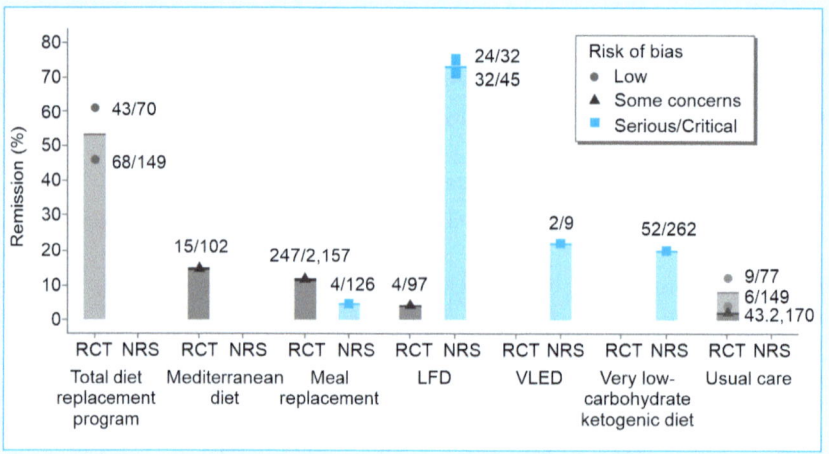

FIG. 1: Percentage of remissions of type 2 diabetes mellitus at 12 months after intervention with different diet types, stratified by study design and risk of bias. Each dot, with varying shapes to reflect risk of bias, indicates the data point for each of the studies mentioned in the main text which provided data in this form at 12 months. The column represents the mean for the diet type. Remission was defined as either HbA1c < 48 mmol/mol (<6.5%) or fasting plasma glucose < 7 mmol/L, with no glucose-lowering medication. Total diet replacement programs included an initial low energy formula diet, prescribed for an 8–12-week induction phase, followed by stepped food reintroduction aimed to achieve energy balance for weight loss maintenance. VLED advised a 2.9 MJ (700 kcal) food-based diet for 1 week, then dietary advice for energy intake that matched for ideal body weight. Very low-carbohydrate ketogenic diet was ad libitum intake, carbohydrate < 30 g/day to achieve ketosis and 3–5 servings of non-starchy vegetables. Usual diet or standard diet interventions included diabetes education support, but no new diet intervention.

(LFD: low-fat diet; NRS: nonrandomized study; RCT: randomized controlled trial; VLED: very low energy diet)

and HbA1c levels as measures of glycemic control. Both interventions resulted in reductions in the daily time with glucose levels above 140 mg/dL (7.8 mmol/L) and HbA1c levels, but the reductions were significantly greater in the PPT group compared to the MED group. The mean 6-month change in "time above 140" was −0.3 ± 0.8 h/day for MED and −1.3 ± 1.5 h/day for PPT, with a significant difference ($p < 0.001$). Similarly, the mean 6-month change in HbA1c was −0.08 ± 0.19% for MED and −0.16 ± 0.24% for PPT, also showing a significant difference ($p = 0.007$).[33]

In a study conducted by de Carvalho et al., the effect of different dietary patterns, including the low-fat vegan diet, MED diet, vegetarian diet, dietary approaches to stop hypertension (DASH) diet, and vegan diet, on glycemic markers in individuals with T2DM was evaluated. The systematic review showed that adopting these dietary patterns resulted in improved glycemic control, primarily through a reduction in %HbA1c, when compared to conventional diets typically used for metabolic treatment of individuals with T2DM. Additionally, the dietary patterns were found to promote a better quality of life among individuals with T2DM, attributed to the nutritional characteristics of these patterns and the presence of bioactive compounds that play important roles in the body.[34]
Table 4 provides an overview of the key nutritional recommendations for patients with T2DM based on guidelines as well as dietary patterns with a high degree of

TABLE 4: Summary of nutritional recommendations for type 2 diabetes mellitus, as derived from international guidelines.

Nutrients	Recommendations
1–2 calorie intake	Reduce energy intake in all individuals with overweight/obesity (calorie deficit of 250–500 kcal/day) to promote weight loss (0.5–1.0 kg/week) to a final body weight within the normal range
1–2 macronutrient distribution	There is insufficient evidence to recommend specific macronutrient distribution, but a moderate carbohydrate reduction might favor glucose control and promote a moderate weight loss
1–2 carbohydrates	Prefer low glycemic index foods (whole grains, fruits, legumes, green salad with olive oil dressing and most vegetables). Limit refined carbohydrates (pasta, white bread, rice, white potatoes, etc.)
1–2 sugars	• Limit intake of sucrose-containing foods and sugary drinks • Prefer non-nutritive sweeteners as substitutes of sugar • Low calorie or unsweetened beverages should be preferred, but their consumption limited
1–2 fibers	30–50 g/day of dietary fibers (at least one-third of soluble origin)
1–2 proteins	As in the general population, 1.0–1.5 g/kg ideal body weight; reduce protein intake to 0.8 g/kg of body weight or lower in patients with chronic kidney disease
1–2 fats	• As in the general population, 20–35% of total kcal/day • Avoid trans-fatty acids and limit saturated fatty acids (SFAs) to 7–9%. Increase foods enriched in long-chain omega-3 polyunsaturated fatty acids (PUFAs) and monounsaturated fatty acids (MUFAs)
1-2 micronutrients and vitamins	• Correct micronutrient and vitamin deficiencies • Consider vitamin supplementation (B-group vitamins or folic acid) in metformin-treated patients
1–2 sodium	Limited as in the general population; consider additional limitations in those with hypertension
1–2 alcohol	Limited as in the general population
1–2 dietary pattern	Favor a dietary model based on Mediterranean style

evidence. These interventions aim to reduce energy intake and promote a weight loss of 5-10% of initial body weight. By achieving this weight loss, individuals can experience improved insulin sensitivity, better control of blood glucose and blood pressure levels, and reduced lipid levels. It is recommended to follow regular mealtimes and adopt a healthy diet in conjunction with increased physical activity. These combined lifestyle changes have been shown to be beneficial for managing T2DM.[35]

PHYSICAL ACTIVITY AND EXERCISE RECOMMENDATIONS

Exercise has been proven to enhance peripheral insulin sensitivity in individuals with T2DM, leading to better glucose control. However, the impact of exercise on beta cell function is still not fully understood. According to Johansen et al., the inclusion of an ILI that includes high volumes of exercise in individuals with

T2DM has the potential to enhance beta cell function. This improvement in beta cell function may be linked to reductions in low-grade inflammation and/or body weight. The study suggests that the combination of exercise and lifestyle modifications could have beneficial effects on beta cell function, which plays a crucial role in glucose regulation in individuals with T2DM.[27]

There is robust and consistent evidence supporting the importance of regular physical activity in maintaining a stable body weight over time, preventing weight gain, and reducing the risks associated with overweight and obesity.[23] When it comes to weight loss and weight maintenance, the evidence suggests that a higher volume of physical activity may be necessary compared to what is required for general health benefits. The specific amount of physical activity needed varies among individuals. To effectively promote weight loss and sustain weight loss, many individuals may need to engage in physical activity at the upper end of the recommended range, which is 150–300 min/week of moderate-intensity physical activity. This higher level of activity helps create an energy deficit and supports successful weight management. Additionally, incorporating resistance exercise into the routine can be beneficial for preserving lean body mass, which can help prevent a positive energy balance.[36]

Exercise exerts both acute and chronic effects on the key determinants of glucose tolerance, namely whole-body insulin sensitivity and pancreatic beta cell function. Increasing physical activity by 500 kcal/week is associated with a significant reduction of approximately 9% in the risk of developing T2DM. The link between physical activity and lower T2DM risk is primarily attributed to the acute and chronic effects of exercise on enhancing insulin sensitivity.[37,38] Acutely, exercise stimulates the transcription and translocation of glucose transporter type 4 (GLUT4) in skeletal muscle, leading to increased glucose uptake. Exercise also reduces postexercise circulating levels of triglycerides.[39] A single bout of exercise typically improves insulin sensitivity by 25% or more, and this effect persists for approximately 72 hours before gradually declining. Both aerobic and resistance exercise improve insulin sensitivity, although aerobic exercise tends to have a more pronounced effect **(Table 5)**.[38,40]

The chronic effects of exercise further enhance insulin sensitivity. Studies on exercise training consistently demonstrate increases in insulin sensitivity ranging from 25 to 50%, particularly when exercise training is accompanied by reductions in adiposity. Chronic exercise enhances insulin sensitivity through various mechanisms, including a reduction in inflammatory cytokines, increased activity of glycogen synthase (associated with greater glycogen storage capacity), and increased capillarization of skeletal muscle, which improves perfusion and glucose extraction by the muscle tissue. RCTs investigating interventions that enhance insulin sensitivity, such as insulin-sensitizing drugs, diet-induced weight loss, bariatric surgery, and exercise training, have shown a reduced burden on pancreatic beta cells and a slowing of the decline in beta cell function. Consequently, these interventions can prevent or delay the onset of prediabetes or T2DM by preserving beta cell function.[41] In summary, exercise exerts both acute and chronic effects that enhance insulin sensitivity, reduce the burden on pancreatic beta cells, and contribute to the prevention or delay of prediabetes and T2DM.

TABLE 5: Summary of aerobic exercise and resistance exercise.

	Aerobic exercise	Resistance exercise
Frequency	*Start*: 3 days/week of moderate intensity exercise and not consecutive days *General population*: Moderate intensity (5 days/week) or vigorous intensity (3 days/week)	2 or 3 nonconsecutive days/week with a minimum of 48–72 hours of rest between each training session
Intensity	*Moderate intensity*: 40–60% heart rate reserve, i.e., brisk walking in type 2 diabetes mellitus (T2DM) *Vigorous intensity*: >60% heart rate reserve	*Moderate intensity*: 50% of an individual's one repetition maximum (1 RM) *Vigorous intensity*: 75–80% of the 1 RM
Duration	*Moderate intensity*: At least 150 min/week; 10-minute bouts	*Large muscle groups exercises*: 5–10 exercises and 10–15 repetitions with 1–4 sets for each exercise
Mode	Exercises using large muscles like swimming, cycling, walking, running, and rowing	Resistance machines and free weights as primary mode of training Functional movement exercises
Rate of progression	10% increase/week in intensity or duration	• Recommended slow • *2-for-2 rule*: Stating that weight increases should occur if the individual can perform 2 more repetitions on his or her final set in 2 consecutive resistance training sessions • Three weekly sessions using three sets of 8–12 repetitions at 75–80% 1 RM

The ATTICA study supports the notion that physical activity plays a crucial role in improving insulin sensitivity, particularly in mitigating the adverse effects of obesity. This population-based, cross-sectional health and nutrition survey involved 1,058 subjects who were categorized as physically active. The study found that individuals who were overweight or obese but engaged in increased levels of physical activity demonstrated health indices comparable to those of individuals with normal body weight. The findings of the ATTICA study emphasize the potential benefits of incorporating physical activity into the lifestyle of overweight or obese individuals. By engaging in regular physical activity, these individuals can experience improvements in insulin sensitivity, counteracting the negative impact of excess weight on metabolic health. This suggests that physical activity has the potential to mitigate the adverse effects of obesity on insulin sensitivity, contributing to better overall health outcomes.[42]

Exercise is essential for achieving optimal blood glucose levels and reducing body weight, BMI, and waist circumference. A systematic review and meta-analysis examined the therapeutic effects of exercise on glycemic control in individuals with T2DM. Out of 21,559 articles, 32 RCTs were included, showing that exercise interventions led to significant improvements in glycated hemoglobin (HbA1c) ($p < 0.0001$), fasting blood glucose ($p = 0.03$), BMI, and waist circumference. These findings highlight the importance of exercise as an adjunct therapy in managing T2DM, contributing to improved glycemic control and overall quality of life.[43]

BEHAVIORAL MODIFICATION AND PSYCHOLOGICAL SUPPORT

Type 2 diabetes mellitus is a multifactorial lifestyle disease, influenced by dietary habits and sedentary behavior. The American Diabetes Association (ADA) emphasizes the importance of supporting behavioral change as a key objective in diabetes care, with lifestyle modifications like increased physical activity, healthy diet, smoking cessation, weight loss, and coping strategies being central to diabetes treatment. Prevention and management of T2DM require individual, environmental, social, and policy-level changes. Research recommends investigating the effects of multiple behavior changes in individuals with T2DM and utilizing behavior change techniques (BCTs) associated with significant improvements in HbA1c.[44] Self-monitoring of diet and physical activity is a proven effective BCT for weight management and is a crucial component of behavioral obesity treatment. Research has consistently demonstrated the association between dietary self-monitoring, including its frequency, and successful weight loss outcomes. When combined with other self-regulation strategies such as goal setting and feedback, self-monitoring further enhances weight loss efforts. Digital self-monitoring methods have shown higher engagement rates compared to traditional paper-based approaches. Key BCTs associated with positive outcomes in changing diet and physical activity behaviors include "instruction on how to perform a behavior", "action planning", "social support", "behavioral practice/rehearsal", "problem solving", "self-monitoring of behavior", "goal setting", "goal review", "prompt practice", "use of follow-up prompts", "prompting generalization of a target behavior", "feedback on behavior", and "demonstration of the behavior".[44,45]

A systematic review and meta-analysis conducted by Cradock et al. demonstrated that diet and physical activity interventions resulted in clinically significant reductions in HbA1c at 3 and 6 months. Specific BCTs and intervention features identified in the study can inform more effective structured lifestyle intervention treatment strategies for T2DM. Meta-analyses revealed that at 3 months, there was an average reduction of −1.11% in HbA1c in the intervention groups compared to the control groups (−0.53% overall reduction, $p < 0.00001$). Additionally, meta-analyses showed a reduction in body weight of −3.18 kg at 24 months (−3.73 kg overall reduction, $p = 0.002$). Four of the 46 identified BCTs were associated with a >0.3% reduction in HbA1c: "Instruction on how to perform a behavior", "behavioral practice/rehearsal", "demonstration of the behavior", and "action planning". "Intervention features such as "supervised physical activity," "group sessions", "contact with an exercise physiologist", "contact with an exercise physiologist and a dietitian", "baseline HbA1c > 8%", and interventions of greater frequency and intensity were also associated with significant HbA1c reduction.[44]

Digital tools, such as online tools, apps, and tracking technologies, are increasingly utilized for long-term behavior change support. In an RCT, Carter et al. compared the acceptability and feasibility of a self-monitoring weight management intervention using a smartphone app, website, and paper diary. Results showed a mean weight change of 4.6 kg with the smartphone app, 2.9 kg with the paper diary, and 1.3 kg with the website at 6 months. The smartphone app intervention received high satisfaction and acceptability ratings. Weight management apps have the potential to positively impact weight-related outcomes, although many studies have low methodological quality. A meta-analysis by Villinger et al., involving over 6,300 participants, demonstrated the effectiveness of app-based mobile interventions in changing nutrition behaviors and improving nutrition-related health outcomes. Digital tools, such as apps, offer a cost-effective and scalable method for collecting health-related data. However, it is crucial to note that evidence-based behavior change strategies are often lacking in digital weight management offerings.[45]

The logical model of the National Health Service–DPP (NHS–DPP) outlines the anticipated mechanisms of action, demonstrating how various constructs are interconnected to achieve the main outcomes of improving dietary behaviors, increasing physical activity, and achieving weight loss/maintenance to reduce the risk of T2DM. The model is based on information and BCTs extracted from the National Institute for Health and Care Excellence (NICE) PH38 guidance. The first component of the model involves providing service users with initial information about their risk of developing T2DM as well as the risks and benefits associated with lifestyle changes. This information aims to create an intention to change behavior (second component). The third component of the model is a self-regulatory cycle that involves setting realistic short-term and long-term goals for diet, physical activity, and weight loss as well as self-monitoring of behaviors, developing coping strategies, reviewing progress, and adjusting goals based on achievements. This cycle facilitates the development and maintenance of self-efficacy, allowing individuals to learn from their experiences and leading to increased autonomy and satisfaction upon achieving their goals. The fourth component represents the expected outcomes of the intervention, which include increased activity levels, improved diet, and corresponding weight loss. **Flowchart 2** shows the visual representation of the logical model.[46]

Psychological Support in Diabetes

Psychological distress is prevalent among individuals with diabetes, affecting over 40% of the population. This distress serves as both a risk factor for and a consequence of diabetes diagnosis. People with diabetes who experience significant psychological ill-health are more likely to have poorer diabetes self-care, leading to adverse biomedical outcomes, increased complications, higher healthcare costs, decreased productivity, and even increased mortality. It is crucial to acknowledge that most distress experienced by individuals with diabetes is not pathological but represents the emotional burdens that come with managing a severe and demanding chronic illness. It is the responsibility of healthcare providers and support networks to recognize and assist individuals in understanding and managing emotional upset, interpersonal tension, and the stress associated with the demands of diabetes management. Research has shown that psychological treatments can improve glycemic control in children and adolescents with type 1 diabetes mellitus (T1DM), while interventions like counseling, cognitive behavioral therapy, family therapy,

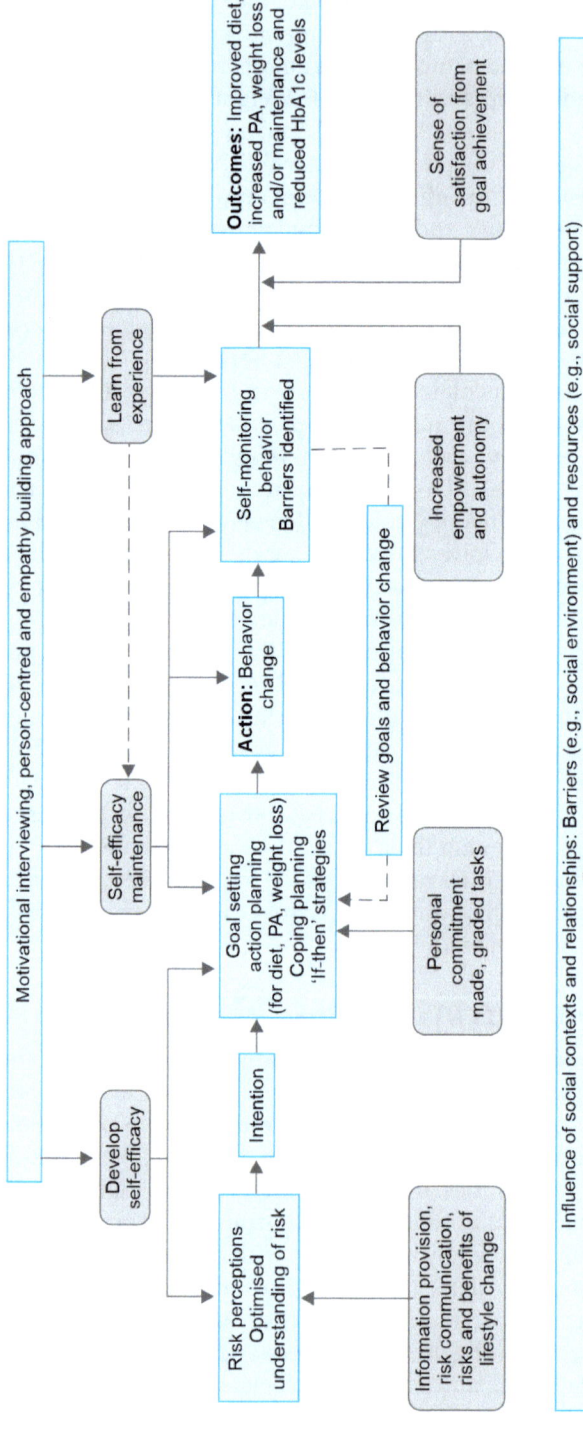

FLOWCHART 2: Logic model showing anticipated mechanisms of action of the NHS-DPP.
(HbA1c: glycated hemoglobin; PA: physical activity; NHS-DPP: National Health Service–Diabetes Prevention Program)

and psychodynamic therapy have been effective in improving long-term glycemic control and reducing psychological distress in individuals with T2DM.[47]

Unfortunately, many guidelines for diabetes care primarily focus on medical aspects and often overlook the psychological needs of patients. This lack of psychological support leads to a poor quality of life and reduced overall well-being for individuals with diabetes. Accepting the need for lifelong medication can be challenging for many individuals, resulting in poor treatment adherence and difficulties with diabetes self-management. These psychosocial challenges can eventually lead to depressive disorders and other psychological issues, which further contribute to poor self-care, adverse health outcomes, increased mortality, functional limitations, higher healthcare costs, reduced quality of life, and diminished productivity. Addressing the emotional and psychological needs of individuals with diabetes is essential, particularly when personal efforts to meet these challenges are unsuccessful, or when diabetes-related complications take a toll on physical and mental health. Recognizing that psychosocial impact is a strong predictor of mortality and morbidity in individuals with diabetes, it is crucial to integrate psychosocial aspects into all levels of diabetes management. By doing so, better treatment adherence and good glycemic control can be achieved. Studies have demonstrated that addressing psychological needs can lead to HbA1c improvements of 0.5-1% in adults with T2DM. Psychosocial interventions such as cognitive–behavioral therapy, motivational therapy, problem-solving therapy, coping skills training, and family behavior therapy have all shown promise in improving treatment adherence and achieving better glycemic control. As a result, psychosocial interventions are now recognized as an integral part of diabetes care, as they play a crucial role in improving glycemic control, self-care behavior, reducing the risk of complications, and enhancing the quality of life for individuals with diabetes.[48]

International guidelines strongly recommend the integration of psychosocial care into collaborative and patient-centered medical care for all individuals with diabetes. The primary objectives of this integrated approach are to optimize health outcomes and improve health-related quality of life. To achieve these goals, healthcare providers are advised to assess symptoms of various psychological factors such as diabetes distress, depression, anxiety, and disordered eating. Additionally, evaluating cognitive capacities using appropriate standardized and validated tools is also recommended. These assessments should be conducted during the initial visit, at regular intervals, and whenever there are significant changes in the disease, treatment, or life circumstances of the individual with diabetes. Furthermore, involving caregivers and family members in the assessment process is highly encouraged, recognizing their potential impact on the patient's well-being and diabetes management.[49] By implementing comprehensive psychosocial assessments and involving the broader support network, healthcare providers can better understand and address the psychological aspects of diabetes care, thereby enhancing the overall treatment experience and health outcomes for individuals with diabetes.

REFERENCES

1. NCD Risk Factor Collaboration (NCD-RisC). Worldwide trends in body-mass index, underweight, overweight, and obesity from 1975 to 2016: a pooled analysis of 2416 population-based measurement studies in 128·9 million children, adolescents, and adults. Lancet. 2017;390(10113):2627-42.
2. Schnurr TM, Jakupović H, Carrasquilla GD, Ängquist L, Grarup N, Sørensen TIA, et al. Obesity, unfavourable lifestyle and genetic risk of type 2 diabetes: a case-cohort study. Diabetologia. 2020;63(7):1324-32.
3. Prospective Studies Collaboration; Whitlock G, Lewington S, Sherliker P, Clarke R, Emberson J, Halsey J, et al. Body-mass index and cause-specific mortality in 900 000 adults: collaborative analyses of 57 prospective studies. Lancet. 2009;373(9669):1083-96.
4. Brunner EJ, Shipley MJ, Witte DR, Fuller JH, Marmot MG. Relation between blood glucose and coronary mortality over 33 years in the Whitehall Study. Diabetes Care. 2006;29(1):26-31.
5. Twig G, Afek A, Derazne E, Tzur D, Cukierman-Yaffe T, Gerstein HC, et al. Diabetes risk among overweight and obese metabolically healthy young adults. Diabetes Care. 2014;37(11):2989-95.
6. Pan XR, Li GW, Hu YH, Wang JX, Yang WY, An ZX, et al. Effects of diet and exercise in preventing NIDDM in people with impaired glucose tolerance. The Da Qing IGT and Diabetes Study. Diabetes Care. 1997;20(4):537-44.
7. Tuomilehto J, Lindström J, Eriksson JG, Valle TT, Hämäläinen H, Ilanne-Parikka P, et al; Finnish Diabetes Prevention Study Group. Prevention of type 2 diabetes mellitus by changes in lifestyle among subjects with impaired glucose tolerance. N Engl J Med. 2001;344(18):1343-50.
8. Knowler WC, Barrett-Connor E, Fowler SE, Hamman RF, Lachin JM, Walker EA, et al; Diabetes Prevention Program Research Group. Reduction in the incidence of type 2 diabetes with lifestyle intervention or metformin. N Engl J Med. 2002;346(6):393-403.
9. Diabetes Prevention Program Research Group; Knowler WC, Fowler SE, Hamman RF, Christophi CA, Hoffman HJ, Brenneman AT, et al. 10-year follow-up of diabetes incidence and weight loss in the Diabetes Prevention Program Outcomes Study. Lancet. 2009;374(9702):1677-86.
10. National Institutes of Health, National Heart Lung Blood Institute. Clinical Guidelines on the Identification, Evaluation, and Treatment of Overweight and Obesity in Adults: The Evidence Report. Rockville, MD: DHHS, Public Health Service; 1998. NIH Publication No. 00-4084.
11. US Preventive Services Task Force. Screening for obesity in adults: recommendations and rationale. Ann Intern Med. 2003;139(11):930-2.
12. Ma J, Yank V, Xiao L, Lavori PW, Wilson SR, Rosas LG, et al. Translating the Diabetes Prevention Program lifestyle intervention for weight loss into primary care: a randomized trial. JAMA Intern Med. 2013;173(2):113-21.
13. The Diabetes Prevention Program Research Group. The Diabetes Prevention Program. Design and methods for a clinical trial in the prevention of type 2 diabetes. Diabetes Care. 1999;22(4):623-34.
14. The Diabetes Prevention Program (DPP) Research Group. The Diabetes Prevention Program (DPP): description of lifestyle intervention. Diabetes Care. 2002;25(12):2165-71.
15. Diabetes Prevention Program Outcomes Study Research Group; Orchard TJ, Temprosa M, Barrett-Connor E, Fowler SE, Goldberg RB, Mather KJ, et al. Long-term effects of the Diabetes Prevention Program interventions on cardiovascular risk factors: a report from the DPP Outcomes Study. Diabet Med. 2013;30(1):46-55.
16. Herman WH, Edelstein SL, Ratner RE, Montez MG, Ackermann RT, Orchard TJ, et al; Diabetes Prevention Program Research Group. Effectiveness and cost-effectiveness of diabetes prevention among adherent participants. Am J Manag Care. 2013;19(3):194-202.
17. Diabetes Prevention Program Research Group. The 10-year cost-effectiveness of lifestyle intervention or metformin for diabetes prevention: an intent-to-treat analysis of the DPP/DPPOS. Diabetes Care. 2012;35(4):723-30.
18. Look AHEAD Research Group. Eight-year weight losses with an intensive lifestyle intervention: the look AHEAD study. Obesity (Silver Spring). 2014;22(1):5-13.
19. Pi-Sunyer X. The Look AHEAD Trial: a review and discussion of its outcomes. Curr Nutr Rep. 2014;3(4):387-91.
20. Rushing J, Wing R, Wadden TA, Knowler WC, Lawlor M, Evans M, et al; The Look AHEAD Research Group. Cost of intervention delivery in a lifestyle weight loss trial in type 2 diabetes: results from the Look AHEAD clinical trial. Obes Sci Pract. 2017;3(1):15-24.
21. Sacks FM, Bray GA, Carey VJ, Knowler WC, Lawlor M, Evans M, et al; Look AHEAD Research Group. Comparison of weight-loss diets with different compositions of fat, protein, and carbohydrates. N Engl J Med. 2009;360(9):859-73.

22. Williamson DA, Anton SD, Han H, Champagne CM, Allen R, Leblanc E, et al. Early behavioral adherence predicts short and long-term weight loss in the POUNDS LOST study. J Behav Med. 2010;33(4):305-14.
23. Rochon J, Bales CW, Ravussin E, Redman LM, Holloszy JO, Racette SB, et al; CALERIE Study Group. Design and conduct of the CALERIE study: comprehensive assessment of the long-term effects of reducing intake of energy. J Gerontol A Biol Sci Med Sci. 2011;66(1):97-108.
24. Ravussin E, Redman LM, Rochon J, Das SK, Fontana L, Kraus WE, et al; CALERIE Study Group. A 2-year randomized controlled trial of human caloric restriction: feasibility and effects on predictors of health span and longevity. J Gerontol A Biol Sci Med Sci. 2015;70(9):1097-104.
25. Webb VL, Wadden TA. Intensive Lifestyle Intervention for Obesity: Principles, Practices, and Results. Gastroenterology. 2017;152(7):1752-64.
26. Jensen MD, Ryan DH, Apovian CM, Ard JD, Comuzzie AG, Donato KA, et al; American College of Cardiology/American Heart Association Task Force on Practice Guidelines; Obesity Society. 2013 AHA/ACC/TOS guideline for the management of overweight and obesity in adults: a report of the American College of Cardiology/American Heart Association Task Force on Practice Guidelines and The Obesity Society [published correction appears in J Am Coll Cardiol. 2014 Jul 1;63(25 Pt B):3029-30]. J Am Coll Cardiol. 2014;63(25 Pt B):2985-3023.
27. Johansen MY, Karstoft K, MacDonald CS, Hansen KB, Ellingsgaard H, Hartmann B, et al. Effects of an intensive lifestyle intervention on the underlying mechanisms of improved glycaemic control in individuals with type 2 diabetes: a secondary analysis of a randomised clinical trial. Diabetologia. 2020;63(11):2410-22.
28. Lean ME, Leslie WS, Barnes AC, Brosnahan N, Thom G, McCombie L, et al. Primary care-led weight management for remission of type 2 diabetes (DiRECT): an open-label, cluster-randomised trial. Lancet. 2018;391(10120):541-51.
29. Lean MEJ, Leslie WS, Barnes AC, Brosnahan N, Thom G, McCombie L, et al. Durability of a primary care-led weight-management intervention for remission of type 2 diabetes: 2-year results of the DiRECT open-label, cluster-randomised trial. Lancet Diabetes Endocrinol. 2019;7(5):344-55.
30. Taheri S, Zaghloul H, Chagoury O, Elhadad S, Ahmed SH, El Khatib N, et al. Effect of intensive lifestyle intervention on bodyweight and glycaemia in early type 2 diabetes (DIADEM-I): an open-label, parallel-group, randomised controlled trial. Lancet Diabetes Endocrinol. 2020;8(6):477-89.
31. de la Iglesia R, Loria-Kohen V, Zulet MA, Martinez JA, Reglero G, Ramirez de Molina A. Dietary Strategies Implicated in the Prevention and Treatment of Metabolic Syndrome. Int J Mol Sci. 2016;17(11):1877.
32. Churuangsuk C, Hall J, Reynolds A, Griffin SJ, Combet E, Lean MEJ. Diets for weight management in adults with type 2 diabetes: an umbrella review of published meta-analyses and systematic review of trials of diets for diabetes remission. Diabetologia. 2022;65(1):14-36.
33. Ben-Yacov O, Godneva A, Rein M, Shilo S, Kolobkov D, Koren N, et al. Personalized Postprandial Glucose Response—Targeting Diet Versus Mediterranean Diet for Glycemic Control in Prediabetes. Diabetes Care. 2021;44(9):1980-91.
34. de Carvalho GB, Dias-Vasconcelos NL, Santos RKF, Brandão-Lima PN, da Silva DG, Pires LV. Effect of different dietary patterns on glycemic control in individuals with type 2 diabetes mellitus: A systematic review. Crit Rev Food Sci Nutr. 2020;60(12):1999-2010.
35. Petroni ML, Brodosi L, Marchignoli F, Sasdelli AS, Caraceni P, Marchesini G, et al. Nutrition in Patients with Type 2 Diabetes: Present Knowledge and Remaining Challenges. Nutrients. 2021;13(8):2748.
36. Kirkpatrick CF, Liday C, Maki KC. The Effects of Carbohydrate-Restricted Dietary Patterns and Physical Activity on Body Weight and Glycemic Control. Curr Atheroscler Rep. 2020;22(6):20.
37. Aune D, Norat T, Leitzmann M, Tonstad S, Vatten LJ. Physical activity and the risk of type 2 diabetes: a systematic review and dose-response meta-analysis. Eur J Epidemiol. 2015;30(7):529-42.
38. Bird SR, Hawley JA. Update on the effects of physical activity on insulin sensitivity in humans. BMJ Open Sport Exerc Med. 2017;2(1):e000143.
39. Ramírez-Vélez R, Correa-Rodríguez M, Tordecilla-Sanders A, Aya-Aldana V, Izquierdo M, Correa-Bautista, et al. Exercise and postprandial lipemia: effects on vascular health in inactive adults. Lipids Health Dis. 2018;17(1):69.
40. Williams JE, Helsel B, Nelson B, Eke R. Exercise considerations for type 1 and type 2 diabetes. ACSMs Health Fit J. 2018;22(1):10-6.
41. DeFronzo RA, Abdul-Ghani MA. Preservation of β-cell function: the key to diabetes prevention. J Clin Endocrinol Metab. 2011;96(8):2354-66.

42. Kavouras SA, Panagiotakos DB, Pitsavos C, Chrysohoou C, Anastasiou CA, Lentzas Y, et al. Physical activity, obesity status, and glycemic control: The ATTICA study [published correction appears in Med Sci Sports Exerc. 2007;39(11):2093]. Med Sci Sports Exerc. 2007;39(4):606-11.
43. Shah SZA, Karam JA, Zeb A, Ullah R, Shah A, Haq IU, et al. Movement is Improvement: The Therapeutic Effects of Exercise and General Physical Activity on Glycemic Control in Patients with Type 2 Diabetes Mellitus: A Systematic Review and Meta-Analysis of Randomized Controlled Trials. Diabetes Ther. 2021;12(3):707-32.
44. Cradock KA, Ó Laighin G, Finucane FM, Gainforth HL, Quinlan LR, Ginis KA. Behaviour change techniques targeting both diet and physical activity in type 2 diabetes: A systematic review and meta-analysis. Int J Behav Nutr Phys Act. 2017;14(1):18.
45. Wiechert M, Holzapfel C. Nutrition Concepts for the Treatment of Obesity in Adults. Nutrients. 2021;14(1):169.
46. Hawkes RE, Miles LM, French DP. The theoretical basis of a nationally implemented type 2 diabetes prevention programme: how is the programme expected to produce changes in behaviour? Int J Behav Nutr Phys Act. 2021;18(1):64.
47. Davies M. Psychological aspects of diabetes management. Medicine (Abingdon). 2019;47(2):131-4.
48. Kalra S, Jena BN, Yeravdekar R. Emotional and Psychological Needs of People with Diabetes. Indian J Endocrinol Metab. 2018;22(5):696-704.
49. Young-Hyman D, de Groot M, Hill-Briggs F, Gonzalez JS, Hood K, Peyrot M. Psychosocial Care for People With Diabetes: A Position Statement of the American Diabetes Association [published correction appears in Diabetes Care. 2017;40(2):287] [published correction appears in Diabetes Care. 2017;40(5):726]. Diabetes Care. 2016;39(12):2126-40.

CHAPTER 6

Nutrition and Obesity/Diabetes

Key Highlights
- Clinical guidelines for diabetes management suggest a distribution of 45–60% carbohydrates, 10–20% protein, and 20–35% fat of total energy, the American Diabetes Association recommends individualized assessment for macronutrient distribution.
- Healthy fats, such as those found in avocados, nuts, seeds, and olive oil, should be included in moderation. These fats provide essential fatty acids and help promote heart health.
- The hypothalamus and brainstem play a crucial role in detecting metabolic signals that initiate specific and coordinated physiological responses, primarily focused on regulating appetite, and energy expenditure.
- A high-fiber diet is beneficial for individuals with obesity and diabetes. It helps regulate blood sugar levels, improves satiety, and promotes healthy digestion.
- Choosing low-glycemic index (GI) foods, such as whole grains, nonstarchy vegetables, lean proteins, and healthy fats, which have a smaller impact on blood sugar levels, can help regulate glucose levels and prevent rapid spikes in blood sugar.

INTRODUCTION

Obesity has become a significant global health concern, with its prevalence rapidly increasing worldwide. According to the World Health Organization (WHO), approximately 700 million adults are currently affected by obesity, and this number continues to rise each year. This alarming trend contributes to a higher incidence of metabolic complications, such as metabolic syndrome, insulin resistance, hypertension, dyslipidemia, and type 2 diabetes mellitus (T2DM). The International Diabetes Federation (IDF) reports that 1 in 11 adults between the ages of 20 and 79 years (equivalent to 463 million individuals) suffer from diabetes, and shockingly, half of them (232 million people) remain undiagnosed. These statistics emphasize the urgent need to address the growing obesity epidemic and its associated health consequences.[1-3]

The substantial increase in prevalence of obesity over the past few decades is primarily attributed to the global phenomenon of urbanization and the accompanying lifestyle changes.[4] Extensive evidence supports the notion that T2DM can be largely prevented by adopting a healthy lifestyle, which includes maintaining a healthy body weight, engaging in regular exercise, and consuming a high-quality diet.[5] The clinical management of T2DM involves a combination of healthy diets, lifestyle modifications, and glucose-lowering medications that aim to prevent or delay both the acute symptoms of hyperglycemia and the long-term complications of the disease. To effectively prevent T2DM, it is recommended to follow a healthy dietary pattern as outlined by the Dietary Guidelines for Americans and the American Diabetes Association (ADA). This dietary pattern emphasizes the consumption of fruits, vegetables (excluding potatoes), whole grains, nuts, and legumes, while limiting the intake of refined grains, red or processed meats, and sugary beverages. Additionally, improving the quality of fats and carbohydrates consumed is crucial.[6-9] This can be achieved by substituting saturated fats and high-glycemic index (GI) carbohydrates with unsaturated fats and carbohydrates that have a lower GI and higher fiber content. By adopting these dietary modifications, individuals can make significant strides in preventing T2DM and promoting overall health.

In the prevention and management of obesity and its associated disorders, nutritionists have been employing medical nutrition therapy (MNT) in conjunction with other medical interventions. Over the past few decades, there has been a concerning trend of increased consumption of unhealthy diets characterized by high fat and sugar content, while the intake of fruits, vegetables, and whole grains has declined due to industrialization. Such dietary patterns significantly contribute to weight gain and various metabolic disorders.[1] While it was initially expected that providing nutritional advice promoting healthy diets and lifestyles, along with relevant interventions, would curb this trend, the rising prevalence of obesity suggests that general recommendations alone may not be sufficient. Instead, there is a growing recognition of the need for personalized nutrition (PN) approaches that take into account individual factors such as genetics, personal differences, environmental conditions, and their interactions.

Personalized nutrition has emerged as a proposed approach for addressing obesity and other metabolic disorders. PN recognizes the complex interplay between genetics, environmental factors, and personal characteristics, such as eating habits, behaviors, physical activity, and gut microbiota. By tailoring nutritional recommendations to an individual's unique profile, PN aims to optimize health outcomes and effectively manage obesity and related conditions.[10]

NUTRITION TRANSITION AND GLOBAL DIETARY TRENDS

The epidemic of T2DM can be attributed to urbanization and environmental transitions, which have brought about significant changes in work patterns, food systems, and dietary habits. As societies have shifted from labor-intensive occupations to sedentary jobs, with increased reliance on computers and machines, physical activity levels have decreased. Furthermore, economic growth and environmental changes have transformed the landscape of food production, processing, and distribution. One major consequence has been the proliferation of fast food establishments worldwide, offering calorie-dense meals, oversized portions, and processed meats, refined carbohydrates, sugary beverages, and unhealthy fats. The expansion of large chain supermarkets has also played a significant role, displacing local food markets and promoting the availability of highly processed foods, high-energy snacks, and sugary drinks in both developed and developing countries. In parallel, regions undergoing epidemiological transition have witnessed a surge in livestock production and consumption, leading to increased intake of beef, pork, dairy products, eggs, and poultry. Developing countries, in particular, have experienced a remarkable change in this regard as the data shown by the United Nations Food and Agriculture Organization **(Fig. 1)**. Additionally, nutrition transition involves the refinement of grain products, where whole grains are processed into refined grains like polished white rice and refined wheat flour. This process diminishes the nutritional value of grains, including their fiber, micronutrients, and phytochemicals. These macro-level changes in urbanization, work patterns, food systems, and dietary choices have collectively contributed to the global rise in T2DM and associated health issues. Understanding these dynamics is crucial for developing effective strategies to address the challenges posed by the current nutrition landscape and to promote healthier lifestyles.[9,11]

Several decades ago, the notion of a global obesity pandemic was met with skepticism. However, in the 1970s, dietary patterns started to change, with a growing reliance on processed foods, increased consumption of meals outside the home, and a rise in the use of edible oils and sugary drinks. This shift was accompanied by a decrease in physical activity and an increase in sedentary behaviors. The adverse consequences of these transformations began to be acknowledged in the early 1990s, particularly in low- and middle-income populations, but it was not until conditions, such as diabetes, hypertension, and obesity became widespread that

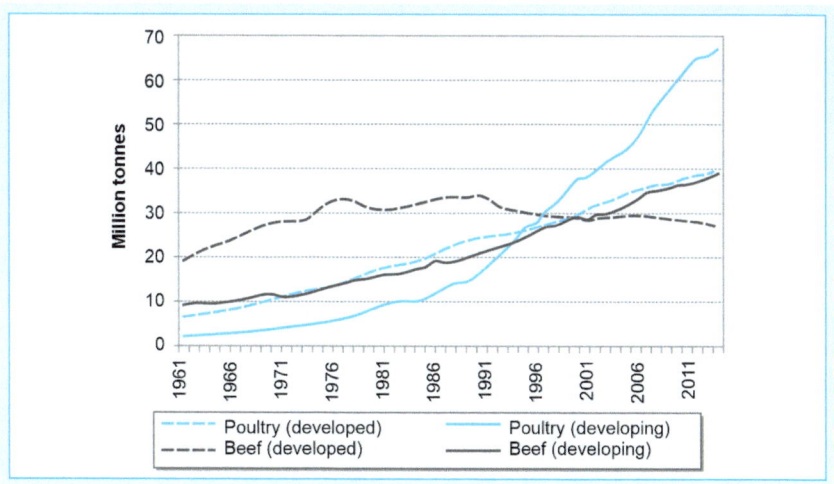

FIG. 1: Trend of consumption of poultry and beef in the developed and developing countries.

their impact became clear. Today, the rapid escalation in obesity and overweight rates is extensively documented, spanning urban and rural regions in the poorest countries of sub-Saharan Africa and South Asia, as well as populations in wealthier nations. Simultaneously, significant changes in dietary patterns and physical activity levels have been observed and well-documented. These interrelated trends emphasize the urgent need for global attention and concerted efforts to address the escalating obesity crisis and its associated health consequences.[12]

Over the past few decades, a wealth of evidence from prospective observational studies and clinical trials has emerged, highlighting the significant role of individual nutrients, specific foods, and overall dietary patterns in the prevention and management of T2DM. It is now recognized that the quality of dietary fats and carbohydrates consumed is of greater importance than the mere quantity of these macronutrients **(Fig. 2)**. Certain dietary approaches have demonstrated favorable outcomes in reducing the risk of diabetes, improving glycemic control, and enhancing blood lipid profiles. These approaches emphasize the consumption of whole grains, fruits, vegetables, legumes, and nuts, while moderating alcohol intake and reducing the consumption of refined grains, red or processed meats, and sugar-sweetened beverages **(Fig. 3)**. By focusing on the overall quality of the diet, various dietary patterns have shown promise in personalizing nutrition recommendations. These include the Mediterranean diet, low-GI diet, moderately low-carbohydrate diet, and vegetarian diet. These dietary patterns can be tailored to individual and cultural food preferences, while considering appropriate calorie needs for weight management, diabetes prevention, and management. Although

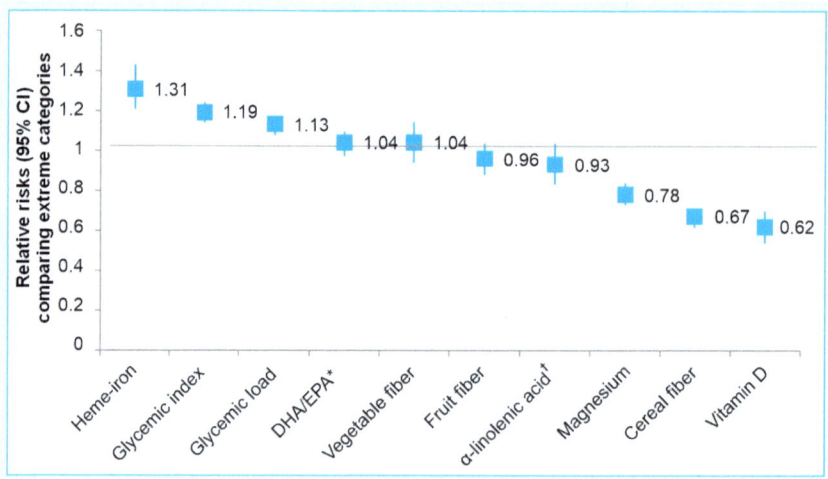

*Relative risks are a comparison of extreme categories, except for DHA/EPA (per 250 mg/day increase).
†α-linolenic acid (per 0.5 g/day).

FIG. 2: Summary of meta-analyses of prospective cohort studies on nutrient intake and type 2 diabetes mellitus.

Note: All nutrients were assessed from dietary intake, except vitamin D for which blood 25-hydroxyvitamin D was used.
(DHA: docosahexaenoic acid; EPA: eicosapentaenoic acid)
Source: With permission from Ley SH et al. (2014).[9]

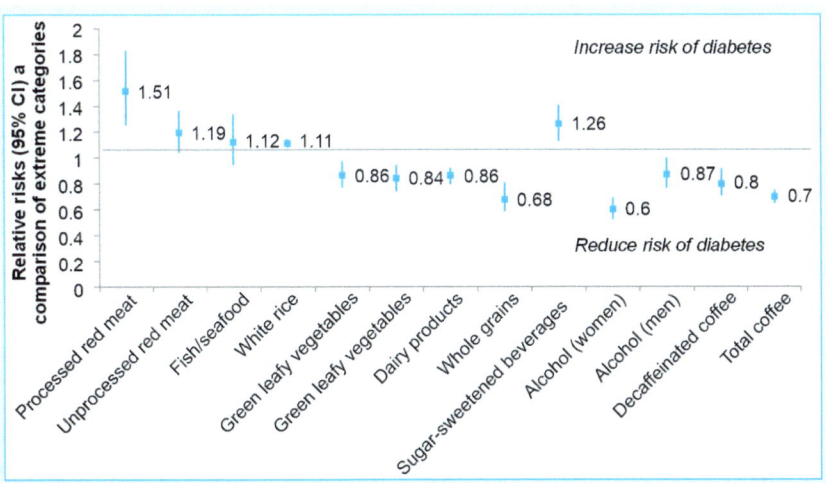

FIG. 3: Summary of meta-analyses of prospective cohort studies on food and beverage intake and type 2 diabetes mellitus.

Note: Relative risks are comparison of extreme categories, except for processed meat (per 50 g/day increase), unprocessed red meat and fish/sea food (per 100 g/day), white rice (per each serving/day), whole grains (per 3 servings/day), sugar-sweetened beverages in European cohorts (per 336g/day), alcohol (abstainers with 22 g/day for men and with 24 g/day for women).

Source: With permission from Ley SH et al. (2014).[9]

substantial progress has been made in developing and implementing evidence-based nutrition recommendations in developed countries, there is a need for concerted efforts and policies on a global scale to address regional disparities. Collaborative endeavors are necessary to ensure that effective strategies for diabetes prevention and management are accessible and relevant across diverse populations and geographic regions.[9]

Macronutrient Balance and Caloric Intake

The Global Nutrient Database has compiled data on the availability of macronutrients and micronutrients in 195 countries from 1980 to 2013. This database utilized information from the Food and Agriculture Organization of the United Nations Supply and Utilization Accounts (SUAs), which included 394 food and agricultural commodities. These commodities were then matched with food items in the United States Department of Agriculture Food Composition Database to obtain nutrient composition data. Globally, the database revealed that in 2013, an average of 2,710 kcal [95% uncertainty interval (UI) 2,660–2,770]/person/day was available. However, there were significant variations in energy availability across different levels of development. Low-SDI (sociodemographic index) countries had an average energy availability of 2,170 kcal (2,090–2,250)/person/day, whereas high-SDI countries had a higher average of 3,270 kcal (3,220–3,310)/person/day. Among the most populous countries, energy availability also varied **(Fig. 4)**. The United States had the highest level of energy availability, with an average of 3,500 kcal (3,450–3,560)/person/day. On the other hand, Ethiopia had the lowest level of

CHAPTER 6: Nutrition and Obesity/Diabetes

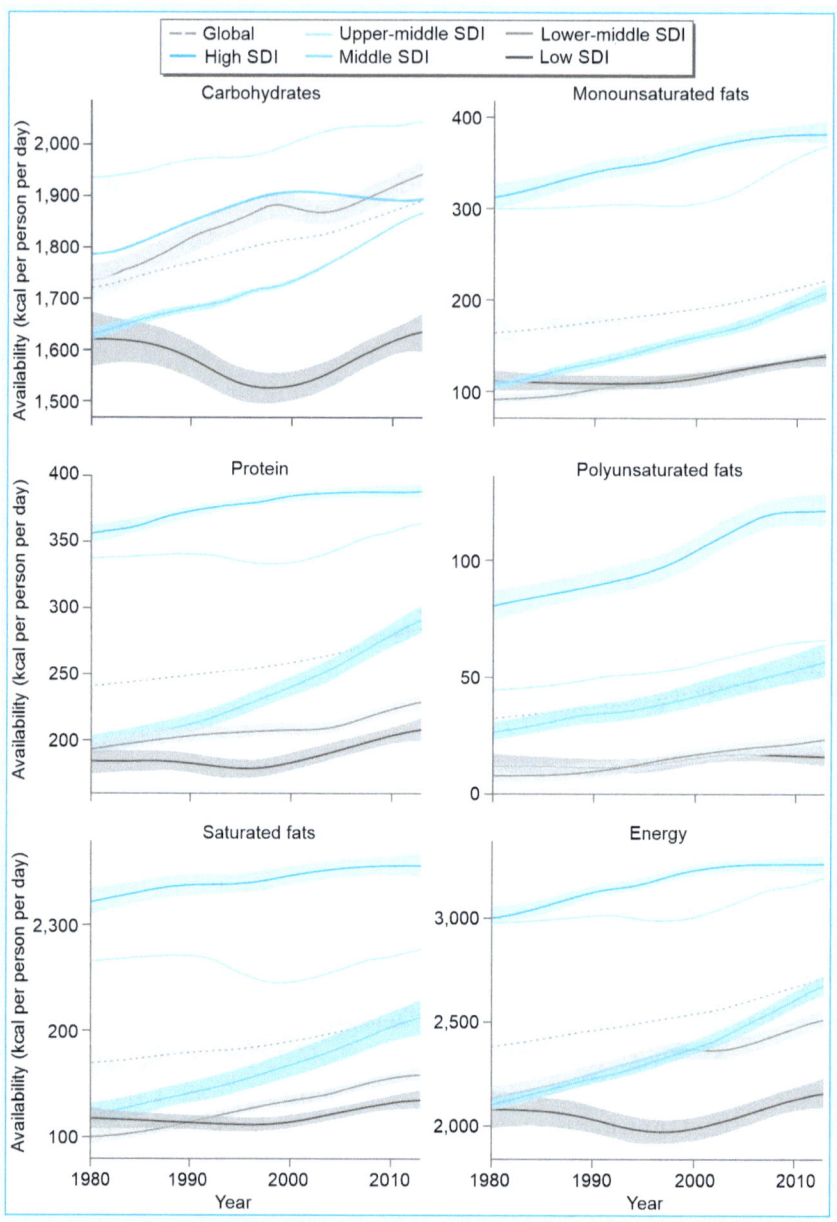

FIG. 4: Trend of energy and macronutrients availability at global and regional level, 1980–2013. *(For color version, see Plate 2)*

(SDI: sociodemographic index)

energy availability, with an average of 1,880 kcal (1,810–1,940)/person/day. These findings highlight the disparities in energy availability across different countries and development levels, indicating the varying access to sufficient calorie intake.[13]

Protein, fat, and carbohydrate are the primary macronutrients that provide energy for the human population. The WHO recommends consuming 55–75%

of daily energy from carbohydrates, 15-30% from fat, and 10-15% from protein. The acceptable macronutrient distribution range (AMDR) in the United States recommends 10-35% of daily energy from protein, 20-35% from fat, and 45-65% from carbohydrates. It is noteworthy that increased intake of all three macronutrients, or certain subtypes has been associated with insulin resistance and diabetes.[14] While many clinical guidelines for diabetes management suggest a distribution of 45-60% carbohydrates, 10-20% protein, and 20-35% fat of total energy, the ADA recommends individualized assessment for macronutrient distribution **(Table 1)**.[8,15-17]

Body weight and adiposity are regulated by the balance between energy intake from macronutrients and energy expenditure, which is controlled by neuroendocrine mechanisms. The intricate interplay of carbohydrates, lipids, and proteins considering both their quantity and quality in the diet, influences energy homeostasis and fuel metabolism. Consuming excessive amounts of simple sugars and certain saturated fatty acids (SFAs) can have negative effects on body adiposity. On the other hand, the consumption of protein and dietary fiber appears to have positive effects on satiety and processes related to energy metabolism.[18]

Carbohydrates

Carbohydrates, the most abundant macronutrient in the human diet, provide 45-70% of daily calories. However, they are not considered essential for humans

TABLE 1: A comparison of nutrition therapy recommendations for patients with type 2 diabetes mellitus.[8,15-17]

	ADA 2013 and 2019	CDA 2018	DNSG-EASD 2023
Energy balance	For overweight or obese adults with type 2 diabetes mellitus, maintain a healthful eating pattern while reducing energy intake to promote weight loss	A nutritionally balanced calorie-reduced diet to achieve and maintain a lower, healthier body weight in people who are overweight or obese	Reduced caloric intake to lose or maintain body weight in people with BMI >25 kg/m²
Macronutrient distribution	No ideal recommended percentage of calories from carbohydrate, protein, and fat; distribution should be based on individualized assessment	Individualization within ranges of 45–60% carbohydrate, 15–20% protein, 20–35% fat of total energy	Ranges of 45–60% carbohydrate, 10–20% protein, ≤35% fat of energy
Dietary eating patterns	A variety of eating patterns are acceptable with consideration for personal preferences and metabolic goals	A variety of dietary patterns are acceptable with consideration for personal preferences, values, and abilities	No specific recommendations
Glycemic index and glycemic load	Substitute low-glycemic load foods for higher glycemic load foods may be beneficial	Choose food sources of a low-glycemic index	Low-glycemic index foods are suitable as carbohydrate-rich choices

Continued

Continued

	ADA 2013 and 2019	**CDA 2018**	**DNSG-EASD 2023**
Dietary fiber and whole grains	Consume at least the amount recommended for the general public (14 g/1,000 kcal or 25 g/day for women and 38 g/day for men)	Consume higher intake than those for the general public (25–50 g/day or 15–25 g/1,000 kcal)	Consume fiber intake >40 g/day (or 20 g/1,000 kcal/day) with half as soluble; choose cereal-based foods high in fiber and whole grains
Sucrose and fructose	Limit or avoid intake of sugar-sweetened beverages	Added sucrose or fructose can be substituted for other carbohydrate as a mixed meal up to a maximum of 10% total daily energy intake	Moderate intake of free sugars (up to 50 g/day) recommended without exceeding 10% total energy
Protein	Reducing the amount of dietary protein below usual intake is not recommended for people with diabetes and kidney disease	Usual intake recommended for those without kidney disease, but consider restricting protein to 0.8 g/kg body weight for people with diabetes and chronic kidney disease	Insufficient evidence to recommend protein restriction for those with type 2 diabetes mellitus and incipient nephropathy
MUFAs and PUFAs	MUFA-rich eating pattern may be beneficial	MUFAs up to 20% of energy and PUFAs up to 10%	10–20% of energy from MUFAs and up to 10% from PUFAs
Omega-3 fatty acids	No support for omega-3 fatty acid supplements	No support for omega-3 fatty acid supplements	No support for omega-3 fatty acid supplements
Saturated fat, dietary cholesterol, and trans fat	Same as recommended for the general public (<10% of energy, aiming for 300 mg dietary cholesterol per day, limiting trans fat as much as possible)	No >7% of energy from saturated fats; limit intake of trans fatty acids to a minimum	Under 10% of energy from saturated and trans fatty acids (<8% if LDL cholesterol is elevated); below 300 mg/day cholesterol
Micronutrient supplements	No support for vitamin or mineral supplements	Routine vitamin and mineral supplementation is generally not recommended	No recommendation for vitamin and mineral supplements
Alcohol	Advised to drink in moderation with consideration for managing delayed hypoglycemia	Same precautions as in the general public with additional consideration for risk of hypoglycemia and weight gain	Moderate use of alcohol is acceptable with consideration for prolonged hypoglycemia and weight control
Sodium	Reduce sodium intake less than 2,300 mg/day in general, and further reduction in sodium is to be individualized	No specific cutoffs recommended for people with type 2 diabetes mellitus	Restrict salt intake under 6 g/day

(ADA: American Diabetes Association; CDA: Canadian Diabetes Association; DNSG-EASD: Diabetes and Nutrition Study Group-European Association for the Study of Diabetes; LDL: low-density lipoprotein; MUFAs: monounsaturated fatty acids; PUFAs: polyunsaturated fatty acids)

Source: Adapted from ADA, CDA, and DNSG-EASD.[8,15-17]

and their increased consumption has been linked to "carbotoxicity." Clinical trials have demonstrated the benefits of reducing carbohydrate intake for metabolic health, particularly in conditions like T2DM, where ketogenic diets limiting carbohydrates to <10% of daily energy have shown effectiveness in promoting weight loss and improving glycemic profiles.[14]

A recent large-scale epidemiological study, the Prospective Urban Rural Epidemiology (PURE) study, revealed an association between high carbohydrate intake (highest quintile vs. lowest quintile) and increased risk of mortality and dyslipidemia. Starch, sucrose, and high-fructose corn syrup (HFCS) are major contributors to carbohydrate-derived calories in adults. Various mechanisms have been proposed to explain the molecular effects of carbohydrate intake, such as rapid digestion of simple carbohydrates leading to insulin spikes, subsequent appetite stimulation, and potential facilitation of fat deposition through lipogenesis promotion and lipolysis inhibition.[14]

Fructose metabolism, in particular, is suggested to have a prolipogenic nature in the liver, making it more detrimental to metabolic health compared to other carbohydrates. A significant portion of fructose absorbed by the intestines is metabolized in the liver, where it undergoes phosphorylation by the enzyme ketohexokinase (KHK) and conversion by aldolase-B into D-glyceraldehyde and dihydroxyacetone phosphate. These three-carbon metabolites can further contribute to fatty acid synthesis or serve as a precursor for triglyceride production. Unlike glucose, fructose metabolism in the liver lacks tight regulation through insulin signaling or negative feedback from adenosine triphosphate (ATP) and citrate. This lack of regulation promotes de novo lipogenesis (DNL), resulting in the generation and release of very low-density lipoprotein (VLDL) particles into the bloodstream, contributing to hypertriglyceridemia and unfavorable lipid profiles. Ectopic lipid accumulation from fructose metabolism is believed to generate toxic lipid species, such as ceramide and diacylglycerol (DAG), which may ultimately impair insulin signaling and lead to insulin resistance **(Fig. 5)**.[14]

Various organizations have recommended reducing the intake of added sugars and sugar-sweetened beverages for diabetes management.[8,15-17] Overconsumption of high fructose-sweetened beverages has negative effects on visceral fat deposition, lipid metabolism, blood pressure, insulin sensitivity, and DNL, particularly in overweight and obese individuals. However, naturally occurring fructose from whole fruits is unlikely to be detrimental due to its slower digestion and absorption. Nevertheless, regular consumption of fruit juices is not recommended.[19] Non-nutritive sweeteners have the potential to reduce overall calorie and carbohydrate intake.[8,15] Short-term studies have indicated that replacing added sugar with non-nutritive sweeteners can lead to weight loss and improved glycemic control. However, the long-term effects of non-nutritive sweeteners need further investigation.[20]

Fat

Dietary fats have been implicated in the development of various metabolic disorders including obesity, insulin resistance, T2DM, and cardiovascular disease. The accumulation of triglycerides in tissues other than adipose tissue has long been recognized as a significant indicator of these medical conditions. Free fatty acids (FFAs) are hydrophobic molecules categorized based on the length and saturation

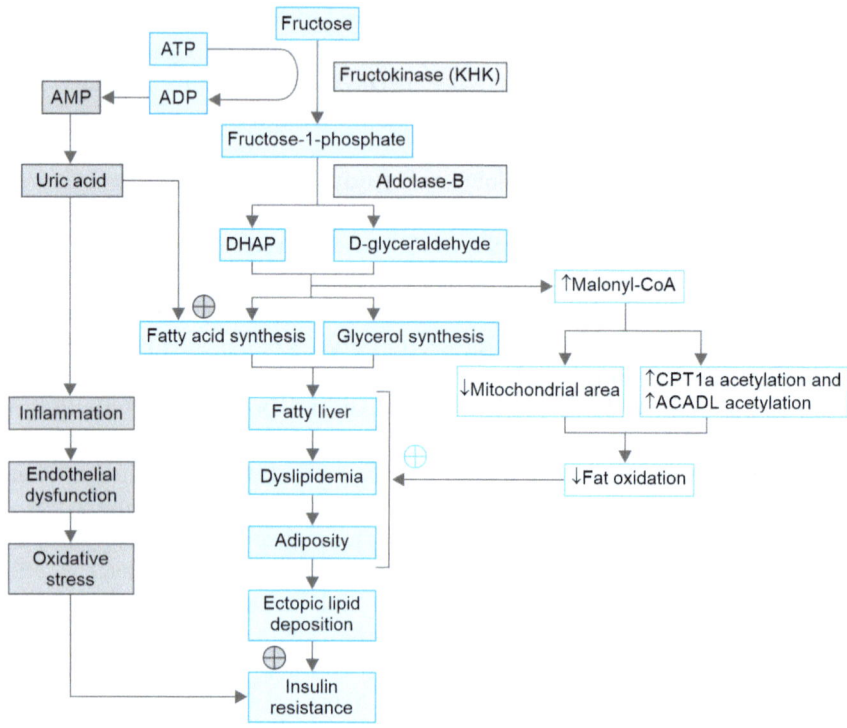

FIG. 5: Potential molecular mechanisms mediating the adverse consequences of high fructose intake.
[ACADL: long-chain specific acyl-CoA dehydrogenase; CPT1a: carnitine palmitoyltransferase 1 (hepatic isoform a); DHAP: dihydroxyacetone phosphate KHK: ketohexokinase]

of their side chains, such as short-chain fatty acid (SCFA), medium-chain fatty acid (MCFA), long-chain fatty acid (LCFA), and very long-chain fatty acid (VLCFA) fatty acids. Elevated dietary and plasma levels of LCFA have been associated with obesity and insulin resistance.[14]

Research has demonstrated that SFAs are linked to unfavorable metabolic and cardiovascular outcomes, while polyunsaturated fats, including omega-3 fatty acids, are associated with better outcomes. Therefore, among the recommended range of 20–35% of calorie intake from fats, emphasis should be placed on consuming sources of "good" fats, such as monounsaturated fats found in avocados, nuts, olive oil, chia seeds, and fatty fish, which are rich in polyunsaturated fat. Increased levels of DAGs have been strongly linked to insulin resistance, and ceramides have been found to be elevated in the muscle and liver of insulin-resistant individuals. Higher fat intake leads to increased mitochondrial metabolism, resulting in enhanced mitochondrial machinery and oxidative capacity in rodents. However, this also leads to the generation of reactive oxygen species (ROS), particularly superoxides, primarily caused by electron leakage from complex 1 and complex 3 of the mitochondrial electron transport chain, which can contribute to muscle dysfunction and insulin resistance **(Fig. 6)**.[14]

Scientific evidence suggests that the quality of dietary fat consumed is more significant than the overall fat intake in achieving metabolic objectives.[8] While

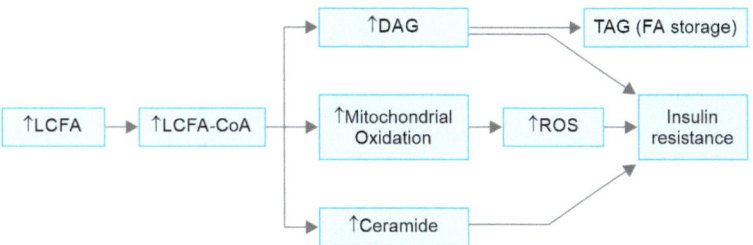

FIG. 6: Potential molecular mechanisms for long-chain fatty acid (LCFA)-induced insulin resistance.
(DAG: diacylglycerol; ROS: reactive oxygen species; TAG: triglyceride)

specific recommendations for the distribution of fat composition may differ, organizations generally endorse reducing the consumption of saturated fat and trans fat derived from industrial hydrogenation to lower the risk of cardiovascular disease **(Table 1)**.[8,15-17]

Protein

Prolonged exposure to high-protein diets has been associated with an increased risk of insulin resistance, T2DM, and elevated mortality in both rodents and humans. Among the essential amino acids, particular attention has been focused on branched-chain amino acids (BCAAs)—isoleucine, leucine, and valine—due to their crucial role in protein synthesis and their influence on key signaling pathways including insulin, mammalian target of rapamycin (mTOR), and fibroblast growth factor 21 (FGF21).

While unraveling the intricate relationship between diet, circulating BCAA levels, and cardiometabolic health is still ongoing, it is evident that the activation of mTOR plays a significant role in connecting protein and BCAAs to metabolic dysfunction **(Fig. 7)**. The mTOR complex exists in two primary forms: mTORC1, which integrates nutritional signals to regulate essential cellular processes like protein synthesis and autophagy, and mTORC2, which modulates hormonal signals such as insulin and IGF-1. The interplay between mTOR and insulin sensitivity involves both these complexes, with hormonal feedback from the insulin/IGF-1 pathway essential for mTORC1 activation. Decreasing overall protein intake or BCAA levels has demonstrated a reduction in mTORC1 activation in the liver, muscle, and white adipose tissue, indicating that chronic hepatic mTORC1 signaling contributes to insulin resistance by inhibiting insulin receptor substrate-1 (IRS-1). Notably, the impact of BCAA-mediated mTOR activation and insulin resistance appears to be influenced by the nutritional composition of the overall diet **(Fig. 7)**.[14]

Organizations provide varying recommendations for protein intake among individuals with diabetic kidney disease including both microalbuminuria and macroalbuminuria **(Table 1)**.[8,15-17]

Calorie Intake

The hypothalamus and brainstem play a crucial role in detecting metabolic signals that provide information about the body's energy status **(Fig. 8)**. These signals are

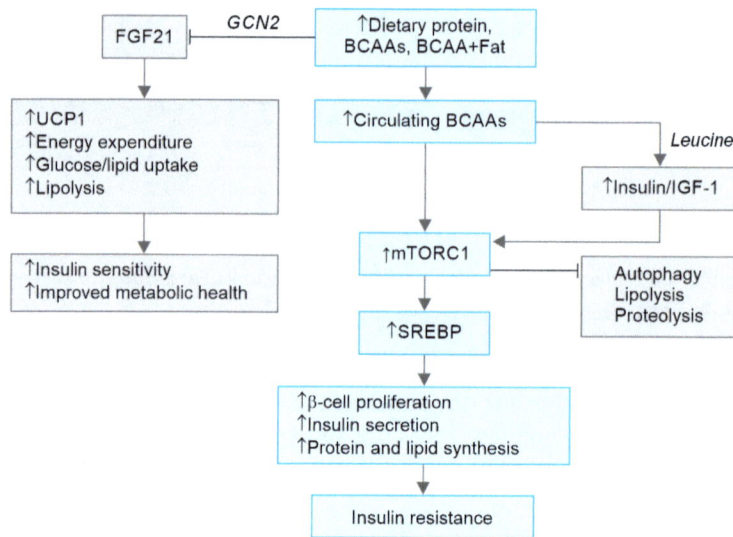

FIG. 7: Potential molecular mechanisms for protein and branched-chain amino acid (BCAA)-induced insulin resistance.

(GCN: general control nonderepressible-kinase; FGF-1: fibroblast growth factor -1; IGF-1: insulin-like growth factor-1; mTORC1: mammalian target of rapamycin complex S6K1: ribosomal S6 kinase 1; 1; SREBP: sterol regulatory element-binding protein; UCP1: uncoupling protein 1)

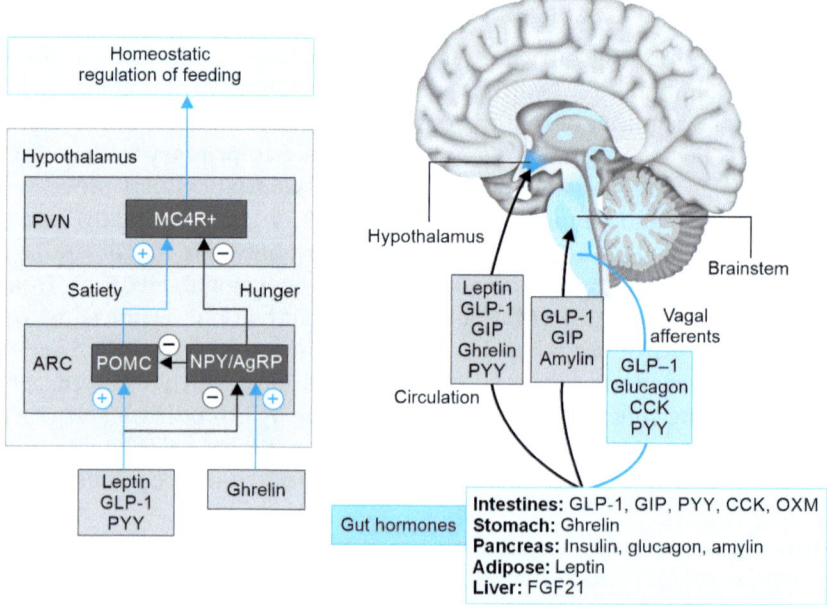

FIG. 8: Gut–brain regulation of food intake.

(AgRP: agouti-related protein; ARC: arcuate nucleus; CCK: cholecystokinin; FGF-1: fibroblast growth factor-1; GIP: glucose-dependent insulinotropic polypeptide; GLP-1: glucagon-like peptide-1; MC4R: melanocortin 4 receptor; OXM: oxyntomodulin; POMC: proopiomelanocortin; PVN: paraventricular nucleus; PYY: peptide tyrosine tyrosine) integrated to initiate specific and coordinated physiological responses, primarily focused on regulating appetite and energy expenditure.[21]

The hypothalamic arcuate nucleus (ARC) is located adjacent to the median eminence, a specialized area that directly receives circulating hormones and nutrients. Within the ARC, two distinct subpopulations of neurons express neuropeptides related to appetite regulation: (1) anorexigenic proopiomelanocortin (POMC) neurons and (2) orexigenic agouti-related protein (AgRP) neurons. AgRP neurons are coexpressed with neuropeptide Y (NPY), another potent orexigenic peptide. Both POMC and AgRP/NPY neurons project their connections to hypothalamic paraventricular nucleus (PVN) neurons expressing melanocortin 4 receptor (MC4R). POMC neurons in the ARC work to reduce food intake and increase energy expenditure by releasing alpha-melanocyte-stimulating hormones (α-MSHs), which then activate MC4R signaling. Serotonin, acting through the 5HT-2C receptor on POMC neurons, plays a role in mediating the anorexic effect of these neurons. In contrast, AgRP/NPY neurons in the ARC inhibit melanocortin signaling by directly inhibiting POMC neurons and indirectly antagonizing the action of α-MSH on MC4R. Experimental evidence shows that loss-of-function mutations in MC4R in rodents result in increased food intake, reduced energy expenditure, and the development of severe obesity. Similarly, in humans, MC4R mutations are the leading cause of severe early-onset obesity, accounting for up to 6% of cases before 10 years of age. These findings underscore the critical involvement of the central melanocortin system in maintaining energy homeostasis.[21]

Glycemic Index and Glycemic Load

Glycemic Index

The GI is a widely used measure to assess the postprandial glycemic response, as it strongly correlates with the rise in blood glucose levels after a meal. According to Atkinson and colleagues, a high-GI is defined as 70 or higher and is associated with certain types of bread, breakfast cereals, or rice. On the other hand, a low-GI is 55 or lower and is associated with various legumes, pasta, fruits, or dairy products.[22]

Sucrose, which is composed of equal parts glucose and fructose, has a medium GI of 65. Fructose follows a different metabolic pathway compared to glucose. It is primarily metabolized in hepatocytes, where it undergoes conversion into glucose (about 50% of the fructose) before being released into the bloodstream. As a result, fructose leads to minimal changes in blood glucose levels and has a very low-GI of 15. In contrast, carbohydrates with longer or more complex chains composed solely of glucose can have a more pronounced impact on the postprandial glycemic response.[22]

Glycemic Load

The GI is a standardized measure that indicates the blood glucose response to a specific carbohydrate-containing food, reflecting its quality. However, GI alone does not account for the amount of carbohydrates consumed. To address this limitation, the concept of glycemic load (GL) was introduced to assess and compare the effects of carbohydrate-containing foods or diets.[22]

Glycemic load is calculated by multiplying the GI of a food by its carbohydrate content and dividing it by the serving size, typically measured in grams (GL = GI × carbohydrate content/serving size in gram). A high-GL is defined as 20 or higher, a low-GL is 10 or lower, and values between 10 and 20 are considered medium. It is important to note that the relationship between GI and GL is not always straightforward. Some foods may have a low-GI but a high-GL, such as certain types of noodles or pasta that are typically consumed in larger quantities. Conversely, there are foods with a low-GL but a high-GI, such as watermelon, which can have a high-GI when consumed in small portion sizes.[22]

Weight Management

Low-GI diets are generally considered beneficial for metabolic health due to their potential to improve glycemic control. There is a potential association between GI and obesity, which is related to the lipogenic effects of high insulin levels. Consequently, it has been suggested that diets that result in a low insulin response, such as low-GI or low-GL diets, may play a significant role in weight loss.[23]

One possible explanation is that high-GI/GL meals trigger a rapid insulin response, leading to a quicker feeling of hunger and subsequent overeating. This occurs as the metabolic fuels in the body are depleted. Another mechanism is the potential for increased satiety and reduced voluntary food intake. These mechanisms are particularly relevant for individuals who are overweight or obese.[23]

Weight Loss in Children and Adolescents

The clinical trials provide compelling evidence that low-GI and low-GL diets are effective in promoting weight loss in children and adolescents, surpassing the outcomes of reduced-fat diets.[24,25] For instance, in a 12-month study by Ebbeling et al., participants following a low-GL diet ad libitum achieved remarkable reductions in fat mass (–3.0 ± 1.0 kg) and body mass index (BMI) (–1.3 ± 0.7 kg/m^2), which were statistically significant when compared to the reduced-fat control group (fat mass: 1.8 ± 1.0 kg, BMI: 0.7 ± 0.5 kg/m^2, $p = 0.01$ and $p = 0.02$, respectively).[24] Similarly, Spieth et al. conducted a study lasting approximately 4.3 months and observed significant weight loss (–2.03 ± 0.59 kg) and BMI reduction in the low-GL group compared to the control group (weight loss: 1.31 ± 0.72 kg, $p < 0.05$). These findings demonstrate the superior efficacy of low-GI and low-GL diets in facilitating weight loss among children and adolescents.[25] Similarly, a study examining the impact of GI on energy intake in children found that there was a tendency toward reduced energy intake at lunch after consuming a low-GI breakfast compared to a high-GI breakfast. However, it is important to note that the mean difference of 75 kJ (18 kcal) was not statistically significant ($p = 0.406$). Interestingly, among boys, there was a noticeable trend toward a decreased energy intake in the low-GI group compared to the high-GI group. This suggests that consuming foods with a low-GI may contribute to better appetite control and reduced overall calorie consumption in children.[26] A recent systematic review and meta-analysis conducted by Schwingshackl et al. has provided compelling evidence supporting the benefits of a low-GI/GL diet in children and adolescents who are overweight or obese. The meta-analysis synthesized data from nine randomized controlled trials (RCTs) and revealed that a low-GI/GL diet had a positive impact on triglyceride levels and the homeostatic model assessment (HOMA)-index (a measure of insulin resistance) when compared to a high-GI/GL dietary approach. The findings demonstrated that compared to high-GI diets, low-GI protocols led to significant reductions in serum triglycerides with a mean difference of –15.14 mg/dL [95% confidence interval –26.26, –4.00]. Additionally, the HOMA-index showed a significant decrease with a mean difference of –0.70 [95% confidence interval –1.37, –0.04] in the fixed-effects model. These results highlight the potential of a low-GI/GL diet to improve metabolic markers in children and adolescents who are overweight or obese.[27]

Weight Loss in Adults

A recent systematic review and meta-analysis conducted by Perin et al. examined randomized clinical trials and provided compelling evidence supporting the effectiveness of low-GI/GL diets in adults with obesity (BMI ≥ 30 kg/m^2). The findings revealed that low-GI/GL diets were associated with significant reductions in fasting glucose and insulin levels, as well as greater body weight reduction compared to high-GI/GL diets. The meta-analysis showed that adults with a BMI ≥30 kg/m^2 following low-GI/GL diets experienced a greater reduction in body weight (–0.93 kg; p = 0.045) compared to those on high-GI/GL diets. Furthermore, low-GI/GL diets were found to be beneficial in reducing fasting glucose levels (–1.97 mg/dL; p = 0.030) and fasting insulin levels (–0.55 µU/mL; p = 0.007) compared to high-GI/GL diets. These results provide strong evidence that low-GI/GL diets can effectively improve metabolic markers and promote weight loss in adults with obesity. Incorporating low-GI/GL foods into dietary strategies may be a valuable approach for individuals aiming to manage their weight and improve glycemic control.[28]

A systematic review conducted by Schwingshackl et al. further supports the beneficial effects of long-term interventions involving a low-GI/GL diet. The review included 14 studies and found compelling evidence for the positive impact of low-GI/GL diets on fasting insulin levels and proinflammatory markers such as C-reactive protein, which can potentially contribute to the primary prevention of obesity-associated diseases. The primary meta-analysis revealed significant findings. Weighted mean differences in the change of C-reactive protein favored the low-GI/GL diets, showing a more pronounced decrease [–0.43 mg/dL, p = 0.01]. Similarly, fasting insulin levels exhibited a greater improvement with low-GI/GL diets compared to other dietary approaches [–5.16 pmol/L, p = 0.002]. Additionally, the review highlighted that low-GI/GL diets led to a more significant reduction in fat-free mass [–1.04 kg, p = 0.003]. While this finding indicates a decrease in lean body mass, it is important to note that the overall benefits of low-GI/GL diets in terms of fasting insulin levels and inflammatory markers outweigh the potential impact on fat-free mass. These findings suggest that long-term adherence to a low-GI/GL diet can contribute to improved metabolic health by reducing fasting insulin levels and proinflammatory markers, such as C-reactive protein. However, individuals should be mindful of preserving muscle mass and consider incorporating strategies to maintain or increase lean body mass while following a low-GI/GL dietary approach.[29]

To gain a comprehensive understanding of the relationship between low-GI/GL diets and weight loss, a pooled analysis of the current data would be valuable. Such an analysis would provide a more robust perspective on the topic. However, it is crucial to acknowledge the need for more long-term, large randomized controlled clinical trials specifically designed to evaluate weight loss, with substantial differences in dietary GI/GL between the test and control groups. Moreover, it is essential to conduct more "real-world" effectiveness studies that assess long-term weight maintenance. These studies would provide valuable insights into the practical application and sustainability of low-GI/GL diets. Additionally, research should aim to determine the possible mechanisms of action underlying the observed effects. It is worth noting that the benefits of low-GI/GL diets extend beyond weight loss. Even if the concept of "a calorie is a calorie" holds true, low-GI/GL diets have favorable effects on obesity-related risk factors such as heart disease and diabetes. These effects are mediated through mechanisms that are independent of weight loss, highlighting the broader health benefits of adopting a low-GI/GL dietary approach.[23]

Diabetes Management

Obesity is closely linked to the development of T2DM, highlighting the significance of weight loss in the nutritional management of individuals who are overweight or obese and have diabetes. In these cases, achieving even a moderate reduction in body weight, typically ranging from 5 to 10% of the initial body weight, can yield substantial benefits. When coupled with increased physical activity, weight loss interventions play a crucial role in improving insulin sensitivity and glycemic control in individuals with T2DM. Moreover, for individuals at high risk of developing T2DM, weight loss interventions can serve as a preventive measure, reducing the likelihood of disease onset. As a result, weight loss becomes an integral part of a comprehensive approach to managing and preventing T2DM.[30]

A substantial body of research has emerged investigating the impact of low-GI diets in the management of diabetes. A previous meta-analysis involving 356 individuals with type 1 diabetes mellitus (T1DM) and T2DM found that low-GI diets can effectively improve blood glucose control, comparable to the effects of medications targeting postmeal blood glucose levels.[31] Another meta-analysis examining 16 studies revealed that low-GI diets lead to significant reductions in fructosamine and glycated hemoglobin (HbA1c) levels in individuals with T2DM, indicating improved carbohydrate and lipid metabolism.[32] A Cochrane systematic review encompassing 11 RCTs lasting 4 weeks or longer confirmed the benefits of a low-GI diet in enhancing glycemic control while reducing the risk of hypoglycemic events. These findings are particularly significant because improving blood glucose levels is often associated with an increased risk of hypoglycemia, posing a major obstacle to achieving optimal glycemic control, especially in individuals with T1DM.[33,34]

Notably, an updated review which included an additional large-scale RCT, reported a significant improvement in HbA1c (with a weighted mean difference of −0.4% across seven studies) and fructosamine (with a weighted mean difference of −0.23 mmol/L across four shorter-term studies) when comparing low-GI diets to control diets. These improvements hold clinical significance and are substantial enough to contribute to a reduced risk of diabetes complications.[35,36]

The management of diabetes continues to prioritize diet and lifestyle interventions, as evidenced by a recent umbrella review that examined published meta-analyses of RCTs. This comprehensive review demonstrated that hypocaloric diets for weight management in individuals with T2DM are superior in achieving remission compared to diets focusing on specific macronutrient profiles or styles including low-GI diets. These findings emphasize the importance of reducing body weight, particularly body fat, through a reduction in total energy intake as the primary goal in T2DM treatment.[37]

However, it is worth noting that a low-GI/GL diet can also provide benefits for overweight and obese patients with T2DM. Overweight and obesity are significant risk factors for the development of T2DM, and incorporating a low-GI/GL diet alongside weight loss efforts may offer additional advantages. While the primary focus should be on reducing body weight, the inclusion of a low-GI/GL diet can further support the management of T2DM in overweight and obese individuals.

Role of Fiber, Micronutrients, and Antioxidants

Role of Fiber

The physiological effects of dietary fiber are illustrated in **Flowchart 1**. Consuming a high-fiber diet has several benefits, including the delay of carbohydrate absorption and digestion, leading to reduced postprandial hyperglycemia. Additionally, it increases satiety, which can contribute to weight loss. In individuals with insulin resistance, the mechanism of action may involve SCFAs. SCFAs are produced when certain microbes in the intestinal colon ferment dietary fiber, and they have anti-inflammatory properties that affect both gut epithelial cells and immune cells.[38]

A high-fiber diet is known to have positive effects on metabolic health, particularly in individuals with T2DM. Fiber-rich foods, which contain complex carbohydrates resistant to digestion, help decrease glucose absorption and insulin secretion. Consuming a high amount of dietary fiber, especially soluble fiber above the recommended level by the ADA, has been shown to improve blood glucose

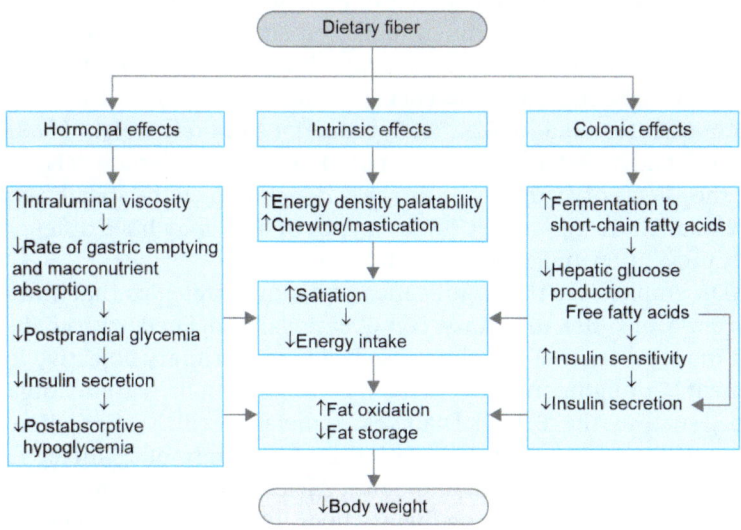

FLOWCHART 1: The physiologic effect of dietary fiber.

control, reduce hyperinsulinemia, and lower plasma lipid levels. Multiple studies have demonstrated a significant reduction in the risk of developing diabetes with increased dietary fiber intake. There is an inverse relationship between fiber consumption and markers of insulin resistance.[38]

Furthermore, in overweight or obese patients with T2DM, following a low-GI, high-fiber diet has been shown to significantly ($p < 0.001$) reduce glucose and insulin area under the curve. These favorable effects on postprandial glucose and insulin levels are sustained throughout the day.[38] A comprehensive meta-analysis of RCTs examining the impact of legumes on glycemic markers revealed that incorporating legumes into a high-fiber diet leads to significant reductions in fasting blood glucose levels and glycated proteins. In addition, a recent meta-analysis of RCTs investigated the effects of high-fiber diets compared to low-fiber diets on markers of glycemia. The findings from this study demonstrated that high-carbohydrate and high-fiber diets have a significant positive impact on glycemic markers including improvements in fasting blood glucose levels, postprandial plasma glucose levels, and HbA1c.[39] Multiple organizations, as shown in **Table 1**, recommend increasing fiber intake as part of diabetes management.[8,15-17] However, the latest guidelines from the ADA do not specifically recommend increasing fiber intake beyond the level already recommended for the general public. This is because the amount of fiber required to achieve modest reductions in HbA1c and preprandial glucose levels was found to be unrealistically high, exceeding 50 g/day.[8,15]

The role of dietary fiber in preventing obesity has been extensively studied through systematic reviews and meta-analyses. In a meta-analysis conducted by Chen et al. (2017), which examined 14 studies (11 cross-sectional studies and 3 cohort studies), dietary fiber was found to have a significant protective effect against the risk of metabolic syndrome. However, four studies showing high heterogeneity and publication bias were removed from the analysis.[40] Another systematic review and meta-analysis by Jovanovski et al. (2021) focused specifically on viscous fiber. This analysis included 15 RCTs investigating the effects of viscous fiber supplementation. The findings suggested significant effects of viscous fiber on body weight, percentage body fat, and BMI, although no significant effect was observed on waist circumference. The analysis showed that viscous fiber supplementation resulted in significant reductions in body weight (−0.81 kg), BMI (−0.25 kg/m^2), and body fat (−1.39%) compared to the control group. It is important to note that the effects of dietary fiber can vary depending on the specific type of fiber and individual characteristics. Different types of fiber may have different impacts on obesity prevention and overall health.[41]

The ADA emphasizes the significance of dietary strategies that aim to control hyperglycemia in order to reduce complications associated with diabetes. They highlight the regulation of blood glucose levels as a primary objective in diabetes management. In alignment with these recommendations, various organizations worldwide, such as the British Diabetes Association (BDA), Canadian Diabetes Association (CDA), European Association for the Study of Diabetes (EASD), as well as agencies in India, Japan, and South Africa, have also provided nutritional guidelines that include increasing dietary fiber intake for individuals with T2DM.

These recommendations underline the importance of dietary fiber as part of a comprehensive approach to diabetes management **(Table 1)**.[8,15-17,39]

Micronutrients and Antioxidants

Diabetes-related hyperglycemia contributes to intracellular oxidative stress, which refers to an imbalance between the production of ROS and the body's antioxidant defense systems. This oxidative stress is closely intertwined with metabolic disturbances, and achieving improved glycemic control is associated with a reduction in prooxidant status. Multiple mechanisms play a role in the development of oxidative stress in the presence of elevated glucose levels. These mechanisms include glucose autoxidation, protein glycation, formation of advanced glycation end products, activation of the polyol pathway, protein kinase C-dependent activation of nicotinamide adenine dinucleotide phosphate (reduced form) (NADPH) oxidase, and increased production of superoxide radicals by mitochondria. ROS function as signaling molecules and can modulate various biological functions by activating specific signal transduction mechanisms. Some of these mechanisms are implicated in the pathogenesis of diabetes and its associated complications.[42]

Enhancing antioxidant status is believed to be one of the mechanisms through which dietary antioxidant treatment can contribute to the prevention and reduction of diabetic complications. Diabetes is associated with increased oxidative stress, which can damage various organs and tissues in the body, leading to complications, such as diabetic retinopathy (which can cause blindness), diabetic nephropathy (kidney failure), peripheral neuropathy (nerve damage), and cardiovascular diseases. Antioxidants help neutralize ROS and reduce oxidative damage, thereby protecting against these complications. By reducing oxidative stress, dietary antioxidants have the potential to mitigate the risk of diabetic complications and improve overall health outcomes for individuals with diabetes.[42]

Micronutrients, including vitamins and minerals, play a vital role in the reduction of oxidative stress in diabetic patients. They act as essential coenzymes or cofactors in metabolic reactions and can indirectly contribute to improved glycemic control and exhibit antioxidant properties. These micronutrients are part of a larger group of essential nutrients listed in the recommended dietary allowances (RDAs) report by the Food and Nutrition Board, National Research Council, USA. It is noteworthy that the ADA recommends obtaining micronutrients from natural food sources rather than relying on supplements for diabetic individuals. Educating diabetic individuals about the importance of consuming sufficient amounts of vitamins and minerals from natural food sources while adhering to recommended sugar and carbohydrate intake is crucial. This approach ensures a balanced and nutrient-rich diet, promoting overall health and well-being in diabetes management.[42]

Obesity is known to disrupt the micronutrient status of individuals, leading to deficiencies in various minerals such as iron, calcium, magnesium, zinc, and copper, as well as vitamins including folate, vitamin A, D, and B12. Micronutrients play essential roles as cofactors for enzymatic reactions and regulate crucial metabolic processes in the body. Imbalances or deficiencies in micronutrients can have severe implications for human health including congenital disabilities, impaired growth,

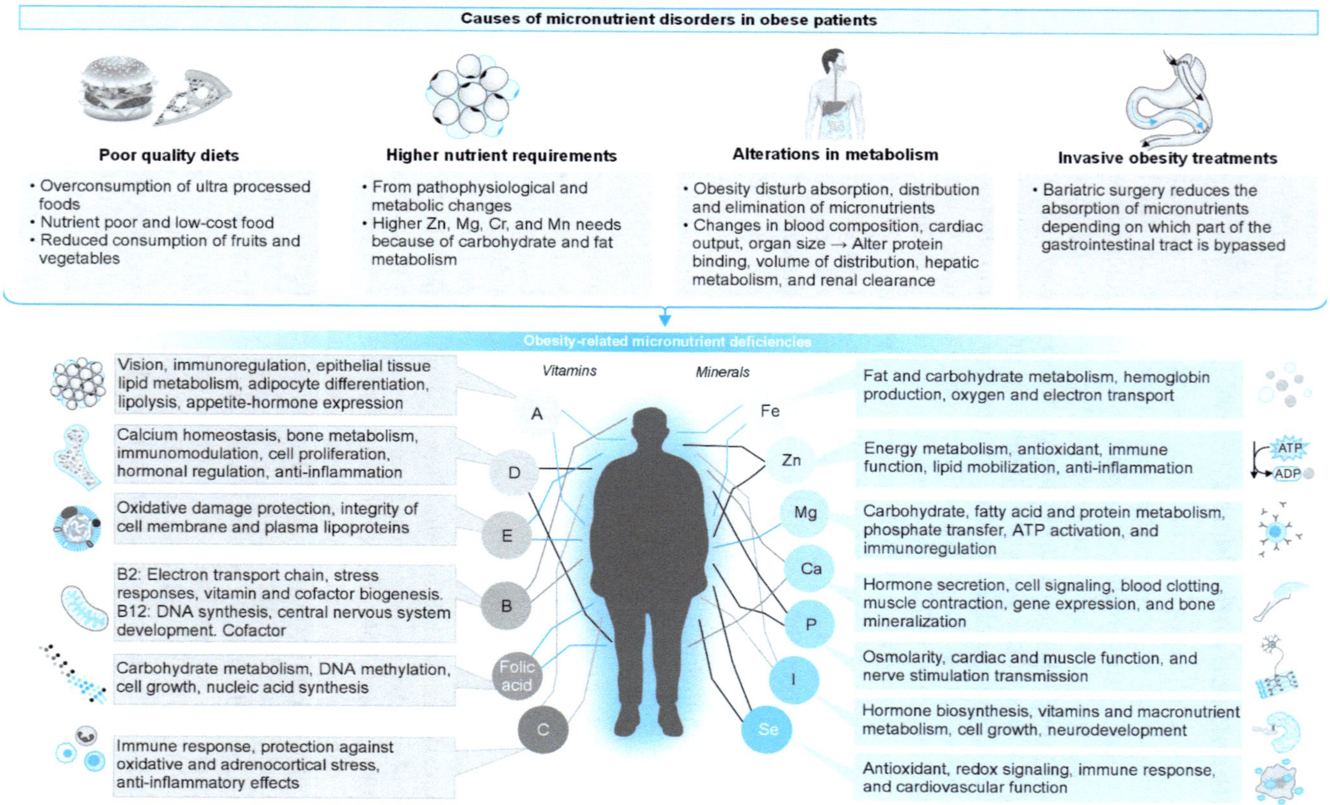

Causes of micronutrient disorders in obese patients

Poor quality diets
- Overconsumption of ultra processed foods
- Nutrient poor and low-cost food
- Reduced consumption of fruits and vegetables

Higher nutrient requirements
- From pathophysiological and metabolic changes
- Higher Zn, Mg, Cr, and Mn needs because of carbohydrate and fat metabolism

Alterations in metabolism
- Obesity disturb absorption, distribution and elimination of micronutrients
- Changes in blood composition, cardiac output, organ size → Alter protein binding, volume of distribution, hepatic metabolism, and renal clearance

Invasive obesity treatments
- Bariatric surgery reduces the absorption of micronutrients depending on which part of the gastrointestinal tract is bypassed

Obesity-related micronutrient deficiencies

Vitamins

- **A**: Vision, immunoregulation, epithelial tissue lipid metabolism, adipocyte differentiation, lipolysis, appetite-hormone expression
- **D**: Calcium homeostasis, bone metabolism, immunomodulation, cell proliferation, hormonal regulation, anti-inflammation
- **E**: Oxidative damage protection, integrity of cell membrane and plasma lipoproteins
- **B**: B2: Electron transport chain, stress responses, vitamin and cofactor biogenesis. B12: DNA synthesis, central nervous system development. Cofactor
- **Folic acid**: Carbohydrate metabolism, DNA methylation, cell growth, nucleic acid synthesis
- **C**: Immune response, protection against oxidative and adrenocortical stress, anti-inflammatory effects

Minerals

- **Fe**: Fat and carbohydrate metabolism, hemoglobin production, oxygen and electron transport
- **Zn**: Energy metabolism, antioxidant, immune function, lipid mobilization, anti-inflammation
- **Mg**: Carbohydrate, fatty acid and protein metabolism, phosphate transfer, ATP activation, and immunoregulation
- **Ca**: Hormone secretion, cell signaling, blood clotting, muscle contraction, gene expression, and bone mineralization
- **P**: Osmolarity, cardiac and muscle function, and nerve stimulation transmission
- **I**: Hormone biosynthesis, vitamins and macronutrient metabolism, cell growth, neurodevelopment
- **Se**: Antioxidant, redox signaling, immune response, and cardiovascular function

FIG. 9: Micronutrient deficiencies associated with obese patients.

(Ca: calcium; Cr: chromium; Fe: iron; I: iodine; Mg: magnesium; Mn: manganese; P: phosphorus; Se: selenium; Zn: zinc) learning disabilities, compromised immune function, increased risk of cancer and cardiovascular disease, impaired antioxidant defense mechanisms, osteoporosis, neurodegenerative disorders, malfunction of the intestinal microbiota, and dysfunction in various organs and systems. Furthermore, micronutrient deficiencies can worsen the development of obesity as they are involved in fat and carbohydrate metabolism, glucose metabolic pathways, the insulin-signaling cascade, and pancreatic β-cell function. Numerous studies have been conducted to investigate micronutrient deficiencies in individuals with obesity, highlighting the importance of addressing these deficiencies **(Fig. 9)**.[43]

Indeed, further in-depth research and a more detailed understanding are necessary to address and clarify the action of antioxidant therapy in the pathophysiology of obesity and complications associated with T2DM. This includes exploring the specific mechanisms by which antioxidants exert their effects, identifying the optimal combination of vitamins and minerals for maximum efficacy, and determining the appropriate dosage for therapeutic use. The development of a standard vitamin mocktail, which refers to a combination of specific vitamins and minerals, and the standardization of their dosage would be valuable in ensuring consistent and effective antioxidant therapy for individuals with obesity and T2DM. Standardization would help healthcare professionals in prescribing and administering the therapy, as well as facilitate research and clinical trials to assess its safety and efficacy. By conducting further research and obtaining a more comprehensive understanding of the role of antioxidants in obesity and T2DM, as well as their interactions with other treatments and medications, we can advance toward the development of evidence-based guidelines and protocols for antioxidant therapy. This will ultimately contribute to improving the management and prevention of complications associated with T2DM.

REFERENCES

1. Zeinalian R, Ahmadikhatir S, Esfahani EN, Namazi N, Larijani B. The roles of personalized nutrition in obesity and diabetes management: a review. J Diabetes Metab Disord. 2022;21(1):1119-27.
2. Blüher M. Obesity: global epidemiology and pathogenesis. Nat Rev Endocrinol. 2019;15(5):288-98.
3. Seidell JC, Halberstadt J. The global burden of obesity and the challenges of prevention. Ann Nutr Metab. 2015;66 Suppl 2:7-12.
4. Zimmet PZ, Magliano DJ, Herman WH, Shaw JE. Diabetes: a 21st century challenge. Lancet Diabetes Endocrinol. 2014;2(1):56-64.
5. Walker KZ, O'Dea K, Gomez M, Girgis S, Colagiuri R. Diet and exercise in the prevention of diabetes. J Hum Nutr Diet. 2010;23(4):344-52.
6. Inzucchi SE, Bergenstal RM, Buse JB, Diamant M, Ferrannini E, Nauck M, et al. Management of hyperglycemia in type 2 diabetes: a patient-centered approach: position statement of the American Diabetes Association (ADA) and the European Association for the Study of Diabetes (EASD). Diabetes Care. 2012;35(6):1364-79. Erratum in: Diabetes Care. 2013;36(2):490.
7. US Department of Health and Human Services, U.S. Department of Agriculture. (2015). Dietary guidelines for Americans 2015–2020. [online] Available from https://health.gov/our-work/nutrition-physical-activity/dietary-guidelines/previous-dietary-guidelines/2015 [Last accessed October, 2023].
8. Evert AB, Boucher JL, Cypress M, Dunbar SA, Franz MJ, Mayer-Davis EJ, et al. Nutrition therapy recommendations for the management of adults with diabetes. Diabetes Care. 2013;36(11):3821-42.
9. Ley SH, Hamdy O, Mohan V, Hu FB. Prevention and management of type 2 diabetes: dietary components and nutritional strategies. Lancet. 2014;383(9933):1999-2007.

10. Ordovas JM, Ferguson LR, Tai ES, Mathers JC. Personalised nutrition and health. BMJ. 2018;361:bmj.k2173.
11. World food consumption patterns – trends and drivers. [online] Available from https://agriculture.ec.europa.eu/system/files/2023-03/agri-market-brief-06_en.pdf. [Last accessed October, 2023].
12. Popkin BM, Adair LS, Ng SW. Global nutrition transition and the pandemic of obesity in developing countries. Nutr Rev. 2012;70(1):3-21.
13. Schmidhuber J, Sur P, Fay K, Huntley B, Salama J, Lee A, et al. The Global Nutrient Database: availability of macronutrients and micronutrients in 195 countries from 1980 to 2013. Lancet Planet Health. 2018;2(8):e353-68.
14. Wali JA, Solon-Biet SM, Freire T, Brandon AE. Macronutrient Determinants of Obesity, Insulin Resistance and Metabolic Health. Biology (Basel). 2021;10(4):336.
15. Evert AB, Dennison M, Gardner CD, Garvey WT, Lau KHK, MacLeod J, et al. Nutrition Therapy for Adults With Diabetes or Prediabetes: A Consensus Report. Diabetes Care. 2019;42(5):731-54.
16. Diabetes Canada Clinical Practice Guidelines Expert Committee; Sievenpiper JL, Chan CB, Dworatzek PD, Freeze C, Williams SL. Nutrition Therapy. Can J Diabetes. 2018;42 Suppl 1:S64-S79.
17. Diabetes and Nutrition Study Group (DNSG) of the European Association for the Study of Diabetes (EASD). Evidence-based European recommendations for the dietary management of diabetes. Diabetologia. 2023;66(6):965-85.
18. San-Cristobal R, Navas-Carretero S, Martínez-González MÁ, Ordovas JM, Martínez JA. Contribution of macronutrients to obesity: implications for precision nutrition. Nat Rev Endocrinol. 2020;16(6):305-20.
19. Stanhope KL, Schwarz JM, Keim NL, Griffen SC, Bremer AA, Graham JL, et al. Consuming fructose-sweetened, not glucose-sweetened, beverages increases visceral adiposity and lipids and decreases insulin sensitivity in overweight/obese humans. J Clin Invest. 2009;119(5):1322-34.
20. Gardner C, Wylie-Rosett J, Gidding SS, Steffen LM, Johnson RK, Reader D, et al. Nonnutritive sweeteners: current use and health perspectives: a scientific statement from the American Heart Association and the American Diabetes Association. Circulation. 2012;126(4):509-19.
21. Roh E, Choi KM. Hormonal Gut-Brain Signaling for the Treatment of Obesity. Int J Mol Sci. 2023;24(4):3384.
22. Veit M, van Asten R, Olie A, Prinz P. The role of dietary sugars, overweight, and obesity in type 2 diabetes mellitus: a narrative review. Eur J Clin Nutr. 2022;76(11):1497-501.
23. Esfahani A, Wong JM, Mirrahimi A, Villa CR, Kendall CW. The application of the glycemic index and glycemic load in weight loss: A review of the clinical evidence. IUBMB Life. 2011;63(1):7-13.
24. Ebbeling CB, Leidig MM, Sinclair KB, Hangen JP, Ludwig DS. A reduced-glycemic load diet in the treatment of adolescent obesity. Arch Pediatr Adolesc Med. 2003;157(8):773-79.
25. Spieth LE, Harnish JD, Lenders CM, Raezer LB, Pereira MA, Hangen SJ, et al. A low-glycemic index diet in the treatment of pediatric obesity. Arch Pediatr Adolesc Med. 2000;154(9):947-51.
26. Henry CJ, Lightowler HJ, Strik CM. Effects of long-term intervention with low- and high-glycaemic-index breakfasts on food intake in children aged 8-11 years. Br J Nutr. 2007;98(3):636-40.
27. Schwingshackl L, Hobl LP, Hoffmann G. Effects of low glycaemic index/low glycaemic load vs. high glycaemic index/ high glycaemic load diets on overweight/obesity and associated risk factors in children and adolescents: a systematic review and meta-analysis. Nutr J. 2015;14:87.
28. Perin L, Camboim IG, Lehnen AM. Low glycaemic index and glycaemic load diets in adults with excess weight: Systematic review and meta-analysis of randomised clinical trials. J Hum Nutr Diet. 2022;35(6):1124-35.
29. Schwingshackl L, Hoffmann G. Long-term effects of low glycemic index/load vs. high glycemic index/load diets on parameters of obesity and obesity-associated risks: a systematic review and meta-analysis. Nutr Metab Cardiovasc Dis. 2013;23(8):699-706.
30. Marsh K, Barclay A, Colagiuri S, Brand-Miller J. Glycemic index and glycemic load of carbohydrates in the diabetes diet. Curr Diab Rep. 2011;11(2):120-7.
31. Brand-Miller J, Hayne S, Petocz P, Colagiuri S. Low-glycemic index diets in the management of diabetes: a meta-analysis of randomized controlled trials. Diabetes Care. 2003;26(8):2261-7.
32. Opperman AM, Venter CS, Oosthuizen W, Thompson RL, Vorster HH. Meta-analysis of the health effects of using the glycaemic index in meal-planning. Br J Nutr. 2004;92(3):367-81.
33. Thomas D, Elliott EJ. Low glycaemic index, or low glycaemic load, diets for diabetes mellitus. Cochrane Database Syst Rev. 2009;2009(1):CD006296.
34. Davis S, Alonso MD. Hypoglycemia as a barrier to glycemic control. J Diabetes Complications. 2004;18(1):60-8.
35. Thomas DE, Elliott EJ. The use of low-glycaemic index diets in diabetes control. Br J Nutr. 2010;104(6):797-802.

36. Stratton IM, Adler AI, Neil HA, Matthews DR, Manley SE, Cull CA, et al. Association of glycaemia with macrovascular and microvascular complications of type 2 diabetes (UKPDS 35): prospective observational study. BMJ. 2000;321(7258):405-12.
37. Churuangsuk C, Hall J, Reynolds A, Griffin SJ, Combet E, Lean MEJ. Diets for weight management in adults with type 2 diabetes: an umbrella review of published meta-analyses and systematic review of trials of diets for diabetes remission. Diabetologia. 2022;65(1):14-36.
38. Saboo B, Misra A, Kalra S, Mohan V, Aravind SR, Joshi S, et al. Role and importance of high fiber in diabetes management in India. Diabetes Metab Syndr. 2022;16(5):102480.
39. Kendall CWC, Esfahani A, Jenkins DJA. The link between dietary fibre and human health. Food Hydrocoll. 2010;24(1):42-8.
40. Waddell IS, Orfila C. Dietary fiber in the prevention of obesity and obesity-related chronic diseases: From epidemiological evidence to potential molecular mechanisms. Crit Rev Food Sci Nutr. 2022;26:1-16.
41. Jovanovski E, Mazhar N, Komishon A, Khayyat R, Li D, Blanco Mejia S, et al. Effect of viscous fiber supplementation on obesity indicators in individuals consuming calorie-restricted diets: a systematic review and meta-analysis of randomized controlled trials. Eur J Nutr. 2021;60(1):101-12.
42. Bonnefont-Rousselot D. The role of antioxidant micronutrients in the prevention of diabetic complications. Treat Endocrinol. 2004;3(1):41-52.
43. Guardiola-Márquez CE, Santos-Ramírez MT, Segura-Jiménez ME, Figueroa-Montes ML, Jacobo-Velázquez DA. Fighting Obesity-Related Micronutrient Deficiencies through Biofortification of Agri-Food Crops with Sustainable Fertilization Practices. Plants (Basel). 2022;11(24):3477.

CHAPTER 7

Pharmacotherapy for Diabetes and Obesity

Key Highlights

- Oral antidiabetic medications, such as metformin, sodium-glucose cotransporter-2 (SGLT-2) inhibitors, are commonly used as first-line treatments for type 2 diabetes mellitus (T2DM).
- Glucagon-like peptide-1 receptor agonists (GLP-1 RAs) have emerged as an effective pharmacotherapy for both diabetes and obesity.
- Insulin therapy is essential for individuals with type 1 diabetes mellitus, as they have an absolute deficiency of insulin. It is also used in some cases of T2DM when oral medications and lifestyle changes are not sufficient to control blood glucose levels.
- The use of anti-obesity medications, such as orlistat, liraglutide, and phentermine/topiramate, in conjunction with lifestyle modifications, can aid in weight loss and management of obesity-related comorbidities.
- Combination therapies have gained attention in the management of diabetes and obesity. The use of dual or triple therapy, such as combining GLP-1 RAs with SGLT-2 inhibitors or with other antidiabetic agents, has shown improved glycemic control and enhanced weight loss compared to monotherapy.
- When managing comorbidities in bariatric patients, choosing medications with weight-neutral or weight-loss potential over those causing weight gain is crucial to mitigate adverse metabolic effects.

INTRODUCTION

Obesity presents itself as a chronic and multifaceted ailment, encompassing a wide range of complexities and variations. Its impact on society is not only disconcerting from a health perspective but also places a substantial economic burden. This condition can lead to over 200 other medical disorders that affect various organ systems, further exacerbating its significance and consequences. Over the years, since 1980, obesity rates have surged twofold in 73 countries. Elevated body mass index (BMI) exceeding 25 kg/m^2 contributes to approximately four million global deaths and imposes a considerable burden on cardiovascular (CV) health. The alarming rise in obesity prevalence, coupled with its profound implications on well-being and the development of comorbidities, underscores the urgent necessity for early identification and intervention. It is crucial to address this issue promptly by utilizing the existing array of therapeutic measures at our disposal.[1]

The foundation of managing weight involves incorporating changes in diet, physical activity, and behavior. However, relying solely on lifestyle modifications for weight loss often proves challenging and yields limited results in the long term. The body responds to reduced caloric intake and increased energy expenditure with adaptive physiological mechanisms that can hinder progress. These responses include an increase in appetite and a disproportionate decrease in resting metabolic rate compared to changes in body composition. This phenomenon, known as adaptive thermogenesis or metabolic adaptation, obstructs weight loss efforts and contributes to weight regain. To address the challenges posed by adaptive changes in appetite and energy expenditure during weight loss, one approach is the utilization of pharmacotherapy for obesity. This strategy aims to counteract these adaptive mechanisms and enhance adherence to lifestyle interventions. According to the guidelines set forth by the American College of Cardiology, American Heart Association, the Obesity Society, and the Endocrine Society, pharmacotherapy for obesity can be considered for individuals with a BMI of 30 kg/m^2 or higher, or a BMI of 27 kg/m^2 or higher with weight-related comorbidities such as hypertension, dyslipidemia, type 2 diabetes mellitus (T2DM), and obstructive sleep apnea. Given the chronic nature of obesity, most anti-obesity medications are approved for long-term use. Until recently, the only anti-obesity medications approved by the Food and Drug Administration (FDA) were phentermine (and other sympathomimetic amines) and orlistat. However, in 2012, phentermine/topiramate extended release (ER) and lorcaserin received FDA approval, followed by naltrexone sustained-release (SR)/bupropion SR and liraglutide 3.0 mg in 2014. These medications offer additional options for long-term treatment of obesity.[2] In the context of long-term weight management, pharmacotherapy is recommended as a supplementary approach alongside a reduced-calorie diet and increased physical activity. This combination of medication, dietary changes, and increased exercise is beneficial for achieving sustainable weight loss. Pharmacotherapy may be considered for adults with a BMI of 30 or higher, or a BMI of 27-29 accompanied by at least one weight-related coexisting condition. It is important to note that pharmacotherapy and lifestyle interventions are most effective when used together, as they have an additive effect on weight loss. By combining medication with lifestyle changes, individuals can experience enhanced results in their weight management journey. Furthermore, pharmacotherapy, when used in conjunction with lifestyle intervention, can also assist in maintaining reduced weight over time, supporting long-term weight management goals.[3]

The worldwide impact of diabetes mellitus (DM) and its associated complications represents a significant threat to global health. Over the past 30 years, the global prevalence of diabetes and impaired glucose tolerance (IGT) has quadrupled. The rapid process of urbanization in many countries has further accelerated the rise in diabetes prevalence. In addition to its health implications, T2DM is also linked to increased healthcare costs, estimated to be around $850 billion globally. The substantial human and financial burdens that accompany T2DM, along with the inherent challenges in effectively treating the condition once diagnosed, make it an ideal target for preventive measures. Recognizing the escalating rates of T2DM and its associated complications, focusing on prevention becomes paramount in mitigating the toll it takes on individuals and societies at large.[4]

Type 2 diabetes mellitus is characterized by a collection of eight core defects, referred to as "the ominous octet," which collectively contribute to its pathophysiology. These defects encompass various aspects of glucose and metabolic regulation. They include decreased insulin secretion, reduced incretin effect (the decrease in insulin release due to impaired gut hormone activity), heightened lipolysis (the breakdown of stored fat), increased glucose reabsorption, decreased glucose uptake by cells, neurotransmitter dysfunction, elevated hepatic glucose production, and augmented glucagon secretion (a hormone that increases blood glucose levels). When considering therapy options for T2DM, it is crucial to target these established pathophysiological defects. Treatment approaches should aim to address each defect to achieve optimal management. Additionally, a patient-centered approach is essential, which involves considering factors beyond glycemic control. This approach takes into account the reduction of overall CV risk, recognizing the interconnected nature of T2DM, and CV health. By addressing both the specific defects contributing to T2DM and individual patient needs, a comprehensive and tailored treatment plan can be developed.[5,6]

The wide range of hypoglycemic agents available offers the opportunity to target multiple pathways involved in the management of T2DM. These medications can effectively control T2DM and alleviate associated symptoms such as hyperglycemia, polyuria, and fatigue. Moreover, they play a crucial role in mitigating the risk of long-term complications associated with T2DM. By utilizing a combination of oral and injectable agents, healthcare providers can tailor individualized treatment approaches for diabetic patients. This approach takes into account various factors such as the efficacy of the medications, potential side effects, costs, presence of comorbidities, tendency for weight gain, and glucose levels. This allows clinicians to design a treatment regimen that best suits the specific needs and circumstances of each patient. By considering these elements and employing a combination of hypoglycemic agents, healthcare providers can optimize the management of diabetes, improve symptom control, and minimize the risk of long-term complications. Individualized therapy plans that address the unique requirements and considerations of each patient can lead to better outcomes in diabetes management.[7]

ORAL ANTIDIABETIC AGENTS AND INSULIN THERAPY

Oral Antidiabetic Agents

Numerous drugs have received approval for the purpose of reducing hyperglycemia associated with DM. Among these agents are biguanides, sulfonylureas (SUs), thiazolidinediones (TZDs), glucagon-like peptide-1 (GLP-1) agonists, dipeptidyl peptidase-4 (DPP-4) inhibitors, α-glucosidase inhibitors (AGIs), amylin mimetic drugs, bile acid binding resins, and SGLT inhibitors.[7] It is important to note that this list is not exhaustive. In addition to their glucose-lowering effects, several FDA-approved medications used in the treatment of T2DM have been recognized for their ability to promote weight loss **(Table 1)**. These include metformin (a biguanide), GLP-1 receptor agonists (GLP-1 RAs), amylin analogs, and SGLT-2 inhibitors.[8] These specific agents offer the dual benefit of improving glycemic control while also supporting weight loss efforts. It is worth mentioning that healthcare providers take into consideration various factors, such as individual patient characteristics, medical history, and treatment goals, when determining the most appropriate glucose-lowering agents to prescribe **(Fig. 1)**.

Biguanides

Metformin is indeed the primary agent used today among the mentioned group of medications. It holds the distinction of being the most commonly prescribed and accepted as a first-line treatment for T2DM. The mechanism of action of metformin involves the activation of AMP-dependent protein kinase [adenosine monophosphate-dependent protein kinase (AMPK)] in situations where cellular energy stores are depleted. This activation leads to increased fatty acid oxidation and inhibition of gluconeogenesis in the liver, thereby reducing blood glucose levels **(Fig. 2)**. Metformin can be administered as a monotherapy or in combination with other hypoglycemic agents. However, caution should be exercised when prescribing metformin to patients with heart failure (HF) or renal failure, as they have an increased risk of lactic acidosis, which is considered the most serious side effect associated with metformin use. Therefore, these patients should receive metformin at low doses and under careful monitoring. An overview of the advantages and disadvantages of metformin can be found in **Table 2**.[5,7,9]

Metformin's favorable characteristics, such as its glycemic efficacy, absence of hypoglycemia, potential for weight loss, tolerability, and cost-effectiveness, have established it as the initial drug of choice for most patients with T2DM. Furthermore, beyond its use in diabetes management, metformin shows promising potential in areas such as antiaging, cancer prevention, and cancer therapeutics, which extends its benefits to individuals without T2DM.[10] Overall, metformin remains a cornerstone in the treatment of T2DM due to its effectiveness, safety profile, and potential for broader applications beyond glycemic control.

Sulfonylureas

Sulfonylureas can be categorized into first and second-generation agents. However, due to their frequent dosing and higher risk of hypoglycemia, the first-generation drugs tolbutamide and tolzamide are no longer used clinically. On the other hand, second-generation SUs such as glibenclamide, gliclazide, and glimepiride are still in use, with some available in ER formulations. The mechanism of action of SUs involves blocking ATP (adenosine triphosphate)-sensitive potassium channels present on pancreatic β-cells. This blockade leads to depolarization of the cells, increased calcium levels, and enhanced secretion of insulin, earning them the

TABLE 1: Profiles of type 2 diabetes mellitus (T2DM) therapy. *(For color version, see Plate 3)*

	Metformin	DPP-4 inhibitor	GLP-1 RA	SGLT-2 inhibitor	TZD	SU and GLN	Pramlintide
Hypoglycemia	Neutral	Neutral	Neutral	Neutral	Neutral	Mild/Moderate	Neutral
Weight	Slight loss	Neutral	Loss	Loss	Gain	Gain	Loss
Renal/GU	Contraindicated if eGFR <30 mL/min/1.73 m²	Dose adjustment is necessary (except linagliptin). Effective in reducing albuminuria	Exenatide not indicated CrCl <30; Possible benefit of liraglutide	Not indicated for eGFR <45 mL/min/1.73 m²; Genital mycotic infection; Possible benefit of empagliflozin	Neutral	More hypo risk	Neutral
GI	Moderate	Neutral	Moderate	Neutral	Neutral	Neutral	Moderate
Cardiac	Neutral	Possible increase in hospitalization with alogliptin and saxagliptin	Liraglutide prevents MACE events	Empagliflozin reduces CV mortality; Canagliflozin reduces MACE events	Moderate risk for CHF; May reduce stroke risk	Possible ASCVD risk	Neutral
Bone	Neutral	Neutral	Neutral	Mild fracture risk	Neutral	Neutral	Neutral
Ketoacidosis	Neutral	Neutral	Neutral	DKA can occur in various stress settings	Neutral	Neutral	Neutral
	Possible benefit			Use with caution		Possible adverse effects	

(ASCVD: atherosclerotic cardiovascular disease; CHF: congestive heart failure; CrCl: creatinine clearance; CV: cardiovascular; DKA: diabetic ketoacidosis; DPP-4: dipeptidyl peptidase-4; eGFR: estimated glomerular filtration rate; GI: gastrointestinal; GLN: glinide; GU: genitourinary; MACE: major adverse cardiac events; SGLT-2: sodium-glucose cotransporter-2; SU: sulfonylurea; TZD: thiazolidinedione)

CHAPTER 7: Pharmacotherapy for Diabetes and Obesity

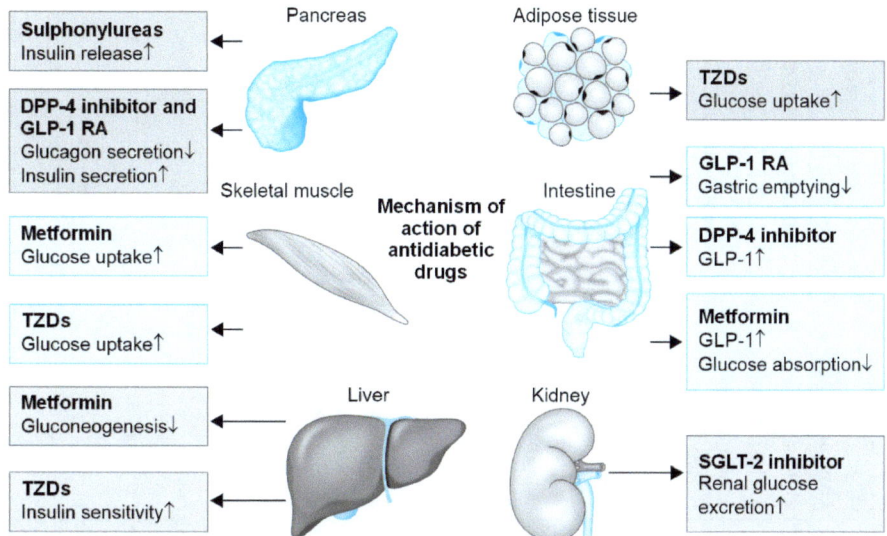

FIG. 1: General mechanism of action of antidiabetic drugs.[5]

(DPP-4: dipeptidyl peptidase-4; GLP-1: glucagon-like peptide-1; GLP-1 RA: glucagon-like peptide-1 receptor agonists; SGLT-2: sodium-glucose cotransporter-2; TZDs: thiazolidinediones)

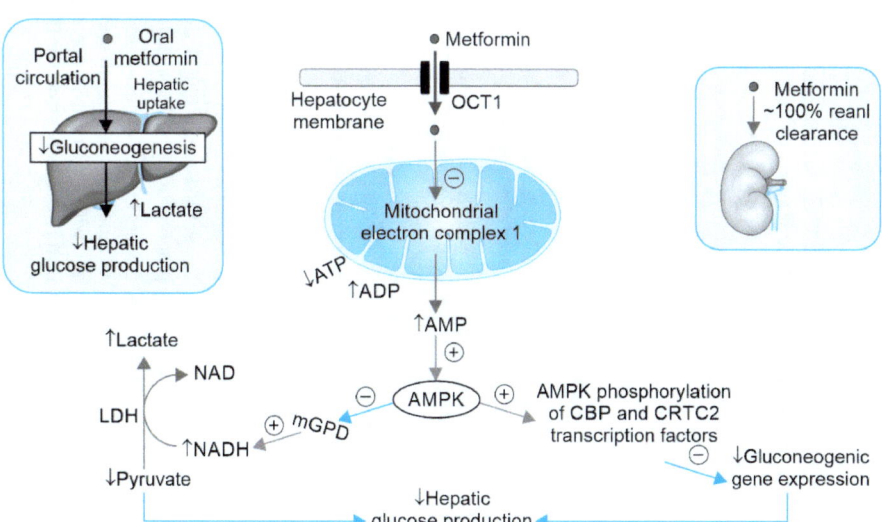

FIG. 2: Metformin acts primarily to suppress glucose production in the liver.[10]

[ADP: adenosine diphosphate; AMP: adenosine monophosphate; ATP: adenosine triphosphate; LDH: lactate dehydrogenase; NAD: nicotinamide adenine dinucleotide; NADH: nicotinamide adenine dinucleotide + hydrogen (H); OCT1: organic cation transporter 1]

TABLE 2: Summary of oral hyperglycemic therapy dosage, advantages, and disadvantages.[5,7,9]

Drug name (expected reduction in HbA1c)	Daily dosage	Advantages	Side effects	Contraindications	Position in the therapeutic armamentarium
Metformin (1.0–2.0%)	500–2,550 mg (depending on immediate vs. extended-release formulations)	• Weight loss • Inexpensive • Extensive experience • Rare hypoglycemia • Low CVD events (UKPDS)	• Diarrhea • Vomiting • Dyspepsia • Flatulence • Metallic taste • Lactic acidosis • Folic acid and vitamin B12 deficiencies	• Renal disease • Heart failure • Liver disease • Hypoxic pulmonary disease	• *2019 joint ESC and EASD*: First-line therapy only in overweight T2DM patients without CVD and not at high risk for CVD • *2022 ADA*: First-line therapy
Sulfonylureas (SU; 1.0–2.0%)	• Glibenclamide (1.25–20 mg) • Glimepiride (1–8 mg) • Gliclazide (30–120 mg)	• Rapid effectiveness • Extensive experience • Low microvascular risk (UKPDS)	• Weight gain • Hypoglycemia • GI distress • Dizziness	• Pregnancy • Ketoacidosis	*2022 ADA*: Added to metformin in patients at low CV risk and no hypoglycemia
Thiazolidinediones (0.5–1.4%)	• Pioglitazone (15–45 mg) • Rosiglitazone (4–8 mg)	• Rare hypoglycemia • Relatively higher HbA1c efficacy • Durability • Lower triglycerides (pioglitazone) • Lower CVD events (PROactive, pioglitazone) • Lowers the risk of stroke and MI inpatients without diabetes and with insulin resistance and history of recent stroke or TIA (IRIS study, pioglitazone)	• Fluid retention • Weight gain • Bone loss • Edema/Heart failure	• Active liver disease • Patients with heart failure (Class III; IV)	*2022 ADA*: As add-on therapy for T2DM

Continued

Continued

Drug name (expected reduction in HbA1c)	Daily dosage	Advantages	Side effects	Contraindications	Position in the therapeutic armamentarium
Meglitinides (0.5–1.5%)	• Repaglinide (0.5–4 mg) • Nateglinide (60–120 mg)	• Ideal for postprandial glucose increase • Ideal for patients with irregular meal schedule	• Weight gain • Hypoglycemia	• Pregnancy • Hypersensitivity • Coadministration of gemfibrozil with repaglinide	• As monotherapy when metformin is contraindicated • 2nd or 3rd-line therapy in combination
Glucagon-like peptide-1 (GLP-1) agonists (0.5–1.0%)	• Exenatide (2 mg) SC • Liraglutide (0.6–3.0 mg) SC • Dulaglutide (0.75–1.5 mg) SC • Semaglutide (0.25–0.5 mg Oral	• Rare hypoglycemia • Decrease weight • Postprandial glucose excursions • Decrease some CV risk factors • Associated with lower CVD event rate and mortality in patients with CVD (PIONEER)	• GI side effects (nausea, vomiting, diarrhea) • increase heart rate • Can cause acute pancreatitis	• Pancreatitis • Renal impairment	*Semaglutide*: Adjunct therapy in adults with T2DM at high CVD risk
Dipeptidyl peptidase-4 (DPP-4) inhibitors (0.5–0.8%)	• Sitagliptin (50–100 mg) • Saxagliptin (2.5–5 mg) • Vildagliptin (50–100 mg) • Linagliptin (5 mg)	• Weight loss • Rare hypoglycemia • Well tolerated	• Hypoglycemia • Pancreatitis • GI distress • Flu-like symptoms • Joint pain	• Pregnancy • Pancreatitis • Heart failure • Angioedema	*ADA and EASD*: 2nd-line therapy in addition to metformin
AGI (0.5–0.8%)	Acarbose (25–300 mg)	Minimal risk of hypoglycemia	GI distress	• Liver cirrhosis • Colonic ulceration • Inflammatory bowel disease	No clear position
SGLT-2 inhibitors (0.7–1.0%)	• Dapagliflozin (5–10 mg) • Empagliflozin (10–25 mg) • Canagliflozin (100–300 mg) • Sotagliflozin (200–400 mg)	• Increase GLP-1 release • Weight loss • Reduce blood pressure • Reduce triglycerides • Decrease blood pressure • Associated with lower CVD event rate and mortality in patients with CVD	• GI distress • Hypoglycemia • Urinary tract infections	• Dialysis • Renal impairment	ADA 2022: Monotherapy or in addition to metformin, in patients with HFrEF (especially with LVEF <45%) and/or CKD, 1st-line therapy in patients with established CVD or at high CVD risk

(ADA: American Diabetes Association; EASD: European Association for the Study of Diabetes; ESC: European Society of Cardiology; HbA1c: glycated hemoglobin)

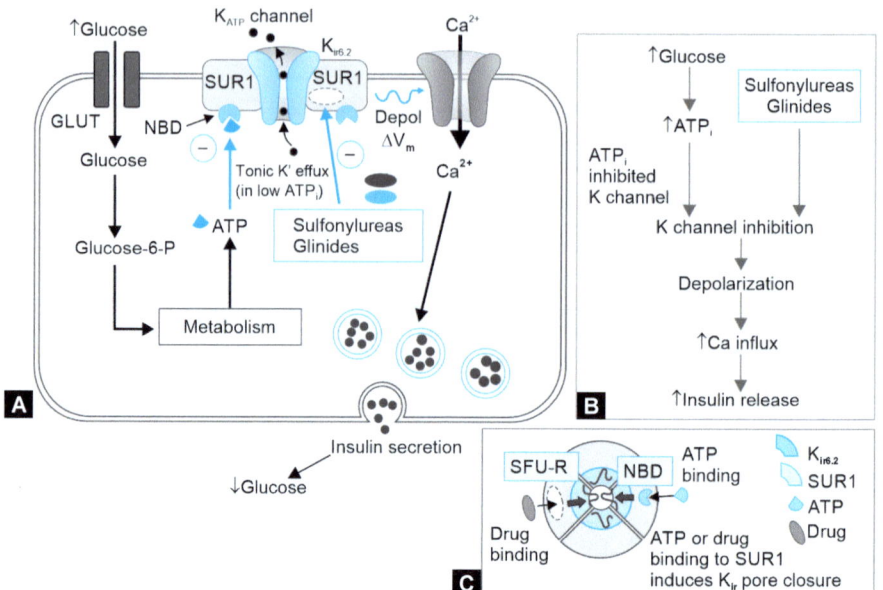

FIGS. 3A TO C: Mechanism of action of sulfonylureas and glinides in pancreatic β-cells and regulation of insulin release by plasma glucose (A to C).[10]

(ATP: adenosine triphosphate)

name "insulin secretagogues" **(Figs. 3A to C)**. SUs are considered highly effective in reducing glycated hemoglobin (HbA1c) levels by approximately 1–1.5%. Their cost-effectiveness has contributed to their widespread use, with SUs currently being employed as a second-line therapy in 50–80% of diabetic patients worldwide.

Among the second-generation SUs, glimepiride and gliclazide demonstrate a more favorable CV profile compared to glyburide, which may be attributed to pharmacodynamic differences among these drugs. Gliclazide, in particular, exhibits a lower incidence of side effects such as hypoglycemia and a more favorable CV profile, making it the preferred choice within the SU category.

Clinical trials such as the UKPDS (UK Prospective Diabetes Study) and the ADVANCE (Action in Diabetes and Vascular Disease: Preterax and Diamicron Modified Release Controlled Evaluation) have revealed that SUs confer microvascular benefits by reducing the incidence and progression of nephropathy and retinopathy without increasing all-cause mortality. However, SUs should be used cautiously in patients with severe hepatic insufficiency and moderate-to-severe renal impairment. The advantages and disadvantages of SUs are outlined in **Table 2**. Despite the proven CV benefits of newer antidiabetic drugs, SUs continue to be frequently utilized in clinical practice due to their affordability, widespread availability, long history of clinical use, and rapid glycemic response. The direct impact of SUs on CV events is yet to be conclusively determined; however, evidence supports the CV safety of glimepiride.[5,7,9,10]

Thiazolidinediones

Thiazolidinediones, also known as glitazones, were initially discovered in the 1980s during attempts to synthesize more potent fibrates. Researchers found that some compounds had hypoglycemic properties in diabetic mice.[9] Currently, two agents from this class, pioglitazone and rosiglitazone, are used clinically. TZDs function as insulin sensitizers by activating the gamma isoform of peroxisome proliferator-activated receptor gamma (PPAR-γ). They enhance glucose uptake by skeletal muscles and adipocytes, improve insulin sensitivity, and subsequently enhance pancreatic beta-cell function.[4] PPAR-γ receptors are primarily expressed in adipose tissue, with lower expression in skeletal muscle, liver, pancreatic β-cells, the central nervous system (CNS), and vascular endothelial cells. The primary effect of TZDs is believed to occur through the activation of PPAR-γ receptors in adipose tissue, promoting the uptake of circulating fatty acids into fat cells, and thereby increasing insulin sensitivity **(Fig. 4)**. TZDs can be used as add-on therapy for T2DM when there is no established cardiovascular disease (CVD), chronic kidney disease (CKD), or high CV risk. They are particularly useful in situations where the risk of hypoglycemia needs to be minimized, or when cost and access to other medications are significant concerns. However, caution should be exercised when using TZDs in patients with diastolic dysfunction or a known history of HF. They are contraindicated in patients with symptomatic HF. It is important to note that TZD-associated HF is primarily caused by fluid retention and not primary cardiac dysfunction, and it is not associated with increased mortality. Common side effects of TZDs include weight gain and edema. These effects are believed to be related to the activation of PPAR-γ receptors in the CNS, leading to increased food intake. Studies have also shown that TZDs may increase the risk of bone fractures in women and can cause a reduction in transaminase levels. Therefore, TZDs should be avoided in patients with liver disease. Rosiglitazone has been associated with an increased incidence of myocardial infarction. An overview of the advantages and disadvantages of TZDs can be found in **Table 2**.[5,7,9,10]

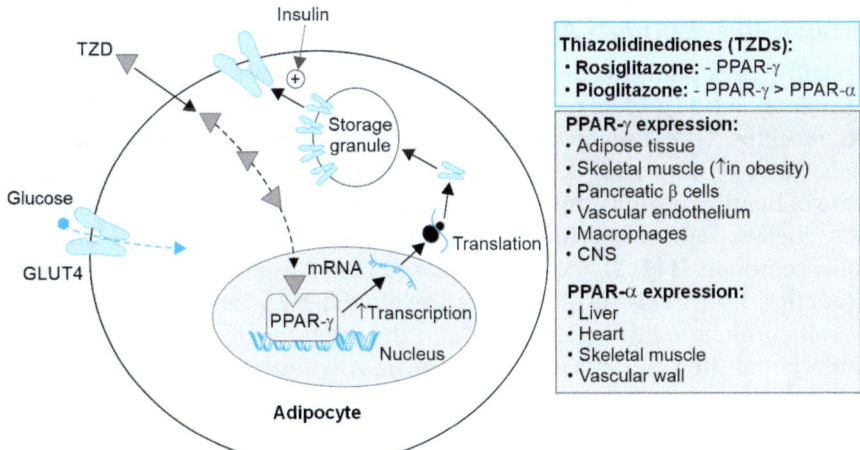

FIG. 4: Glycemic mechanism of action of thiazolidinedione "insulin sensitizers" (using an adipocyte for illustration purposes).[10]

(GLUT4: glucose transporter 4; mRNA: messenger ribonucleic acid; PPAR-α: peroxisome proliferator-activated receptor alpha; PPAR-γ: peroxisome proliferator-activated receptor gamma)

Meglitinides

Meglitinides, such as repaglinide and nateglinide, belong to a class of insulin secretagogue agents that work by blocking the ATP-sensitive potassium channels in pancreatic β-cells **(Figs. 3A to C)**. Unlike SUs, meglitinides have a rapid onset of action but a short duration. These characteristics make them suitable for patients with irregular meal schedules and those who experience rapid postprandial hyperglycemia.[7] Repaglinide, the first member of this group, was approved by the FDA in December 1997, followed by the approval of nateglinide in December 2000.[11] Repaglinide exhibits a dose-dependent, rapid onset mechanism of action when taken 15 minutes before meals. Within 30 minutes of starting a meal, repaglinide can increase insulin levels by up to 150%, with no lingering effects 4 hours later. It has shown effectiveness as monotherapy, reducing HbA1c levels by 1.14% in a 16-week trial with flexible meal dosing.[11] Large-scale prospective studies to confirm the CV safety of meglitinides have not been conducted. However, a nationwide study involving over 100,000 subjects found that the mortality and vascular risk associated with repaglinide monotherapy did not statistically differ from metformin, both in patients with and without previous myocardial infarction.[12] Meglitinides, including repaglinide and nateglinide, do not have a significant impact on high-density lipoprotein (HDL), low-density lipoprotein (LDL), or triglyceride (TG) levels. Meglitinides are oral antidiabetic medications that are affordable, although they may be more expensive than SUs. They are generally well-tolerated and widely available globally. One of the key benefits of meglitinides is their ability to effectively lower postprandial (after-meal) glucose levels. These medications have a rapid onset of action and a short duration, making them particularly suitable for individuals who experience rapid increases in blood glucose after meals. By stimulating insulin release from pancreatic β-cells, meglitinides help to control post-meal glucose spikes and promote better glycemic control. The advantages and disadvantages of meglitinides are outlined in **Table 2**.[7,9,10]

Glucagon-like Peptide-1 Agonists

Glucagon-like peptide-1 is an incretin secreted from the distal ileum in response to nutrients such as proteins and carbohydrates. Following its release, GLP-1 binds to its receptor, GLP-1 receptor (GLP-1R), which is expressed on the pancreatic β-cells, thereby activating a cascade of intracellular events that increases the release of insulin, inhibits the release of glucagon, reduces food intake by causing satiety, delays food emptying and normalizes both postprandial and fasting insulin secretion **(Fig. 5)**.[7,10] GLP-1 RAs are GLP-1 analogs that are resistant to degradation by DPP-4, resulting in an extended half-life compared to natural GLP-1. By prolonging the action of GLP-1, these medications provide a sustained stimulation of the GLP-1R. GLP-1Rs are primarily found in pancreatic beta cells and play a crucial role in regulating blood glucose homeostasis through various mechanisms. GLP-1 RAs, by acting on GLP-1R, can enhance insulin secretion, inhibit glucagon release, slow gastric emptying, promote satiety, and improve glucose control. These medications can achieve "supraphysiologic" GLP-1 levels, surpassing the levels typically seen in the body, leading to potent glucose-lowering effects.[9]

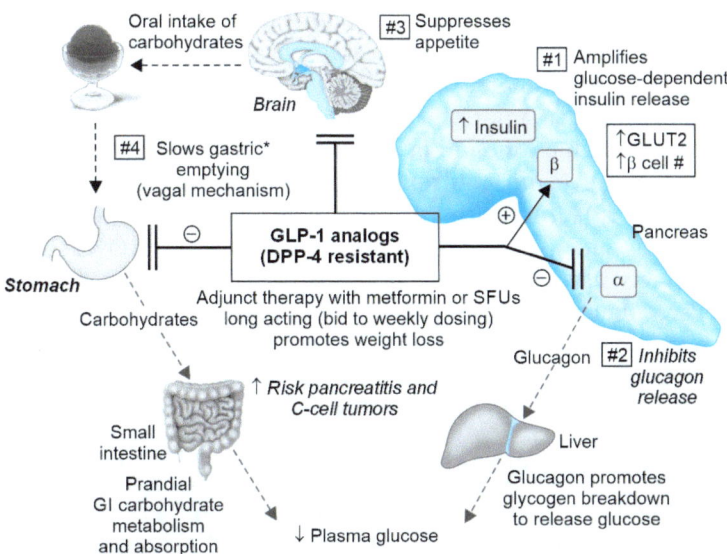

* Not significant for long-acting GLP-1 agonists due to tachyphylaxis.
FIG. 5: Potent GLP-1 agonists exert effects by multiple mechanisms.[10]
(DPP-4: dipeptidyl peptidase-4; GLP-1: glucagon-like peptide-1; GLUT2: glucose transporter 2)

There are two main classes of GLP-1 RAs based on their molecular structure—exendin-4-based GLP-1 RAs and human GLP-1-based GLP-1 RAs. Exendin-4-based GLP-1 RAs, such as exenatide and lixisenatide, are synthetic versions of the exendin-4 molecule found in the venom of the Gila monster lizard. These medications are designed to mimic the actions of GLP-1 and have been modified to resist degradation by DPP-4 enzymes, resulting in a longer duration of action. On the other hand, human GLP-1-based GLP-1 RAs, including liraglutide, dulaglutide, and semaglutide, are structurally similar to the endogenous human GLP-1 hormone. They have been engineered to have increased stability and resistance to DPP-4 degradation, leading to a prolonged effect on GLP-1Rs. All GLP-1 RAs are typically administered via subcutaneous injections, except for oral semaglutide, which is a recent development and can be taken orally. The subcutaneous injections are self-administered by patients and are usually given once daily or once weekly, depending on the specific medication.[9]

Semaglutide is indeed the first oral drug in the GLP-1 RA class approved for the treatment of T2DM. The PIONEER (Peptide Innovation for Early Diabetes Treatment) trial series, which evaluated the efficacy and safety of semaglutide, demonstrated its effectiveness in lowering HbA1c (a measure of long-term blood glucose control) and body weight compared to other antidiabetic drugs. Specifically, the PIONEER-6 trial included 3,183 patients with T2DM who were at high CVD risk. The trial showed that oral semaglutide was non-inferior to placebo in terms of reducing HbA1c levels (3.8% vs. 4.8%, respectively) with a hazard ratio (HR) of 0.79 and a 95% confidence interval (CI) of 0.57–1.11, indicating noninferiority. Importantly, oral semaglutide also resulted in a significant decrease in all-cause mortality (1.4% vs. 2.8% in the oral semaglutide and placebo groups, respectively), with an HR of 0.51 and a 95% CI of 0.31–0.84. Additionally, the use of oral semaglutide was associated with a reduction in systolic blood pressure, despite a slight increase in resting pulse rate. These findings highlight the benefits of oral semaglutide in terms of glycemic control, body weight reduction, CV risk reduction, and overall mortality. Semaglutide is indicated as adjunct therapy for glycemic control improvement in patients with T2DM and to reduce CV events in adults with T2DM at high CVD risk.[9] The advantages and disadvantages of semaglutide are detailed in **Table 2**.[7,9,10] Overall, GLP-1 RAs represent a widely used treatment option of T2DM with high glycemic efficacy through several mechanisms including enhancement of insulin secretion in a glucose dependent way, suppressing glucagon secretion, reducing appetite, and slowing gastric emptying. This class of medications typically does not cause hypoglycemia, unless combined with other agents.

Dipeptidyl Peptidase-4 Inhibitors

Dipeptidyl peptidase-4, found on endothelial cells and T-lymphocytes, acts as a serine protease that primarily inactivates GLP-1 and gastric inhibitory peptide (GIP), incretin hormones involved in insulin secretion, glucagon inhibition, and nutrient absorption. GLP-1 and GIP, known as incretins, play a crucial role in metabolic regulation. By inhibiting DPP-4, DPP-4 inhibitors serve as widely used oral hypoglycemic agents in the management of DM **(Fig. 6)**.[7,10] Common DPP-4 inhibitors include sitagliptin, linagliptin, saxagliptin, vildagliptin, and alogliptin. They can be used alone or in combination, resulting in a reduction of HbA1c by 0.48–0.6% and over 95% inhibition of DPP-4 activity for up to 12 hours, as demonstrated in studies.[7,13,14]

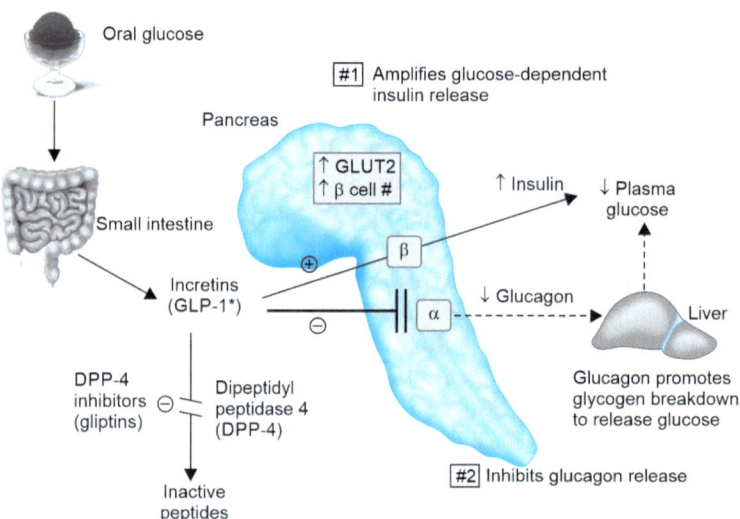

*Physiological t1/2 = 2 minutes due to rapid inactivation by DPP-4.
FIG. 6: Mechanism of action of DPP-4 inhibitors.[10]
(GLP-1: glucagon-like peptide-1; GLUT2: glucose transporter 2)

Dipeptidyl peptidase-4 inhibitors, unlike other antidiabetic agents, do not affect insulin sensitivity or secretion, resulting in no weight gain as an adverse effect. Sitagliptin, saxagliptin, and vildagliptin are renally excreted, requiring dose adjustment in diabetic patients with moderate-to-severe renal disease. In contrast, linagliptin is excreted through the enterohepatic system, making it suitable for use in renal impairment. Although DPP-4 inhibitors have minimal to no weight gain and a low risk of hypoglycemia, they may cause side effects such as nasopharyngitis, upper respiratory tract infections, and headaches. Prolonged use of these agents has been associated with pancreatitis and hepatic dysfunction.[7,9,10]

Dipeptidyl peptidase-4 inhibitors reduce HbA1c levels by approximately 0.5–1% and improve markers of insulin secretion and beta cell function. The beneficial effects of DPP-4 inhibitors persist for at least 2 years. They may also have a modest blood pressure-lowering effect (2–3 mm Hg) and decrease total cholesterol levels. CV outcome trials such as EXAMINE, SAVOR-TIMI 53, TECOS, and CARMELINA have demonstrated the CV safety of DPP-4 inhibitors. These agents are commonly used in clinical practice due to their favorable side effect profile and neutral CV effects **(Table 2)**. Linagliptin has shown renal benefits. However, the main obstacle to the use of DPP-4 inhibitors is their relatively high cost.[9]

Alpha-glucosidase Inhibitors

Acarbose and miglitol are two clinically available agents of the AGI class. These drugs inhibit the enzyme α-glucosidase, which is responsible for breaking down oligosaccharides into monosaccharides in the small intestine. By delaying carbohydrate digestion, they reduce intestinal glucose absorption, resulting in lower postprandial glucose and insulin levels. Recent studies have shown that AGIs also increase gut incretin levels and stimulate the release of GLP-1, further contributing to their HbA1c-lowering effects (0.5–0.8%). In Asia, AGIs are more commonly used as first-line therapy compared to the US. Acarbose has a unique indication for treating post-bariatric hypoglycemia in individuals who have undergone Roux-en-Y gastric bypass (RYGBP), as it helps stabilize glucose levels and prevent postprandial hypoglycemia.[7,9] Strong evidence supports the use of AGIs in reducing the progression from IGT to T2DM in patients with prediabetes. The STOP-NIDDM trial demonstrated that acarbose significantly lowers the risk of CV events by 49%, while the ACE trial showed neutral effects on major adverse CV events.[15-17] Flatulence, diarrhea, and abdominal pain are the major side effects associated with this class of drugs. The advantages and disadvantages of AGIs are summarized in **Table 2**.[7,9,10]

In conclusion, according to current treatment algorithms recommended by societies such as the American Diabetes Association (ADA) and the European Association for the Study of Diabetes (EASD), AGIs do not have a well-defined position. However, in Western populations, the literature indicates that these drugs may be considered for patients who are at risk of hypoglycemia or lactic acidosis, particularly when metformin or SUs are not preferred options.[9]

Sodium-glucose Cotransporter-2 Inhibitors

It is a newer class of antidiabetic medications, known as SGLT-2 inhibitors, was introduced clinically in 2013 with the approval of canagliflozin by the FDA.

These drugs work by targeting the renal SGLT-2 in the proximal renal tubules, which is responsible for glucose reabsorption **(Fig. 7)**.[7,10] Currently, three SGLT-2 inhibitors have been approved in the United States—dapagliflozin, empagliflozin, and canagliflozin. SGLT-2 inhibitors have demonstrated the ability to stimulate glucose excretion, leading to weight loss effects and minimal risk of hypoglycemia. Canagliflozin, for example, has shown a significant reduction in HbA1c levels ranging from 0.77 to 1.03%, and similar results have been observed with dapagliflozin in both short- and long-term treatments. Major cardiovascular outcome trials (CVOTs) have indicated that the CV benefits of SGLT-2 inhibitors may vary depending on the severity of CVD. For instance, the DECLARE-TIMI 58 trial, which enrolled a large number of patients without established CVD, showed a lower reduction in CV events. However, the CVD-REAL 2 study demonstrated a significant risk reduction in hospitalization for heart failure (hHF) and all-cause mortality in the SGLT-2 inhibitor treatment group among a large population of patients. SGLT-2 inhibitors have proven to be valuable antidiabetic drugs that not only reduce glucose levels but also improve cardiorenal outcomes in patients with T2DM. Empagliflozin and dapagliflozin are indicated for use in patients with HF with reduced ejection fraction (HFrEF), regardless of T2DM status. Empagliflozin is currently the only SGLT-2 inhibitor with an indication for use in patients with HF with preserved ejection fraction (HFpEF), irrespective of T2DM. Additionally, dapagliflozin is indicated for use in patients with CKD, with or without T2DM, while canagliflozin is indicated for T2DM patients with diabetic kidney disease. Based on the above evidence, current guidelines recommend initiating SGLT-2

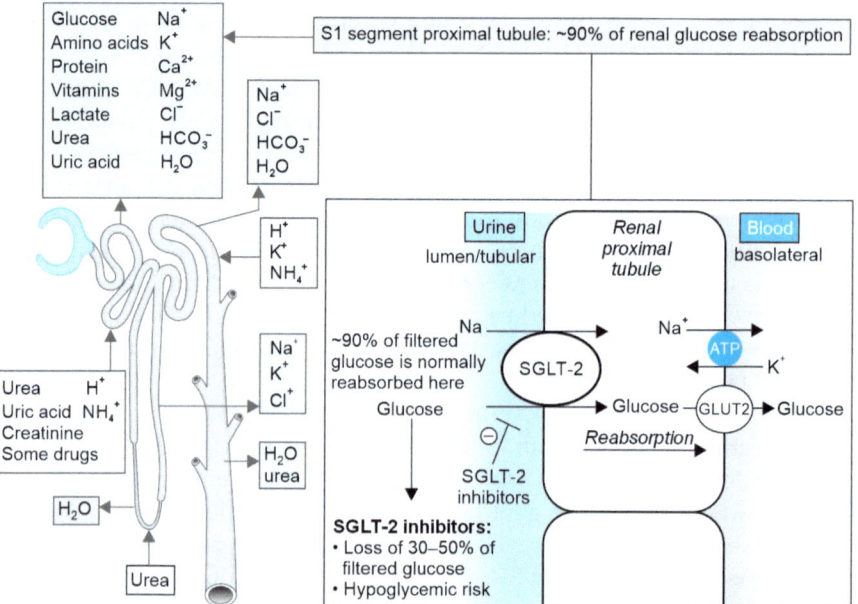

FIG. 7: Sodium-glucose cotransporter-2 (SGLT-2): Glucose is filtered by the renal glomeruli and is reabsorbed in the proximal tubule.[10]

(ATP: adenosine triphosphate; GLUT2: glucose transporter 2)

inhibitor treatment immediately upon the diagnosis of T2DM in patients with established cardiorenal disease or those at high CV risk. This recommendation is independent of baseline HbA1c levels, HbA1c targets, or metformin use **(Flowchart 1 and Table 2)**.[7,9,18]

Insulin Therapy

Insulin, first successfully used in 1922, revolutionized the prognosis of type 1 diabetes mellitus (T1DM) and remains the primary treatment for T1DM and many individuals with T2DM.[7] Over the past century, various types of insulin have been developed, categorized by their source (animal-derived, human insulins produced using recombinant deoxyribonucleic acid (DNA) technology, genetically modified insulin analogues), drug properties (basal, prandial, premixed), or route of administration (subcutaneous injection, inhaled). Insulin facilitates the uptake of peripheral glucose by skeletal muscle and fat, stimulates lipogenesis and protein synthesis, and inhibits lipolysis, proteolysis, hepatic glycogenolysis, and gluconeogenesis.[19] When lifestyle interventions and noninsulin agents (such as oral antidiabetic drugs and incretin therapies) fail to achieve adequate blood glucose control, insulin therapy becomes necessary. While the use of insulin in T2DM is uncommon for newly diagnosed patients, there are several situations where insulin is considered, including severe hyperglycemia, gestational diabetes, significant weight loss, and ketonuria.[20,21]

Insulin preparations are classified based on their onset and duration of action **(Table 3)**. This classification includes short-acting, intermediate-acting, and long-acting analogs. The distinct pharmacokinetic properties of these formulations determine the frequency of dosing and the appropriate timing of administration. Long-acting agents such as glargine and levemir are typically administered at bedtime to meet basal insulin requirements and are associated with a lower risk of hypoglycemia. Short-acting insulin preparations such as glulisine, aspart, and lispro are administered before meals to control postprandial spikes in glucose levels. Insulin regular is another formulation used in emergency situations.[19,22] Basal insulin is commonly the initial regimen added to current therapies, and if necessary, it can be intensified to a full basal-bolus insulin regimen. Adverse events associated with insulin therapy include dose-dependent hypoglycemia, which may necessitate dose reduction. The risk of hypoglycemia is higher in individuals with renal insufficiency, hypothyroidism, hypoadrenalism, as well as in elderly, thin individuals, and those with irregular food intake. Other potential adverse effects include weight gain, fluid retention, local injection site reactions (such as rash, pruritus, lipodystrophy), and hypokalemia.[23,24]

WEIGHT LOSS MEDICATIONS AND BARIATRIC SURGERY

To achieve and sustain weight reduction, clinical interventions encompass a range of approaches including behavior-based interventions, pharmacotherapy, and surgery. Behavior-based interventions focus on inducing lifestyle changes through various means such as dietary restriction, increased physical activity, and reducing sedentary behaviors. These interventions ideally combine information on safe physical activity and healthy eating with cognitive and behavior-based strategies

CHAPTER 7: Pharmacotherapy for Diabetes and Obesity

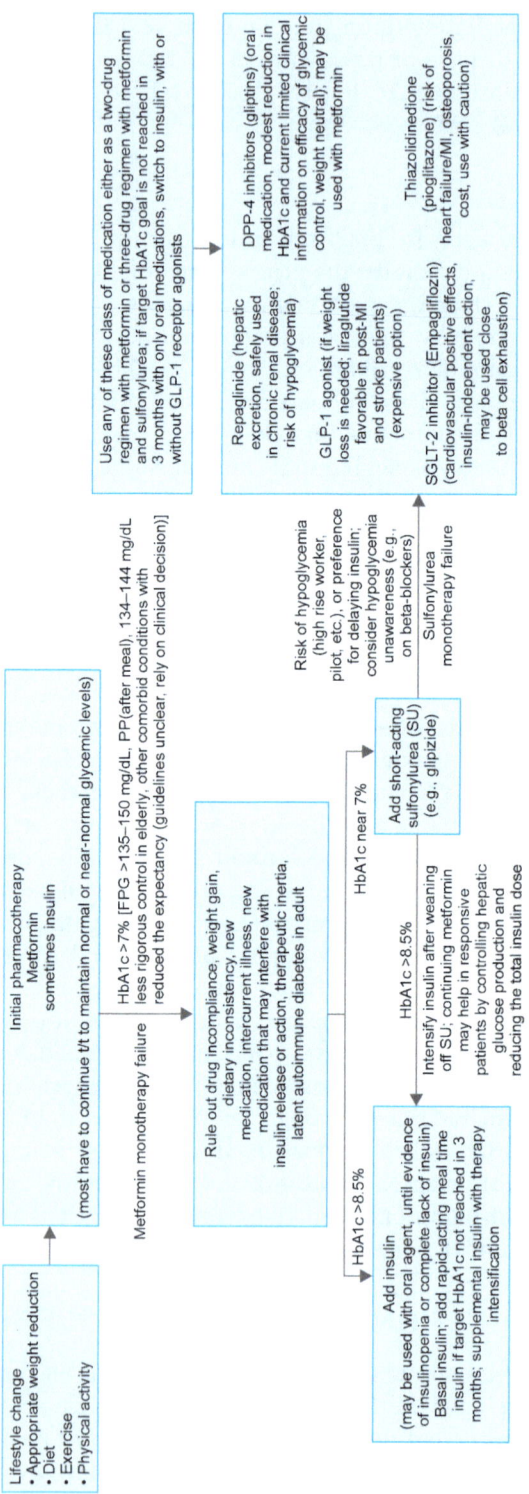

FLOWCHART 1: An algorithm for use of drug regimen in treating diabetes mellitus. *(For color version, see Plate 4)*

(DPP-4: dipeptidyl peptidase-4; GLP-1: glucagon-like peptide-1; HbA1C: glycated hemoglobin; SGLT-2: sodium-glucose cotransporter-2)

Note: Several concepts presented here are adapted from American Diabetes Association/European Association for the study of diabetes. Medication in green causes weight loss, in red causes weight gain.

TABLE 3: Types of insulin preparations and their pharmacokinetic profile.[7]

Insulin type	Onset of action (hours)	Peak of action (hours)	Duration of action (hours)	Maximal duration (hours)
Rapid-acting				
Lispro	1/4–1/2	1–2	3–5	4–6
Aspart	1/4–1/2	1–2	3–6	5–8
Glulisine	0.25–0.5	0.5–1	3–4	4
Short-acting				
Regular	1/2–1	2–4	3–6	6–8
Intermediate-acting				
NPH human	2–4	8–12	12–20	14–22
Long-acting				
Glargine	1–2	None	19–24	24
Detemir	3–4	6–8	20–24	24
Degludec	1	9	24–42	42
Insulin combinations				
Protamine/Lispro	0.25–0.4	0.5–3	14–24	24
Protamine/Aspart	0.1–0.2	1–4	18–24	24

to support participants in making and maintaining lifestyle changes. Behavior-based clinical interventions commonly employ techniques to promote behavior change. These may include facilitating goal setting, encouraging self-monitoring, evaluating the pros and cons of behaviors, emphasizing the health benefits associated with weight loss, and fostering social support. These interventions can be delivered through different formats, including individual counseling sessions conducted in person or remotely, group counseling sessions, technology-based modalities such as computer-based modules and smartphone applications, as well as text messages and print materials. Often, a combination of these formats is utilized to enhance the effectiveness of the interventions.[25]

Therapeutic interventions focused on lifestyle and diet changes have demonstrated modest outcomes in terms of weight loss. As a result, there is a growing interest in the development of drug therapies that can aid and facilitate weight loss. Pharmacotherapy in this context typically involves two approaches—enhancing satiety and suppressing hunger or increasing catabolism, which refers to the breakdown of molecules, including fats, and carbohydrates. These pharmacological interventions aim to regulate appetite and energy balance, ultimately supporting individuals in achieving their weight loss goals. By targeting physiological mechanisms related to hunger and satiety or metabolic processes, these medications can assist in controlling food intake, improving dietary adherence, and promoting a more efficient use of energy within the body. However, it is important to note that the effectiveness of pharmacotherapy for weight loss varies among individuals, and these medications are typically prescribed as part of a comprehensive weight management plan that includes lifestyle modifications and behavioral interventions.[26]

In the United States, there are several medications that have received approval for the treatment of obesity. These medications are intended to aid in weight loss and the maintenance of weight loss when used alongside a reduced calorie diet. The US Food and Drug Administration (USFDA) has established criteria to determine the effectiveness of drugs for obesity treatment. According to the FDA, a medication is considered effective for obesity treatment if it meets either of the following criteria:
- The average weight loss achieved with the medication is at least 5% greater than that observed in control groups.
- The proportion of individuals who lose at least 5% of their baseline body weight is at least 35% and approximately double the proportion seen in the control group.

These criteria serve as benchmarks to assess the efficacy of obesity medications and ensure that they provide significant weight loss benefits compared to control groups. It is important to note that these medications are intended to be used as part of a comprehensive weight management approach, which includes lifestyle modifications and dietary changes.[25] Currently seven major anti-obesity medications are approved by the USFDA **(Table 4)**. Apart from orlistat, liraglutide, and the recently approved semaglutide, the remaining approved medications primarily target CNS pathways that work to reduce appetite or enhance satiety. These drugs act on specific mechanisms in the brain to help regulate food intake and promote feelings of fullness, contributing to weight loss efforts. The therapeutic effects of these medications are centered around their influence on appetite control and satiety signaling, providing additional options for patients seeking pharmacological support in their weight management journey **(Fig. 8)**.[26,27] Weight loss medications are indicated for individuals with obesity who have an initial BMI ≥30 kg/m^2, or a BMI ≥27 kg/m^2 in the presence of other risk factors such as diabetes, dyslipidemia, or controlled hypertension. These medications can be considered as part of a comprehensive treatment approach to help individuals achieve weight loss and improve their overall health. It is important to evaluate each patient's specific medical condition and risk factors before prescribing weight loss medications to ensure their suitability and safety for the individual.[28-30]

In a meta-analysis conducted by Khera et al., the study examined the median percentages of participants achieving weight loss of at least 5% or 10% with five medications approved for long-term weight management. The analysis utilized a systematic review and network meta-analysis to compare weight loss outcomes and adverse events among different drug treatments for obesity. The study included randomized clinical trials involving overweight and obese adults who were treated with long-term weight loss agents approved by the USFDA (orlistat, lorcaserin, naltrexone-bupropion, phentermine-topiramate, or liraglutide) for a minimum duration of 1 year. These trials compared the efficacy of the active agents against either another active agent or a placebo. A total of 28 randomized clinical trials with 29,018 patients were included in the analysis. The findings demonstrated that all the active agents resulted in significant weight loss compared to placebo at the end of 1 year. Specifically, phentermine-topiramate showed a median excess weight loss of 8.8 kg, liraglutide 5.3 kg, naltrexone-bupropion 5.0 kg, lorcaserin 3.2 kg, and orlistat 2.6 kg. In terms of the percentage of participants achieving at least 5% weight loss, the results were as follows—placebo 23%, phentermine-topiramate 75% [odds ratio (OR) 9.22], liraglutide 63% (OR 5.54), naltrexone-bupropion 55%

TABLE 4: Overview of the Food and Drug Administration (FDA)/European Medicines Agency (EMA) approved pharmacotherapy options.[26,27,34]

Drug	Dose	Mean weight loss at ≥1 year, placebo-subtracted	Side effects	Precaution
Phentermine/Topiramate ER	• 3.75 mg/23 mg (14 days) • 7.5 mg/46 mg (thereafter)	9.8 kg	Insomnia, dizziness, paresthesia, depression, anxiety, and memory problems	Abrupt withdrawal of topiramate increases the risk of seizures
Naltrexone/Bupropion	32 mg/360 mg (achieved after 4 weeks)	4.4 kg	Nausea, constipation, headaches, vomiting, dizziness, and dry mouth	Not recommended for patients with seizures, drug addiction, bulimia, anorexia nervosa or in combination with opiates
Liraglutide	3.0 mg	5.3–5.9 kg	Nausea, diarrhea, constipation, vomiting, dyspepsia, and abdominal pain	Contraindicated in patients with a family or personal history of medullary thyroid carcinoma or with MEN2 syndrome (rats and mice developed thyroid C-cell carcinomas; unclear implication for humans)
Semaglutide	0.25 mg, and the dose is titrated every 4 weeks until reaching 2.4 mg	6.6–15.8 kg	Nausea, diarrhea, vomiting, constipation, abdominal pain, headache, fatigue, dyspepsia, dizziness, hypoglycemia for diabetic patients, flatulence, and gastroenteritis	Potential risk of thyroid C-cell tumors. It is contraindicated for patients with a personal or family history of medullary thyroid carcinoma or MEN2
Orlistat	120 mg TID	3.1 kg	Vitamin deficiency, steatorrhea, fecal urgency, and fecal incontinence	Daily multivitamin intake is recommended because of malabsorption of fat-soluble vitamins
Setmelanotide	NA	2.6 kg in MC4R deficiency, 51 and 20.5 kg in two patients with POMC deficiency	Injection site reactions, skin hyperpigmentation, headache, nausea, diarrhea, and abdominal pain	Approved for monogenic forms of obesity
Lorcaserin	10 mg twice a day	3.2 kg	• Without diabetes—headache, dizziness, fatigue, nausea, dry mouth, constipation • With diabetes—hypoglycemia, headache, back pain, fatigue	Pregnancy

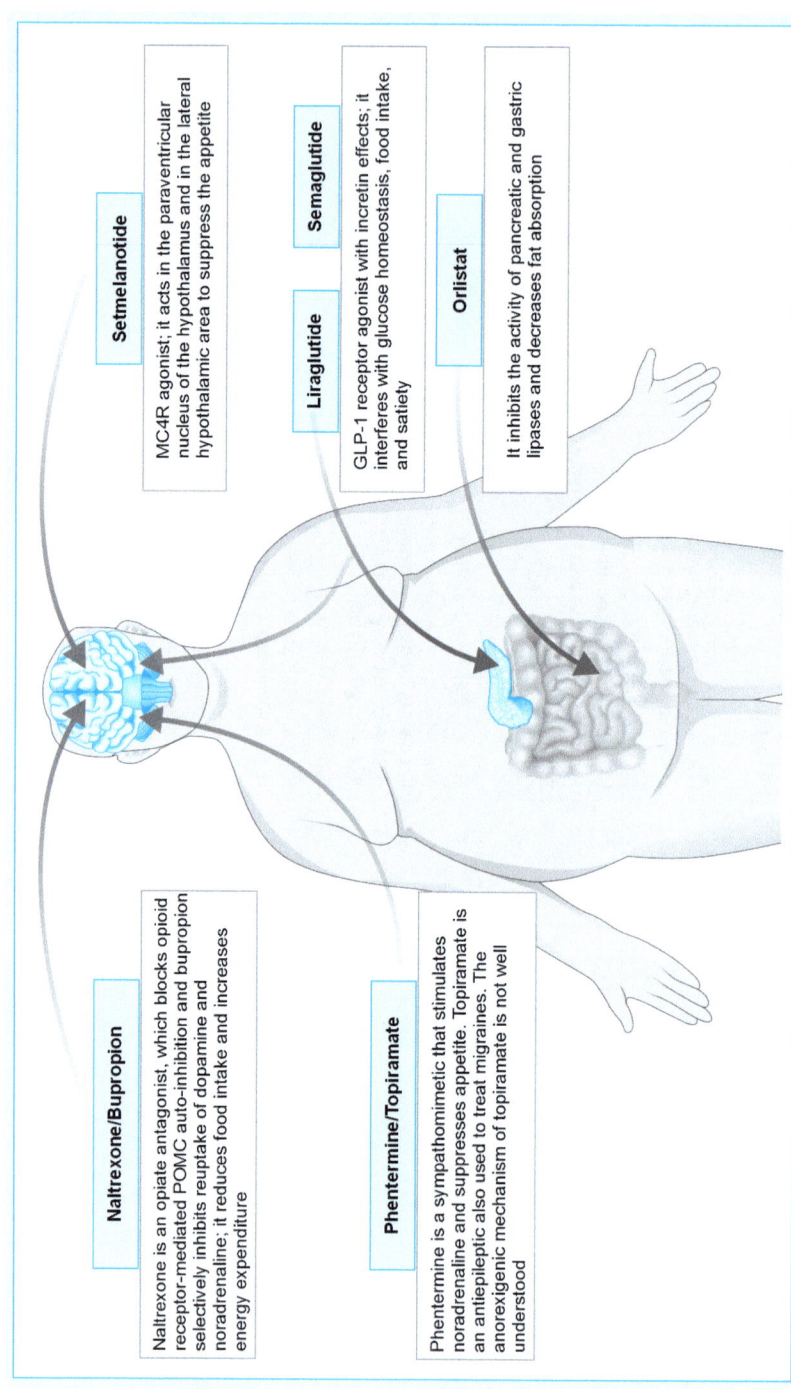

FIG. 8: Summary of the mechanism of action for Food and Drug Administration (FDA)/European Medicines Agency (EMA) approved antiobesity drugs.

(GLP-1: glucagon-like peptide-1; POMC: proopiomelanocortin)

(OR 3.96), lorcaserin 49% (OR 3.10), and orlistat 44% (OR 2.70). This meta-analysis provides valuable insights into the comparative effectiveness of these medications in promoting weight loss among individuals with obesity.[31]

Phentermine

Phentermine, initially approved in 1959 for individuals aged over 16 years, remains the most commonly prescribed anti-obesity medication in the USA and many other countries, except the European Union where it has limitations due to potential adverse effects. Functioning as a sympathomimetic amine, phentermine is known to suppress appetite and has a lower abuse potential compared to amphetamines, primarily due to its minimal release of dopamine. Its weight loss effects are believed to be mediated by the release of catecholamines in the hypothalamus, resulting in reduced appetite and decreased food consumption.[1]

Common treatment-emergent adverse events (TEAEs) associated with phentermine include dizziness, dry mouth, difficulty sleeping, irritability, nausea and/or vomiting, diarrhea, and constipation. Patients with CV disease, hyperthyroidism, glaucoma, a history of drug abuse, or those who are pregnant should not be prescribed phentermine due to contraindications.[1]

The recommended dosage of phentermine is 15–37.5 mg orally once daily, taken 1–2 hours before breakfast. It is important to avoid prescribing phentermine later in the evening to minimize the risk of insomnia. Dosage adjustments should be individualized to achieve an optimal treatment response with the lowest effective dose. In cases where the short-acting effect is preferred, the 8-mg formulation of phentermine can be administered orally two or three times daily, at least 30 minutes before meals.[1]

Orlistat

Orlistat is indicated for weight loss when used in combination with a reduced-calorie diet. Its mechanism of action involves inhibiting the activity of pancreatic and gastric lipases, leading to a reduction in fat absorption by approximately 30%.

The most commonly reported TEAEs associated with orlistat, occurring with an incidence of 5% or more and at least twice that of placebo, include flatulence, oily spotting, fecal urgency, fatty/oily stool, oily defecation, increased defecation, and fecal incontinence. Additionally, there have been reports of other adverse effects such as nephrotoxicity, hepatotoxicity, nephrolithiasis, and pancreatitis.

Orlistat is available in two formulations—a non-prescription, over-the-counter version with a lower dose of 60 mg, and a prescription-strength formulation of 120 mg. Both formulations are taken orally three times a day according to the recommended dosage.[1,32]

Phentermine and Topiramate Extended-release

The precise anorexigenic mechanism of topiramate is not fully understood, but it is believed to involve the modulation of various neurotransmitters. This includes the inhibition of voltage-dependent sodium channels, glutamate receptors, and carbonic anhydrase, as well as the potentiation of γ-aminobutyrate activity.

Topiramate has received FDA approval for the treatment of seizures since 1996 and for migraine prevention since 2004. When combined with low doses of phentermine in a slow-release or ER capsule, known as phentermine and topiramate ER, it has shown superior weight loss efficacy compared to either drug used alone, with fewer side effects. While phentermine-topiramate ER is associated with several side effects, the primary concern is the potential risk of oral clefts in infants exposed to topiramate during pregnancy. Therefore, women of childbearing age using this drug combination should employ reliable contraception and undergo regular monitoring to ensure they do not become pregnant. Additionally, although rare, topiramate has been linked to the development of acute angle-closure glaucoma.

Phentermine-topiramate ER is considered the most effective anti-obesity medication currently available. Although topiramate itself is not classified as a controlled substance, the inclusion of phentermine places the drug combination under the Schedule IV Controlled Substances Act. Phentermine/topiramate ER is taken once daily in the morning, with or without food. It requires gradual titration, starting with an initial dose of 3.75/23 mg once daily for 14 days, followed by an increase to 7.5/46 mg daily. Further dosage escalation to 11.25/69 mg and then to 15/92 mg is recommended for nonresponders who have achieved <3% weight loss at 12 weeks on the middle dose (7.5/46 mg) or <5% weight loss at 12 weeks on the maximum dose (15/92 mg). To mitigate the increased risk of seizures associated with abrupt topiramate withdrawal, a gradual downward titration over 3–5 days is recommended.[1,32]

Lorcaserin

Lorcaserin was specifically developed as an agonist of the serotonin 2C receptor, which is primarily found in the brain. This selectivity minimizes the risk of valvular heart disease associated with other weight loss medications. In 2016, the FDA approved an ER formulation of lorcaserin, which is taken once daily at a dose of 20 mg.

The most commonly reported adverse effects, occurring in >2% of patients without DM and more frequently than in those on placebo, include headache, dizziness, fatigue, nausea, dry mouth, and constipation. In patients with DM taking lorcaserin, the most commonly reported adverse effects include hypoglycemia (blood glucose levels <65 mg/dL), headache, back pain, nasopharyngitis, cough, and fatigue.

Lorcaserin should be taken orally at a dose of 10 mg twice daily or as a once-daily 20 mg ER formulation, with or without food. If a weight loss of less than 5% is achieved after 12 weeks of treatment, lorcaserin should be discontinued. It is important to note that lorcaserin should not be taken in combination with other drugs belonging to the serotonin class, as this may increase the risk of developing a condition resembling neuroleptic malignant syndrome.[1,32]

Naltrexone Sustained-release/Bupropion Sustained-release

Bupropion was originally approved by the FDA in 1985 for the treatment of depression and continues to be widely prescribed as an antidepressant. Unlike many other antidepressants, bupropion is associated with minimal weight gain. Additionally, it has received approval for smoking cessation therapy. Naltrexone, on the other hand, was approved by the FDA in 1984 for the treatment of opioid dependence and alcohol dependence.

The combination of naltrexone SR and bupropion SR, known as NB, has shown synergistic effects in preclinical animal models. This combination enhances the activity of pro-opiomelanocortin (POMC), resulting in reduced food intake and increased satiety. Naltrexone acts by blocking opioid receptor-mediated POMC auto-inhibition, while bupropion selectively inhibits the reuptake of dopamine and noradrenaline.

During the initial 3-week period of dose escalation, transient nausea is the most commonly reported adverse effect, affecting approximately one-third of patients. Other adverse events reported with an incidence of at least 2% among patients treated with NB, compared to those on placebo, include nausea, constipation, headaches, vomiting, dizziness, and dry mouth.

The current formulation of NB consists of 8 mg of naltrexone SR and 90 mg of bupropion in a combined dose. The dosage is gradually increased over a 4-week period. The recommended titration schedule involves taking one tablet once daily in the morning during the first week, one tablet twice daily during the second week, two tablets in the morning and one tablet in the evening during the third week, and finally, two tablets twice daily during the fourth week.[1,32]

Liraglutide

Liraglutide 3 mg has received approval as an anti-obesity medication in the United States, the European Union, and Australia. It belongs to the class of GLP-1 RAs, which are derived from incretin hormones. Liraglutide acts on both peripheral and central receptor pathways, affecting glucose homeostasis, food intake, and satiety. Due to its incretin properties, it is particularly beneficial for patients with T2DM and obesity. Notably, liraglutide is the only injectable anti-obesity drug available, while all others are taken orally.

The most commonly reported TEAEs across the clinical trials were primarily gastrointestinal in nature, including nausea, diarrhea, constipation, vomiting, dyspepsia, and abdominal pain. These side effects were generally transient and of mild-to-moderate intensity. In the past, there have been spontaneous post-marketing reports linking liraglutide, an incretin-based agent, to pancreatitis.

Liraglutide is administered via subcutaneous injection once daily. The dosage is gradually titrated over a period of 5 weeks, reaching a final dose of 3.0 mg. Additionally, liraglutide provides particular benefits for patients with T2DM or those with severe insulin resistance.[1,32]

Semaglutide

Semaglutide is a human glucagon-like peptide 1 (GLP-1) analogue that shares 94% structural similarity with native human GLP-1. It has been modified to enhance its stability and prolong its half-life for once-weekly administration. An amino acid substitution at position 8 makes semaglutide less susceptible to degradation by

DPP-4, and acylation of the peptide backbone with a spacer and C-18 fatty di-acid chain allows specific binding to albumin.

One of the unique features of semaglutide is its ability to directly access the brainstem, septal nucleus, and hypothalamus. It interacts with the brain through the circumventricular organs and adjacent sites near the ventricles. This direct interaction in the CNS contributes to its effects on appetite suppression, reduction in food cravings, improved control of eating, and decreased preference for fatty, energy-dense foods.

Gastrointestinal disorders, including nausea, constipation, and diarrhea, were the most frequently reported adverse effects in participants receiving both semaglutide and liraglutide. Approximately 84.1% of participants receiving semaglutide and 82.7% receiving liraglutide reported gastrointestinal disorders, compared to 55.3% in the placebo group. The contraindications for semaglutide use are the same as those for liraglutide and other GLP-1 analogs.

The recommended starting dose of semaglutide is 0.25 mg, and the dose is titrated every 4 weeks until reaching 2.4 mg, typically within a span of approximately 16 weeks. This gradual titration allows for individualized dosing and helps manage potential side effects during the adjustment period.[33,34]

COMBINATION THERAPY AND NOVEL APPROACHES

Combination therapies for obesity offer the advantage of targeting different mechanisms involved in weight management. Several examples highlight the benefits of combining different components in pharmacotherapy. In human studies, the combination of pramlintide and phentermine demonstrated superior results compared to pramlintide alone. Over a 24-week period, the combination therapy led to an average reduction in body weight of approximately 10.5%, whereas pramlintide alone resulted in a mean reduction of only about 2.5%. Rodent models have also shown interactive effects on food intake and body weight when combining amylin with bupropion-naltrexone. This suggests that the combined therapy can have a synergistic impact on weight management. Another example involves patients with T2DM. Combining exenatide once weekly (a GLP-1 RA) with daily dapagliflozin (an SGLT-2 inhibitor) resulted in significantly greater weight loss compared to using either treatment individually. Over a 28-week period, patients receiving the combination therapy experienced an average weight loss of 3.55 kg, whereas weight loss with daily dapagliflozin alone was 2.0 kg and with exenatide once weekly alone was 1.5 kg. These findings were sustained over a year of treatment. The sustained weight loss observed over a year emphasizes the importance of long-term weight management when evaluating the effectiveness of combination therapies compared to single therapies. This highlights the potential utility of combination therapies in achieving and maintaining weight loss goals.[35]

Tesofensine (with metoprolol): Tesofensine is a medication that acts as a presynaptic uptake inhibitor of noradrenaline, dopamine, and serotonin. In a phase II clinical trial involving 203 obese patients with a BMI between 30 and ≤40 kg/m², tesofensine was evaluated as an adjunct to an energy-restricted diet. The trial was randomized, double-blind, and placebo-controlled, with a treatment duration of 24 weeks. Participants in the trial were divided into two groups—one receiving tesofensine at doses ranging from 0.25 to 1.0 mg once daily, and the other receiving a placebo. Common side effects reported in both groups included nausea, dizziness, and headache. However, these side effects were more frequently reported in the group receiving the active treatment. In addition to its potential for obesity treatment, there is ongoing development of a combination product containing tesofensine 0.25 mg and metoprolol 50 mg for the treatment of Prader–Willi syndrome and other hypothalamic obesities. Prader–Willi syndrome is a genetic disorder associated with obesity and various other symptoms, and tesofensine combined with metoprolol is being investigated as a potential treatment option for individuals with this condition.[33]

Amylin + Semaglutide: A phase 1 trial has assessed the combination of cagrilintide, an amylin analogue, and semaglutide. The combination is thought to have enhanced or synergistic efficacy due to two complementary mechanisms—appetite reduction through the activation of hypothalamic homeostatic pathways and modulation of meal-generated signals via the hindbrain.[33]

Gut peptide hormone co-agonists: Peptide multi-agonists are being developed based on the understanding that gut endocrine cells produce multiple hormones involved in regulating glucose metabolism and appetite. These hormones include proglucagon and its cleavage products GLP-1, glucagon, oxyntomodulin, as well as peptide tyrosine tyrosine (PYY) and GIP. These compounds, also known as co-agonists, aim to target multiple pathways simultaneously. Examples of such co-agonists in development include GLP-1/GIP, GLP-1/glucagon, and GLP-1/GIP/glucagon agonists. However, designing these compounds to achieve optimal ratios for both efficacy and safety poses a significant challenge in drug development.[33]

GIP/GLP-1 co-agonists: Tirzepatide is an innovative GIP/GLP-1 co-agonist, distinguished as the first of its kind. It is composed of a 39 amino acid peptide linked to a fatty acid, enabling it to effectively bind to both GIP and GLP-1 receptors. Its binding potency to GIP receptors is 5, while to GLP-1 receptors it is 1. The formulation of tirzepatide allows for convenient once-weekly administration through a single dose injection device. However, it is worth noting that subjects receiving the highest dose of tirzepatide commonly reported gastrointestinal side effects, leading to withdrawal from treatment.[33]

GLP-1/glucagon/GIP tri-agonists: Tri-agonists that simultaneously target the GLP-1, glucagon, and GIP receptors have been developed with the aim of augmenting weight loss and improving glycemic control. The rationale behind these tri-agonists is to harness the combined effects of all three gut hormone receptors in order to achieve enhanced therapeutic outcomes.[33]

In the realm of medical advancements this year, a notable breakthrough emerged during the 83rd Annual Scientific Sessions of the ADA meeting. Subsequently, significant findings from phase II clinical trials of retatrutide, a novel GIP/GLP-1 and glucagon receptor agonist, were published in prestigious medical journals. Notably, earlier phase I trials also yielded highly promising results.[36]

The diabetes-focused study encompassed a cohort of 281 individuals grappling with T2DM, who were subjected to a random allocation of varying doses of retatrutide (ranging from 0.5 to 12 mg), a 1.5 mg dosage of dulaglutide (an established diabetes medication), or a placebo over a span of 36 weeks. Strikingly, the group administered 4 mg to 12 mg of retatrutide exhibited a substantial reduction in HbA1c levels, ranging from 1.3 to 2.0%, after approximately 6 months. This is in stark contrast to the placebo group, which displayed negligible changes, and dulaglutide, which led to a 1.4% reduction in HbA1c levels. Furthermore, participants who received retatrutide experienced significant weight loss, with the 12 mg dosage group achieving an average weight reduction of 16.9%, equivalent to approximately 17.2 kg. In contrast, the placebo group saw a mere 3.0% reduction, amounting to around 3.3 kg. Encouragingly, retatrutide demonstrated an overall safety and tolerability profile that aligns with established incretin-based therapies like dulaglutide.[37]

Simultaneously, in the study addressing obesity, 388 participants afflicted with obesity, but without diabetes, received various dosages of retatrutide (ranging from 1 to 12 mg) over a duration of 48 weeks. Notably, those administered the two highest dosages experienced remarkable weight loss, exceeding 24% of their total body weight. Impressively, all participants achieved a minimum of 5% reduction in their body weight.[38]

These findings underscore the significant promise of retatrutide as a potential therapeutic option for both diabetes and obesity. Its ability to effectively lower HbA1c levels and induce substantial weight loss in study participants signifies its potential as an innovative treatment approach. However, further extensive research, including larger clinical trials, will be imperative to validate its long-term safety and efficacy, with the ultimate goal of introducing it as a groundbreaking treatment for these conditions.

New Targets in Preclinical or Phase 1 Development

The development of anti-obesity drugs based on the orexigenic hormone ghrelin highlights the complexities involved. One approach involves the addition of a fatty acid to the ghrelin peptide using ghrelin O-acyltransferase to activate the hormone. Another avenue of exploration focuses on ghrelin receptor antagonists, although limited information is currently available on their effectiveness. Various strategies such as vaccines targeting ghrelin (e.g., NOX-B11), ghrelin-neutralizing molecules, and inhibitors of ghrelin O-acyltransferase have been developed and tested, but with modest reported effects thus far. In addition, fibroblast growth factor 21 (FGF21) has shown potential in enhancing insulin sensitivity and promoting beneficial changes in adipose tissue in animal studies. The FGF21 analogue LY240531985 has demonstrated positive effects on lipid concentrations, glucose metabolism, and body weight in early clinical trials. Setmelanotide, an MC4R agonist, has shown weight loss benefits in a phase 2 study involving two patients with POMC deficiency. However, a common pattern has emerged in the development of new candidate drugs for obesity treatment. Promising targets are identified through basic research, molecules are discovered to modulate these targets, and successful animal studies are conducted. Yet, progress often stalls during initial human studies, and many potential drugs fail to progress further. The dwindling number of randomized controlled trials for weight-loss drugs in recent years reflects the challenges faced in the field of anti-obesity drug development, with fewer studies being published and progress being limited.[32]

WEIGHT IMPACT OF ENDOCRINOTROPIC DRUGS

Many medications used to address comorbidities exert an endocrinotropic effect, influencing the endocrine system and potentially contributing to hyperglycemia and subsequently T2DM, dyslipidemia, as well as body fat redistribution favoring central and visceral obesity, sometimes accompanied by subcutaneous fat atrophy (lipodystrophy), non-alcoholic steatohepatitis (NASH), and metabolic syndrome. While managing coexisting conditions in the pre- and post-bariatric surgery phases, healthcare providers should carefully select long-term medications while considering the potential for weight gain. Medications commonly associated with weight gain include antipsychotics, antidiabetics, antihypertensives, antidepressants, and antihistaminics. Preference should be given to medications for comorbid conditions that are either weight-neutral or promote weight loss as a side effect, as indicated in **Table 5**. It is essential to note that medications prescribed for their weight-loss effects should not be used solely for weight reduction purposes **(Fig. 9)**.[39]

TABLE 5: Medications action on weight profile.[39]

Medications	Weight profile
Antidiabetic	• GLP-1 analogs (e.g., exenatide, albiglutide, dulaglutide, semaglutide, and liraglutide) or SGLT-2 inhibitors (dapagliflozin, empagliflozin, and canagliflozin) promote weight loss • Basal insulin causes less weight gain than other insulin types
Antihypertensives	Angiotensin-converting enzyme (ACE) inhibitors, angiotensin receptor blockers (ARBs), and calcium channel blockers should be preferred over β-adrenergic blockers which cause weight gain
Antidepressants	• Paroxetine, amitriptyline, mirtazapine, and nortriptyline are linked to weight gain • Bupropion causes weight loss
Antipsychotics	Clozapine and olanzapine have a greater likelihood for weight gain, while ziprasidone appears to have the lowest risk for weight gain
Antiepileptics	Felbamate, topiramate, and zonisamide may be preferred over other antiepileptics as they cause weight loss
Antihistamines	Choose one with less sedation
Antiretroviral	Most antiretrovirals cause weight gain, weight monitoring is important
(GLP-1: glucagon-like peptide-1; SGLT-2: sodium-glucose cotransporter-2)	

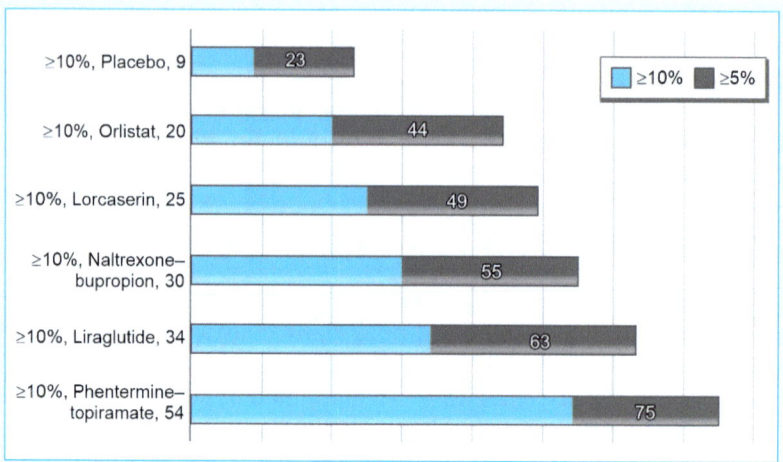

FIG. 9: Weight loss at 1 year with pharmacotherapy combined with low-to-moderate intensity lifestyle counseling.

REFERENCES

1. Srivastava G, Apovian CM. Current pharmacotherapy for obesity. Nat Rev Endocrinol. 2018;14(1):12-24.
2. Saunders KH, Umashanker D, Igel LI, Kumar RB, Aronne LJ. Obesity pharmacotherapy. Med Clin North Am. 2018;102(1):135-48.
3. Heymsfield SB, Wadden TA. Mechanisms, pathophysiology, and management of obesity. N Engl J Med. 2017;376(3):254-66.
4. Majety P, Lozada Orquera FA, Edem D, Hamdy O. Pharmacological approaches to the prevention of type 2 diabetes mellitus. Front Endocrinol (Lausanne). 2023;14:1118848.
5. Thrasher J. Pharmacologic management of type 2 diabetes mellitus: available therapies. Am J Cardiol. 2017;120(1S):S4-16.
6. Dallavalasa S, Tulimilli SV, Prakash J, Ramachandra R, Madhunapantula SV, Veeranna RP. COVID-19: Diabetes perspective-pathophysiology and management. Pathogens. 2023;12(2):184.
7. Mahgoub MO, Ali II, Adeghate JO, Tekes K, Kalász H, Adeghate EA. An update on the molecular and cellular basis of pharmacotherapy in type 2 diabetes mellitus. Int J Mol Sci. 2023;24(11):9328.
8. Artasensi A, Mazzolari A, Pedretti A, Vistoli G, Fumagalli L. Obesity and type 2 diabetes: adiposopathy as a triggering factor and therapeutic options. molecules. 2023;28(7):3094.
9. DeMarsilis A, Reddy N, Boutari C, Filippaios A, Sternthal E, Katsiki N, et al. Pharmacotherapy of type 2 diabetes: An update and future directions. Metabolism. 2022;137:155332.
10. TUSOM Pharmwiki. (2023). Treatment of diabetes. [online] Available from https://tmedweb.tulane.edu/pharmwiki/doku.php/rx_of_diabetes [Last accessed October, 2023].
11. Alhadramy MS. Diabetes and oral therapies. J Taibah Univ Med Sci. 2016;11(4):317-29.
12. Schramm TK, Gislason GH, Vaag A, Rasmussen JN, Folke F, Hansen ML, et al. Mortality and CV risk associated with different insulin secretagogues compared with metformin in type 2 diabetes, with or without a previous myocardial infarction: a nationwide study [published correction appears in Eur Heart J. 2012 May;33(10):1183]. Eur Heart J. 2011;32(15):1900-08.
13. Lotfy M, Singh J, Kalász H, Tekes K, Adeghate E. Medicinal chemistry and applications of incretins and DPP-4 Inhibitors in the treatment of type 2 diabetes mellitus. Open Med Chem J. 2011;5(Suppl 2):82-92.
14. Ishii H, Hayashino Y, Akai Y, Yabuta M, Tsujii S. Dipeptidyl peptidase-4 inhibitors as preferable oral hypoglycemic agents in terms of treatment satisfaction: Results from a multicenter, 12-week, open label, randomized controlled study in Japan (PREFERENCE 4 study). J Diabetes Investig. 2018;9(1):137-45.
15. Coleman RL, Scott CAB, Lang Z, Bethel MA, Tuomilehto J, Holman RR. Meta-analysis of the impact of alpha-glucosidase inhibitors on incident diabetes and cardiovascular outcomes. Cardiovasc Diabetol. 2019;18(1):135.

16. Chiasson JL, Josse RG, Gomis R, Hanefeld M, Karasik A, Laakso M, et al. Acarbose treatment and the risk of cardiovascular disease and hypertension in patients with impaired glucose tolerance: the STOP-NIDDM trial. JAMA. 2003;290(4):486-94.
17. Holman RR, Coleman RL, Chan JCN, Chiasson JL, Feng H, Ge J, et al. Effects of acarbose on cardiovascular and diabetes outcomes in patients with coronary heart disease and impaired glucose tolerance (ACE): a randomised, double-blind, placebo-controlled trial. Lancet Diabetes Endocrinol. 2017;5(11):877-86.
18. Chaudhury A, Duvoor C, Reddy Dendi VS, Kraleti S, Chada A, Ravilla R, et al. Clinical Review of Antidiabetic Drugs: Implications for Type 2 Diabetes Mellitus Management. Front Endocrinol (Lausanne). 2017;8:6.
19. Cheng AYY, Patel DK, Reid TS, Wyne K. Differentiating basal insulin preparations: Understanding how they work explains why they are different. Adv Ther. 2019;36(5):1018-30.
20. American Diabetes Association Professional Practice Committee. 9. Pharmacologic approaches to glycemic treatment: Standards of Medical Care in diabetes-2022. Diabetes Care. 2022;45(Suppl 1):S125-43.
21. Cheng AYY, Wong J, Freemantle N, Acharya SH, Ekinci E. The safety and efficacy of second-generation basal insulin analogues in adults with type 2 diabetes at risk of hypoglycemia and use in other special populations: A narrative review. Diabetes Ther. 2020;11(11):2555-93.
22. Chawla R, Makkar BM, Aggarwal S, Bajaj S, Das AK, Ghosh S, et al. RSSDI consensus recommendations on insulin therapy in the management of diabetes. Int J Diabetes Dev Ctries. 2019;39(S2):43-92.
23. Meneghini LF. Insulin therapy for type 2 diabetes. Endocrine. 2013;43(3):529-34.
24. Davies MJ, D'Alessio DA, Fradkin J, Kernan WN, Mathieu C, Mingrone G, et al. Management of hyperglycemia in type 2 diabetes, 2018. A consensus report by the American Diabetes Association (ADA) and the European Association for the Study of diabetes (EASD). Diabetes Care. 2018;41(12):2669-2701.
25. LeBlanc EL, Patnode CD, Webber EM, Redmond N, Rushkin M, O'Connor EA. Behavioral and pharmacotherapy weight loss interventions to prevent obesity-related morbidity and mortality in adults: an updated systematic review for the U.S. Preventive Services Task Force. JAMA. 2018;320(11):1172-91.
26. Gjermeni E, Kirstein AS, Kolbig F, Kirchhof M, Bundalian L, Katzmann JL, et al. Obesity-An Update on the Basic Pathophysiology and Review of Recent Therapeutic Advances. Biomolecules. 2021;11(10):1426.
27. Lee SJ, Shin SW. Mechanisms, pathophysiology, and management of obesity. N Engl J Med. 2017;376(15):1491-2.
28. Jensen MD, Ryan DH, Apovian CM, Ard JD, Comuzzie AG, Donato KA, et al. 2013 AHA/ACC/TOS guideline for the management of overweight and obesity in adults: a report of the American College of Cardiology/American Heart Association Task Force on Practice Guidelines and The Obesity Society [published correction appears in J Am Coll Cardiol. 2014 Jul 1;63(25 Pt B):3029-3030]. J Am Coll Cardiol. 2014;63(25 Pt B):2985-3023.
29. Yumuk V, Tsigos C, Fried M, Schindler K, Busetto L, Micic D, et al. European Guidelines for Obesity Management in Adults [published correction appears in Obes Facts. 2016;9(1):64]. Obes Facts. 2015;8(6):402-24.
30. Markovic TP, Proietto J, Dixon JB, Rigas G, Deed G, Hamdorf JM, et al. The Australian Obesity Management Algorithm: A simple tool to guide the management of obesity in primary care. Obes Res Clin Pract. 2022;16(5):353-63.
31. Khera R, Murad MH, Chandar AK, Dulai PS, Wang Z, Prokop LJ, et al. Association of Pharmacological Treatments for Obesity With Weight Loss and Adverse Events: A Systematic Review and Meta-analysis [published correction appears in JAMA. 2016;316(9):995]. JAMA. 2016;315(22):2424-34.
32. Bessesen DH, Van Gaal LF. Progress and challenges in anti-obesity pharmacotherapy. Lancet Diabetes Endocrinol. 2018;6(3):237-48.
33. Finer N. Future directions in obesity pharmacotherapy. Eur J Intern Med. 2021;93:13-20.
34. Telci Caklili O, Cesur M, Mikhailidis DP, Rizzo M. Novel anti-obesity therapies and their different effects and safety profiles: a critical overview. Diabetes Metab Syndr Obes. 2023;16:1767-74.
35. Camilleri M, Acosta A. Combination therapies for obesity. Metab Syndr Relat Disord. 2018;16(8):390-4.
36. Urva S, Coskun T, Loh MT, Du Y, Thomas MK, Gurbuz S, et al. LY3437943, a novel triple GIP, GLP-1, and glucagon receptor agonist in people with type 2 diabetes: a phase 1b, multicentre, double-blind, placebo-controlled, randomised, multiple-ascending dose trial. Lancet. 2022;400(10366):1869-81.
37. Rosenstock J, Frias J, Jastreboff AM, Du Y, Lou J, Gurbuz S, et al. Retatrutide, a GIP, GLP-1 and glucagon receptor agonist, for people with type 2 diabetes: a randomised, double-blind, placebo and active-controlled, parallel-group, phase 2 trial conducted in the USA. Lancet. 2023;402(10401):529-44.
38. Jastreboff AM, Kaplan LM, Frías JP, Wu Q, Du Y, Gurbuz S, et al. Triple-hormone-receptor agonist retatrutide for obesity - a phase 2 trial. N Engl J Med. 2023;389(6):514-26.
39. Kalra S, Kapoor N, Bhattacharya S, Aydin H, Coetzee A. Barocrinology: the endocrinology of obesity from bench to bedside. Med Sci (Basel). 2020;8(4):51.

CHAPTER

8

Management of Diabetes and Obesity Complications

Key Highlights

- Liraglutide, a glucagon-like peptide-1 receptor agonist (GLP-1 RA), has shown improvements in cardiovascular risk factors and type 2 diabetes mellitus (T2DM) risk.
- Sodium-glucose cotransporter-2 inhibitors (SGLT-2is) have demonstrated remarkable benefits in individuals with T2DM and established cardiovascular disease (CVD) or risk factors for CVD, particularly in the prevention of heart failure.
- First-line therapy for painful neuropathy recommendations from major guidelines strongly endorse three drug classes—(i) tricyclic antidepressants (especially amitriptyline), (ii) serotonin-norepinephrine reuptake inhibitors (SNRIs) like duloxetine, and (iii) calcium channel alpha-2-delta ligands such as gabapentin and pregabalin.
- The lifestyle changes with metformin are preferred in diabetes patients with diabetic kidney disease (DKD) whereas in managing blood pressure angiotensin-converting enzyme (ACE) inhibitors and angiotensin receptor blockers (ARBs) are recommended. Statins especially atorvastatin recommended in management of lipid profile in these patients.
- A panel of international experts proposed a new term, metabolic dysfunction-associated fatty liver disease (MAFLD), to better encompass the underlying mechanisms involved.
- Medications for MAFLD commonly used for cardiovascular risk reduction and renoprotection in T2DM, such as statins and renin–angiotensin system (RAS) blocking drugs, may have additional anti-fibrotic properties.
- Use pharmacotherapy such as slow-acting drugs for osteoarthritis when necessary.
- Consider advanced pharmacotherapy options for osteoarthritis like nonsteroidal anti-inflammatory drugs (NSAIDs) or intraarticular injections if initial treatments are ineffective.
- Consider positive airway pressure (PAP) therapy as the primary treatment for symptomatic obstructive sleep apnea (OSA).

INTRODUCTION

Obesity-related Complications and Prevalence

According to the World Health Organization (WHO), the prevalence of obesity has nearly tripled between 1975 and 2016.[1] In 2016, there were over 1.9 billion overweight adults aged 18 years and older, with >650 million of them being obese.[1] If current trends continue, it is projected that by 2025, there will be approximately 2.7 billion overweight adults, over 1 billion obese adults, and 177 million severely obese adults.[2]

Based on the analysis of the Global Burden of Disease (GBD) Study 2019, the estimated disability-adjusted life year (DALY) figures related to obesity were 1933 (95% UI 1277–2640).[3] From 2000 to 2019, obesity-related DALYs increased by an average of 0.48% per year and are predicted to rise by 39.8% from 2020 to 2030. The Eastern Mediterranean region and countries with middle socio-demographic indexes experienced the highest burden of obesity-related DALYs.[3] The healthcare system has faced significant financial implications due to obesity.[4] Its increasing prevalence has led to the development of various medical complications, including type 2 diabetes mellitus (T2DM), hypertension, dementia, nonalcoholic fatty liver disease (NAFLD), polycystic ovarian syndrome (PCOS), dyslipidemia, and cancer.

Obesity has also been linked to increased mortality rates, with nearly one in five deaths attributed to obesity, a number three times higher than previous estimates.[5] The obesity epidemic poses a threat to the progress made in life expectancy over the past century, particularly in high-income countries. Recent studies have shown that the impact of obesity on mortality rates is greater in individuals born more recently.[5] In the United States alone, the estimated annual number of deaths attributed to obesity exceeds 280,000. Individuals aged 35–59 years with morbid obesity [body mass index (BMI) 40–50] were found to be five times more likely to die from ischemic heart disease, 6.5 times more at risk of dying from stroke, and 22.5 times more at risk of dying from diabetes compared to those with lower BMI. Morbid obesity has such a severe impact on health that the median survival of affected individuals is reduced by approximately 8–10 years.[6]

Diabetes Complications and Prevalence

The impact of T2DM and its complications on global mortality and disability is significant. According to the GBD Study 2013, diabetes mellitus (DM) in all its forms was ranked as the ninth leading cause of reduced life expectancy.[7] In 2010, it was estimated that DM was responsible for 3.96 million deaths among adults aged 20–79 years, accounting for 6.8% of global mortality.[8] However, a more recent report from the International Diabetes Federation (IDF) in 2021 raised this estimate to 5.0 million deaths attributed to DM and its complications, equivalent to one death occurring every 5 seconds.[9] The incidence of disability associated with DM has seen a significant increase since 1990, particularly among individuals aged 15–69 years.[10] The GBD, Injuries, and Risk Factors Study 2015 highlighted that high fasting glucose levels ranked as the tenth most prevalent global risk factor for DALYs in 1990. By 2005, it had risen to the fourth most common risk factor, and by 2015, it became the third most common. In 2015 alone, this condition accounted for 143 million DALYs, signifying a 22% increase in DALYs from 2005 to 2015.[11]

The complications of DM have traditionally been classified into two categories—macrovascular complications, such as cardiovascular disease (CVD), and microvascular complications, which affect the kidney, retina, and nervous system. An observational study conducted in 28 countries across Asia, Africa, South America, and Europe revealed that half of the patients with T2DM experienced microvascular complications, while 27% of patients had macrovascular complications.[12] Cohort studies conducted in developed countries have indicated that individuals with DM are at least 10–20 times more likely to develop microvascular disorders and 2–4 times more likely to develop macrovascular disorders compared to those without DM.[13] In many developing countries, patients with DM face an increased risk of kidney complications and stroke, although they have a reduced risk of coronary heart disease compared to patients in developed countries.[14]

The increasing prevalence of DM, including undiagnosed cases, along with advancements in the treatment of T2DM, leading to longer lifespans for individuals with the condition, has resulted in a significant rise in the incidence of diabetic complications. In the United States, for instance, approximately 53% of the lifetime medical costs associated with T2DM can be attributed to the treatment of major complications such as nephropathy, neuropathy, retinopathy, stroke, and coronary heart disease.[15] The patient-centered management of T2DM involves implementing lifestyle modifications and combination therapy with medications.[16] While certain developed countries have made advancements in T2DM management through glycemic control and cardiovascular risk management, data regarding such progress in the rest of the world are limited.[13]

CARDIOVASCULAR DISEASE AND HYPERTENSION

Cardiovascular disease is a significant factor leading to death and disability in individuals with diabetes. As the diabetic population is projected to grow, it is expected that the number of people affected by CVD will also rise. Nonetheless, multiple studies indicate a decrease in the risk of CVD among individuals with diabetes since the 1990s. Despite these advancements, people with diabetes still face a two- to fourfold higher likelihood of hospitalization for major CVD events and CVD-related clinical procedures compared to those without diabetes. In most high-income countries, mortality rates due to CVD have decreased among the general population. However, globally, CVD remains a leading cause of death for both individuals with and without diabetes, and those with diabetes continue to experience a two- to fourfold higher mortality rate from CVD than those without diabetes. Several studies provide evidence of a decline in CVD-related mortality among people with diabetes.[17]

Cardiovascular disease, encompassing conditions such as coronary heart disease, peripheral vascular disease, and cerebrovascular disease, stands as the primary cause of illness and death in the United States. In patients diagnosed with T2DM, CVD tends to manifest approximately 14.6 years earlier and with increased severity compared to individuals without diabetes. Additionally, individuals with T2DM have twice the likelihood of developing CVD compared to those without

T2DM, regardless of factors such as age, smoking status, BMI, and systolic blood pressure (SBP). Diabetes mellitus has been linked to more than a twofold increased risk of death due to vascular causes. This heightened risk particularly affects women, to the extent that diabetes eliminates or weakens the typically observed decreased risk of CVD in premenopausal women.[18]

Diabetic heart disease (DHD) encompasses various cardiovascular conditions that arise as a result of DM, including coronary artery disease (CAD) and cardiomyopathy. CAD and cardiomyopathy are often addressed separately as microvascular and macrovascular diseases, but DM can increase the risk of both. In clinical settings, these conditions are often considered together as they contribute to adverse outcomes and an increased risk of death in individuals with CVD.[19]

In patients with diabetes, functional changes in the myocardial microvasculature occur before structural changes. These changes eventually lead to significant macrovascular atherosclerosis.[18] When diabetes is complicated by coronary atherosclerotic heart disease, it presents with the involvement of numerous vascular branches distributed throughout the entire coronary artery system, with evident atherosclerosis.[20]

Diabetic cardiomyopathy (DCM) refers to specific structural and functional abnormalities of the myocardium that occur in patients without CAD or other cardiac risk factors such as hypertension. It primarily manifests as heart failure (HF) and represents a chronic cardiovascular complication of DM. The main pathological features of DCM include left ventricular hypertrophy, myocardial fibrosis, cell necrosis, and other structural changes in the myocardium.[21,22] The myocardium's involvement in the secretion of vasoactive metabolites or neuromodulation leads to changes in coronary artery wall pressure and endothelial shear stress. Pericoronary adipose tissue surrounding the coronary arteries can secrete adipokines, vasoactive mediators, and oxidative products, which directly influence the characteristics of nearby adipocytes.

In diabetic patients, coronary atherosclerosis is primarily driven by chronic inflammation, abnormal lipid metabolism, and secondary autoimmunity. These mechanisms play significant roles in the development and progression of atherosclerosis (AS) in individuals with diabetes (**Fig. 1**). Hyperglycemic conditions can further contribute to autoimmune responses, exacerbating the inflammatory process. The impact of diabetes on cardiomyopathy has also special attention, particularly with regard to abnormal cardiac metabolism, glycotoxicity, lipotoxicity, and impaired mitochondrial function. These factors collectively lead to oxidative stress and inflammation within the heart, contributing to the pathogenesis of cardiomyopathy.[23]

Cardiovascular disease stands as the primary cause of death among individuals with obesity, responsible for approximately 60% of fatalities. Obesity escalates the risk of atherosclerotic disease and HF. Epidemiological studies consistently demonstrate that obesity increases the likelihood of developing ischemic heart disease and experiencing cardiovascular-related mortality. When it comes to predicting the risk of ischemic heart disease, waist-hip ratio emerges as a stronger factor compared to BMI. The influence of waist-hip ratio on disease risk is likely mediated by factors such as T2DM, dyslipidemia, inflammation, and hypertension. Additionally, genetic variants associated with BMI-adjusted waist-hip ratio not

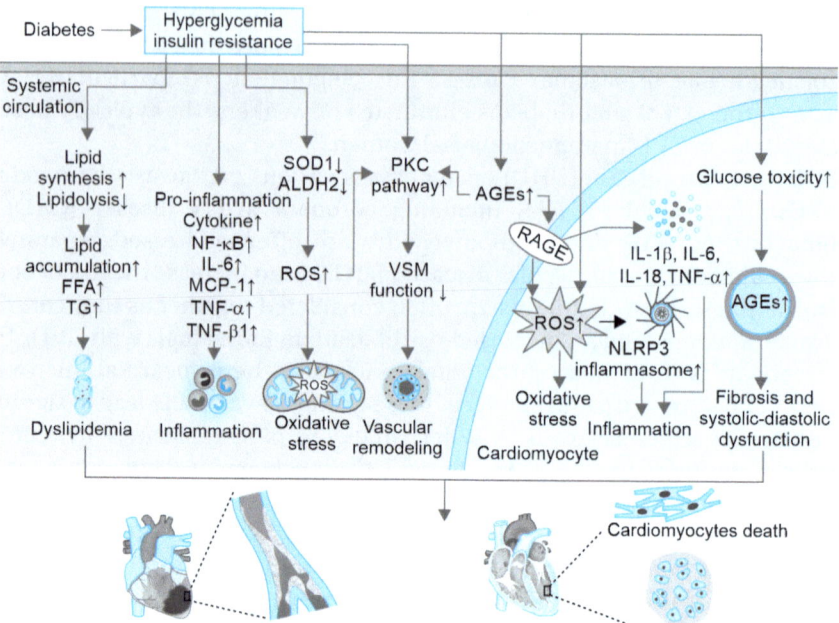

FIG. 1: Pathology and molecular mechanisms of diabetic heart disease.[23] The mechanisms of diabetic heart disease are complex, including oxidative stress, inflammation, and altered metabolic pathways [advanced glycosylation end products (AGEs) formation, PKC pathway], which intersect and work together to ultimately lead to myocardial remodeling and dysfunction.

(ALDH2: aldehyde dehydrogenase-2; ER: endoplasmic reticulum; FFA: free fatty acid; IL: interleukin; MCP-1: membrane cofactor protein-1; NF-κB: nuclear factor kappa B; NLRP3: NOD-like receptor thermal protein domain associated protein 3; PKC: protein kinase C; RAGEs: receptors of AGEs; SDH: sorbitol dehydrogenase; TG: triglyceride; ROS: reactive oxygen species; TNF-α: tumor necrosis factor-alpha; VSM: vascular smooth muscle)[23]

only relate to insulin resistance but also heighten the risk of developing T2DM, dyslipidemia, hypertension, and ischemic heart disease, suggesting a causal link.[24]

The term "obesity cardiomyopathy" is used to describe cardiac abnormalities in terms of morphology, function, and metabolism that arise solely from obesity. In certain cases, the term "metabolic cardiomyopathy" may be employed to encompass a broader range of metabolic disorders, including insulin resistance, DM, and obesity. Overall, chronic obesity is closely linked to cardiac remodeling, which is characterized by left ventricular hypertrophy, cardiac fibrosis, and diastolic dysfunction. Over time, these changes can progress to overt HF **(Fig. 2)**.[25]

Weight loss has been shown to have beneficial effects on traditional CVD risk factors, including hypertension, atherogenic dyslipidemia, and T2DM. However, long-term treatment and support are necessary to prevent relapse. Lifestyle interventions that promote weight reduction have been found to reduce the progression to T2DM and the long-term incidence of cardiovascular mortality in individuals with prediabetes. Emphasizing the importance of diet and food choices, such as following a Mediterranean diet, is crucial for maintaining cardiovascular health and primary prevention of CVD. The Look AHEAD (Action

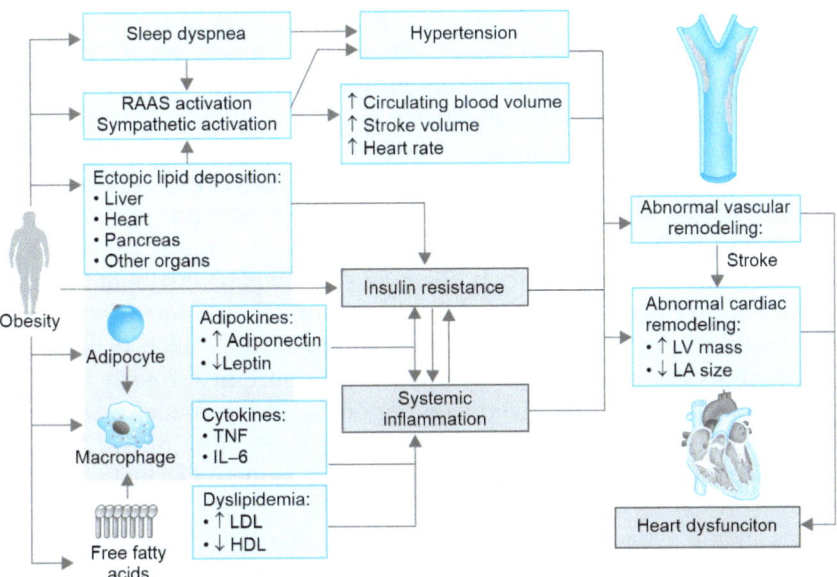

FIG. 2: Overall impact of excessive adipose accumulation on cardiac hemodynamic and ventricular function.

for Health in Diabetes) trial, which examined intensive lifestyle-based weight loss interventions in people with T2DM, did not show a significant benefit for the primary outcome. However, a secondary analysis revealed a 21% lower incidence of cardiovascular death, nonfatal acute myocardial infarction, nonfatal stroke, or hospital admission for angina among individuals who lost more than 10% of their body weight during the first year. This suggests that reaching a certain weight threshold is necessary to achieve a mortality benefit. The nutritional quality of the diet is also a critical factor to consider when counseling individuals on methods of weight loss, with diets rich in vegetables, fruits, and fiber and lower amounts of red meat being generally considered better for cardiovascular health.[26]

Approved pharmacological treatments for weight reduction vary in their efficacy and are limited by cost and safety concerns. For example, drugs such as phentermine and topiramate, used in combination, require careful monitoring of heart rate and creatinine levels due to potential cardiac and cerebrovascular risks. Liraglutide, a glucagon-like peptide-1 receptor agonist (GLP-1 RA), has shown improvements in cardiovascular risk factors and T2DM risk, although dedicated cardiovascular outcome trials have not yet been conducted. Historically, cardiovascular outcome trials for anti-obesity drugs have faced challenges in study design, premature termination due to safety issues, or failure to demonstrate cardiovascular benefits. However, more recent and ongoing trials are expected to provide valuable insights for the future management of obesity-related cardiovascular risk. Semaglutide, a GLP-1 RA, has shown promising results in terms of weight loss and improvements in cardiovascular risk factors. Ongoing trials are evaluating the impact of oral semaglutide on patients with T2DM and the effects of subcutaneous semaglutide on individuals with obesity and established CVD. The SURPASS program is also assessing the efficacy and safety of tirzepatide, a dual glucose-dependent insulinotropic polypeptide (GIP)/GLP-1 RA therapy, in people with T2DM. These trials will help enhance understanding of the relationship between intentional weight loss and cardiovascular outcomes.[26]

Sodium-glucose cotransporter-2 inhibitors (SGLT-2is) have demonstrated remarkable benefits in individuals with T2DM and established CVD or risk factors for CVD, particularly in the prevention of HF. Some SGLT-2i agents have even been approved for the treatment of HF in individuals without T2DM. Although these drugs cause weight loss, their effect on CVD may be attributed to multiple mechanisms, and they are not specifically recommended for the treatment of obesity. However, any weight loss achieved with their use is likely to be beneficial. Regular monitoring of blood glucose levels is important for early detection of T2DM in individuals who are overweight or obese. This provides an opportunity for timely intervention with treatments such as GLP-1 RAs or SGLT-2is, which have shown effectiveness in slowing T2DM progression and reducing the burden of CVD.[26]

Observational data on surgical interventions, such as bariatric procedures, have shown improvements in weight loss and a decreased incidence of T2DM, cardiovascular death, myocardial infarction, and stroke over a 15-year follow-up period. Bariatric surgery has also been associated with a larger potential reduction in cardiorenal complications, particularly HF, compared to atherosclerotic CVD outcomes in individuals with T2DM and obesity. While bariatric surgery is highly effective for weight loss and has demonstrated the potential benefits for CVD prevention, the current accessibility to surgery is limited. It is unlikely to be widely used in the general population, especially as pharmacotherapy options are becoming increasingly effective, approaching the efficacy of bariatric surgery.[26]

NEUROPATHY, NEPHROPATHY, AND RETINOPATHY

Neuropathy

In 2016, an estimated 131.0 million individuals (1.77% of the global population) were affected by diabetes-related lower-extremity complications (DRLECs). This included 105.6 million individuals with neuropathy only, 18.6 million with foot ulcers, 4.3 million with amputation without prosthesis, and 2.5 million with amputation with prosthesis. The age-standardized prevalence rates showed that 1,848 per 100,000 individuals were affected, including 1,480 with neuropathy only, 270 with foot ulcers, 60.6 with amputation without prosthesis, and 36.7 with amputation with prosthesis.[27]

Diabetes-related lower-extremity complications caused an estimated 16.8 million years lived with disability (YLDs) (2.07% of global YLDs) in 2016. This included 12.9 million YLDs from neuropathy only, 2.5 million from foot ulcers, 1.1 million from amputation without prosthesis, and 0.4 million from amputation with prosthesis. The age-standardized YLD rates for DRLECs were 237 per 100,000, including 180 from neuropathy only, 36.3 from foot ulcers, 15.1 from amputation without prosthesis, and 5.4 from amputation with prosthesis. The highest YLD rates for overall DRLECs were observed in North Africa and the Middle East (1,848 per

100,000) and Central Latin America (1,610 per 100,000), while the lowest rates were seen in East Asia (150 per 100,000), Western Sub-Saharan Africa (170 per 100,000), Australasia (190 per 100,000), and Western Europe (220 per 100,000).[27]

Diabetic peripheral neuropathy (DPN) can manifest with a wide range of clinical symptoms and signs. While some individuals may not experience any symptoms and remain asymptomatic, others may present with various manifestations. These can include paresthesia, characterized by tingling or a sensation of pins and needles, as well as numbness and neuropathic pain (NP). The pain is often described as burning, lancinating, shooting, or aching, and its severity can range from mild to severe, causing significant distress. Typically, sensory symptoms and clinical examination signs initially emerge in a symmetric pattern, starting from the toes and extending to the distal foot.[28]

The diagnosis of DPN is commonly established through diabetic foot screening. When DPN is suspected, a comprehensive clinical assessment is essential to exclude other potential causes of neuropathy. This assessment should involve a thorough history-taking and examination, which includes various components. To evaluate small-fiber function, tests such as temperature and pinprick sensation testing are performed. Large fiber function is assessed through vibration sensation testing using a 128-Hz tuning fork and examination of ankle reflexes. Furthermore, the assessment of protective sensation involves the use of a 10-g monofilament. Clinical scoring systems, like the Toronto Clinical Scoring System, may also be employed as diagnostic aids for DPN. While nerve conduction studies are considered the gold standard for evaluating large fiber function, quantitative sensory testing (QST) and skin biopsy can be utilized for diagnosing small fiber neuropathy.[28]

Diabetic neuropathy is a complex syndrome that affects both the somatic and autonomic divisions of the peripheral nervous system. In individuals with severe diabetes, longer nerve fibers tend to experience an early decline in nerve conduction velocity, resulting in the loss of nerve terminals. This damage to nerve terminals contributes to symptoms such as tingling sensations and diminished sensation, while reflex abnormalities often manifest first in the feet before progressing to other areas. The generation of reactive oxygen species (ROS) plays a significant role in the development of these complications, which are initiated and intensified under chronic hyperglycemic conditions. Additionally, several classical hyperglycemic pathways, including the polyol pathway, protein kinase C (PKC) pathway, formation of advanced glycation end products (AGE pathway), and activation of the hexosamine pathway, contribute to the worsening of symptoms, as illustrated in **Figure 3**. Moreover, the excessive oxidation of fatty acids resulting from hyperglycemia and insulin resistance appears to contribute to the pathogenesis of diabetic complications.[29]

Treatment of Diabetic Neuropathy

Peripheral neuropathy is a prevalent form of diabetic NP, characterized by moderate to severe pain, and it is the most common symptom and indication of this condition. Managing NP, including painful diabetic neuropathy (pDN), poses a significant challenge. Numerous clinical practice guidelines from reputable organizations, such as the International Association for the Study of Pain (IASP), the European

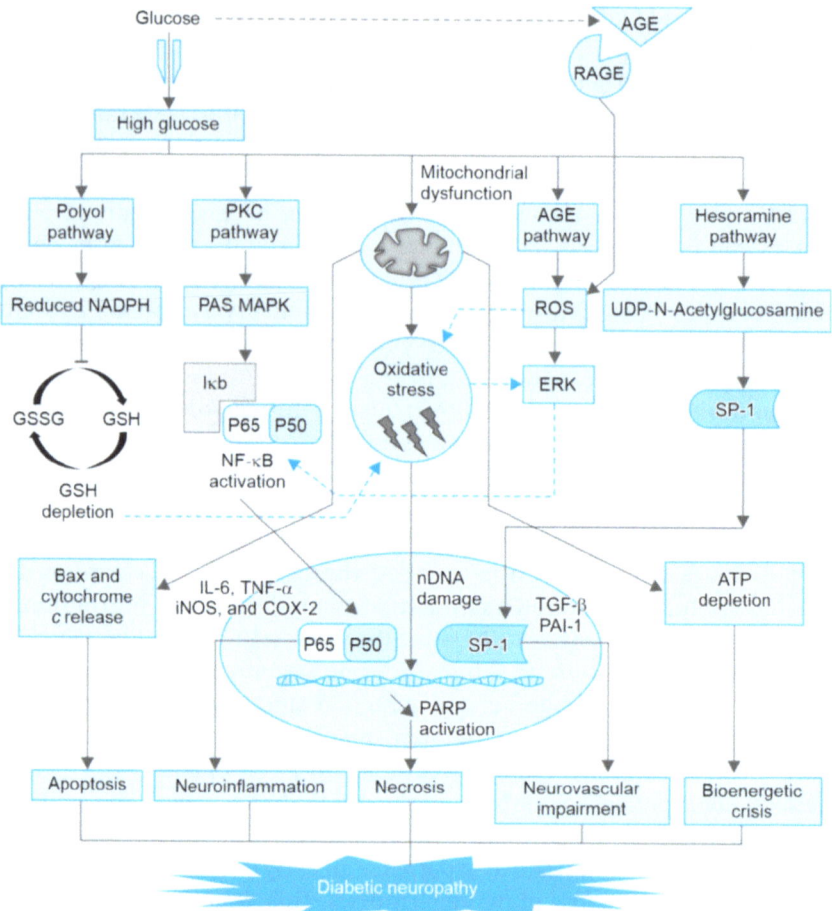

FIG. 3: Pathophysiology of diabetic neuropathy. Hyperglycemia activates numerous metabolic pathways like polyol pathway, protein kinase c (PKC) pathway, advanced glycation end products (AGE) pathway, and hexosamine pathway. All these pathways are known to integrate through hyperglycemia mediated mitochondrial ROS production. Oxidative stress and these classical pathways in combination activate transcription factors such as nuclear factor kappa enhancer of B cells (NF-κB) and speciality protein-1 (SP-1), resulting in neuroinflammation and vascular impairment. Further, these pathways combined with dysfunctional mitochondria mediated apoptosis or bioenergetic depletion can lead to neuronal damage lading to DN. Poly-ADP ribose polymerase (PARP) mediated NADH/ATP depletion can lead to neuronal dysfunction due to failure of various energy dependent processes in neurons.

(COX-2: cyclooxygenase-2; ERK: extracellular signal-regulated kinase; IL-6: interleukin-6; iNOS: inducible nitric oxide synthase; PAI-1: plasminogen activator inhibitor-1; TGF-β: transforming growth factor-β)

Federation of Neurological Societies (EFNS), the National Institute for Health and Care Excellence (NICE) of the UK, the Canadian Pain Society (CPS), the German Society for Neurology (DGN), and the German National Disease Management Guideline for Diabetic Neuropathy, have been published to assist in the assessment and treatment of NP, particularly in individuals with diabetes. The management of NP is based on three main pillars—diabetes management, diabetic neuropathy management, and symptomatic treatment of NP.[30]

There is a broad consensus among these guidelines regarding the pharmacological management of NP. First-line therapy recommendations from all guidelines strongly endorse three drug classes—tricyclic antidepressants (especially amitriptyline), serotonin-norepinephrine reuptake inhibitors (SNRIs) like duloxetine, and calcium channel alpha-2-delta ligands such as gabapentin and pregabalin. Tramadol (a weak opioid + SNRI) is recommended as a second-line option by most guidelines, although NICE suggests its use only as a rescue therapy due to higher withdrawal rates and limited evidence. Third- and fourth-line treatments typically include strong opioids, anticonvulsants (excluding gabapentinoids), and cannabinoids.[30]

For specific syndromes, there are tailored recommendations. For instance, carbamazepine is recommended for trigeminal neuralgia, and topical agents such as lidocaine or capsaicin patches and subcutaneous injections of botulinum toxin may be used for localized NP. Opioids should be reserved for patients who do not respond to other treatment options due to their high risk of adverse effects, and they are only effective in the long term for a small number of patients who may benefit from multimodal pain management. Nonsteroidal anti-inflammatory drugs (NSAIDs) have limited efficacy in purely NP but may be helpful in mixed pain syndromes. It is important to consider these guidelines and tailor the treatment approach to the specific needs and circumstances of each individual, aiming to achieve optimal management of NP while minimizing potential risks and adverse effects. The guidelines discussed do not specifically address the underlying causes or etiologies of NP. Instead, they approach NP as a distinct entity since the efficacy of systemic treatments does not appear to be significantly influenced by the specific etiology. This unified perspective on NP has been adopted by the European Medicines Agency (EMA) for the licensing of medications in Europe. **Table 1** likely illustrates this unifying concept and provides information on the recommended treatments for NP, regardless of the underlying cause.[30]

Pharmacological treatment remains the primary approach for managing DPN. First-line therapies such as pregabalin, gabapentin, and SNRIs are commonly prescribed. However, it is important to note that many of these pharmacological options provide palliative relief by alleviating symptoms without directly targeting the underlying mechanisms that cause pain.[30,31]

Nephropathy

Diabetic nephropathy (DN) is a clinical syndrome characterized by persistent albuminuria and a progressive decline in renal function. It exhibits a distinct pattern of glomerular disease. DN involves both structural and functional changes in the kidneys. Structurally, the pathological features of DN include glomerular mesangial expansion, thickening of the basement membrane, loss of podocytes, nodular glomerulosclerosis, and destruction of endothelial cells. In the early stages of DN, there is tubular hypertrophy, which eventually progresses to interstitial fibrosis with tubular atrophy. In the advanced stages, the injured kidney experiences infiltration by immune cells. Functionally, DN is characterized

TABLE 1: Pharmacotherapy for neuropathic pain.

Drug class	Mechanism of action	Representatives	License[a]	Strength of recommendation[b]	NNT[c]	Additional benefits[d]
Anticonvulsants						
	Calcium channel alpha-2-delta ligand, reduces the synaptic release of several neurotransmitters, channel modulator	Gabapentin	General NP	Strong; 1st line	• 6.3 (5.0–8.3) • 3.3–7.2	No clinically significant drug interactions additionally for pregabalin: Improvement of anxiety and sleep
		ER/enacarbil	General NP	Strong; 1st line	• 8.3 (6.2–13.0) • 3.3–8.3	
		Pregabalin	General NP FDA: pDN	Strong; 1st line	• 7.7 (6.5–9.4) • 3.3–8.3	
	Sodium channel blocker	• Carbamazepine • Oxcarbazepine		Inconclusive	Not reported	
Antidepressants						
TCA	Norepinephrine and serotonin reuptake inhibitor, block of voltage-gated sodium channels, anticholinergic effects	• Amitriptyline • Nortriptyline • Desipramine • Imipramine	General NP	Strong; 1st line	• 3.6 (3.0–4.4) • 2.1–4.2	Improvement of depression and sleep disturbances
SNRI	Norepinephrine and serotonin reuptake inhibitor	Venlafaxine		Strong; 1st line	• 6.4 (5.2–8.4) • 5.2–8.4	Improvement of depression and general anxiety (for both listed drugs)
		Duloxetine	• pDN • FDA: pDN	Strong; 1st line	• 6.4 (5.2–8.4) • 3.8–11.0	
Local therapeutics						
Local anesthetics	Sodium channel blocker	Lidocaine (patch, 5%)	Peripheral NP	Weak; 2nd line (1st line option in elderly and frail patients)	Not reported	No systemic side effects

Continued

Continued

Drug class	Mechanism of action	Representatives	License[a]	Strength of recommendation[b]	NNT[c]	Additional benefits[d]
Local capsaicin	TRPV1 agonist reversible defunctionalization of nociceptor fibers	Capsaicin (patch, 8%)	Peripheral NP	Weak; 2nd line	10.6 (7.4–18.8)	No systemic side effects
Botulinum toxin type A	Acetylcholine release inhibitor, neuromuscular blocking, potentially also mechanotransduction and central effects of NP	BOTOX		Weak, 3rd line	1.9 (1.5–2.4)	Potential effect on neurogenic inflammation
Opioids						
	μ-Receptor agonist, norepinephrine and serotonin reuptake inhibitor	Tramadol		Weak, 2nd line	• 4.7 (3.6–6.7) • 3.1–6.4	Also against inflammatory pain; rapid onset
	μ-Receptor antagonist, noradrenaline reuptake inhibitor	Tapentadol	FDA: pDN		Not reported	Rapid onset
Strong opioids	μ-Receptor agonist κ-Receptor antagonist	Morphine		Weak, 3rd line	4.3 (3.4–5.8)	Rapid onset
	μ-Receptor agonist	Oxycodone		Weak, 3rd line	4.3 (3.4–5.8)	Rapid onset
Cannabinoids						
	CB1 receptor agonists	Nabiximols	NP	Weak against	Not reported	

[a] License according to EMA, if licensed by the FDA for the indication pDN = FDA: pDN.
[b] NeuPSIG GRADE recommendations for NP in general (Finnerup et al. 2015).
[c] For NP in general: Finnerup et al. (2015) (95% CI in brackets), for the indication pDN if reported: Pop-Busui et al. (2017).
[d] Additional benefits adapted from Baron et al. (2010).
(NP: neuropathic pain; pDN: painful diabetic neuropathy; TN: trigeminal neuralgia)

by increased albumin excretion and impaired glomerular filtration rate (GFR).[32] Diabetic nephropathy is the primary cause of chronic kidney disease (CKD) among patients who require renal replacement therapy. Additionally, it is associated with a higher risk of cardiovascular mortality. Traditionally, diabetic nephropathy has been characterized by the presence of significant proteinuria exceeding 0.5 g/24 hours. This stage is commonly referred to as overt nephropathy, clinical nephropathy, proteinuria, or macroalbuminuria.[33]

In 2019, diabetes and CKD emerged as significant noncommunicable diseases, ranking seventh worldwide. They became the fourth leading cause of death and the sixth leading cause of disability. CKD associated with type 1 diabetes mellitus (CKD-T1DM) accounted for 12.9 thousand new cases, 5.02 million patients, 8.20 thousand deaths, and 3.22 million DALYs in 2019. These figures represented a substantial increase of 75.09%, 88.41%, 89.73%, and 72.63% respectively, over a span of 30 years. Similarly, CKD linked to type 2 diabetes mellitus (CKD-T2DM) was responsible for 2.5 million new cases, 129.56 million patients, 405.99 thousand deaths, and 9.87 million DALYs, showing an increase of 156.49%, 94.78%, 172.39%, and 141.73% respectively. T2DM had become the second leading cause of CKD and CKD-related deaths, as well as the third leading cause of CKD-related DALYs in 2019. Throughout this period, Asia, particularly regions such as South and East Asia, carried the greatest burden of CKD associated with diabetes. The region with the highest age-standardized incidence rate (ASIR) of CKD-T1DM shifted from High-income North America in 1990 (ASIR 2.34; age-standardized prevalence rate (ASPR) 104.38) to Eastern Europe in 2019 (ASIR 3.24; ASPR 156.02). Similarly, the region with the highest ASIR of CKD-T2DM changed from High-income North America in 1990 (38.80) to North Africa and the Middle East in 2019 (61.33).[34]

The pathogenesis of kidney damage caused by diabetes mellitus involves a complex interplay of hemodynamic, metabolic, and inflammatory pathways **(Figs. 4A and B)**. Within a hyperglycemic environment, hypertension is induced, leading to disturbed renal perfusion pressure and subsequent microvascular damage in renal arteries, glomerular and tubulointerstitial capillaries. This damage is characterized by arterial wall thickening and lumen narrowing. The upregulation of sodium-glucose cotransporters (SGLTs) promotes glucose uptake, affecting the tubular-glomerular feedback mechanism and resulting in glomerular hypertension. Hyperglycemic states also elevate plasma levels of kallikrein, thrombin, and coagulation factors, contributing to a chronically activated coagulation system associated with vascular injury in diabetic kidney disease (DKD). The immune-mediated pathogenesis of DN is intricate and involves the interaction of multiple pathways. Hyperglycemia and high lipid levels, including oxidative stress, ROS, and oxidized lipids, inflict damage on kidney cells, leading to the release of damage-associated molecular patterns (DAMPs). These, in turn, trigger pro-inflammatory signaling pathways.[23]

Additionally, glycated proteins such as AGEs can directly activate the complement system and initiate pro-inflammatory signaling. Prolonged hyperglycemia stands as a significant determinant of DKD, with additional risk factors including hypertension, smoking, obesity, physical inactivity, and dyslipidemia. Genetic susceptibility is believed to be a crucial factor contributing to the development of DKD **(Flowchart 1)**.[23]

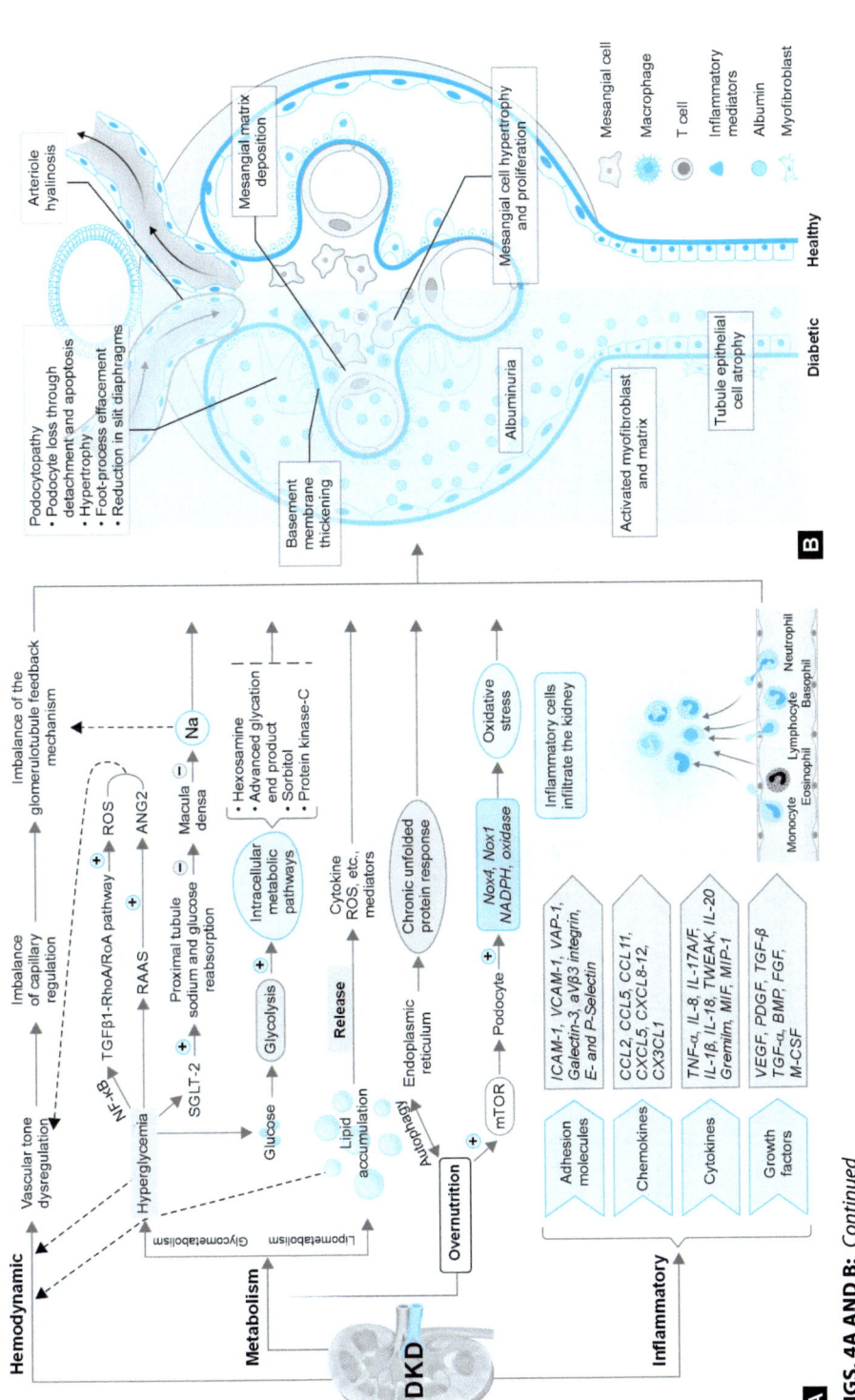

FIGS. 4A AND B: *Continued*

FIGS. 4A AND B: Pathology of the glomerulus and tubules in DKD; (A) The classical pathological mechanisms of DKD. It mainly includes hemodynamic, metabolic disturbances, and inflammation, which often interact with each other. (1) Hemodynamic disturbances lead to dysregulation of tubulobulbar feedback balance. (2) Metabolic disorders are crucial to the pathogenesis of DKD. Hyperglycemia affects pathways such as TGFβ1-RhoA/Roa pathway, RAAS, proximal tubular sodium and glucose reabsorption, and intracellular metabolism; abnormal lipid metabolism can affect the release of mediators such as cytokines and ROS; in the presence of nutrient overload in the organism, endoplasmic reticulum autophagy leads to a chronic unfolded protein response, and mTOR also disturbs the podocytes leading to oxidative stress. (3) Inflammation promotes the release of inflammatory mediators such as adhesion molecules, chemokines, cytokines, and growth factors, causing renal infiltration of inflammatory cells; (B) Schematic representation of the pathological damage of DKD: differences in structural changes of glomeruli and tubules in the diabetic setting and in the healthy state. Diabetic glomerulopathy is characterized by arterial hyalinization, thylakoid stromal deposition, basement membrane thickening, glomerular thylakoid cell hypertrophy and proliferation, podocytosis, proteinuria, tubular epithelial atrophy, activated myofibroblasts, and stromal accumulation.

(ANG2: angiotensin II; BMP: bone morphogenetic protein; CCL: CC chemokine ligand; CXCL: C-X-C motif chemokine ligand; FGF: fibroblast growth factor; ICAM-1: intercellular cell adhesion molecule-1; IL: interleukin; M-CSF: macrophage colony-stimulating factor; MIF: macrophage migration inhibitory factor; MIP-1: macrophage inflammatory protein-1; mTOR: mammalian target of rapamycin; NADPH: nicotinamide adenine dinucleotide phosphate; NF-κB: nuclear factor kappa B; NOX: NADPH oxidase; PDGF: platelet-derived growth factor; RAAS: renin–angiotensin–aldosterone system; ROS: reactive oxygen species; SGLT-2: sodium-glucose cotransporter-2; TGFβ: transforming growth factor-β; TNF: tumor necrosis factor; TWEAK: tumor necrosis factor-like weak inducer of apoptosis; VAP-1: vascular adhesion protein-1; VCAM-1: vascular cell adhesion molecule-1; VEGF: vascular endothelial growth factor)

CHAPTER 8: Management of Diabetes and Obesity Complications

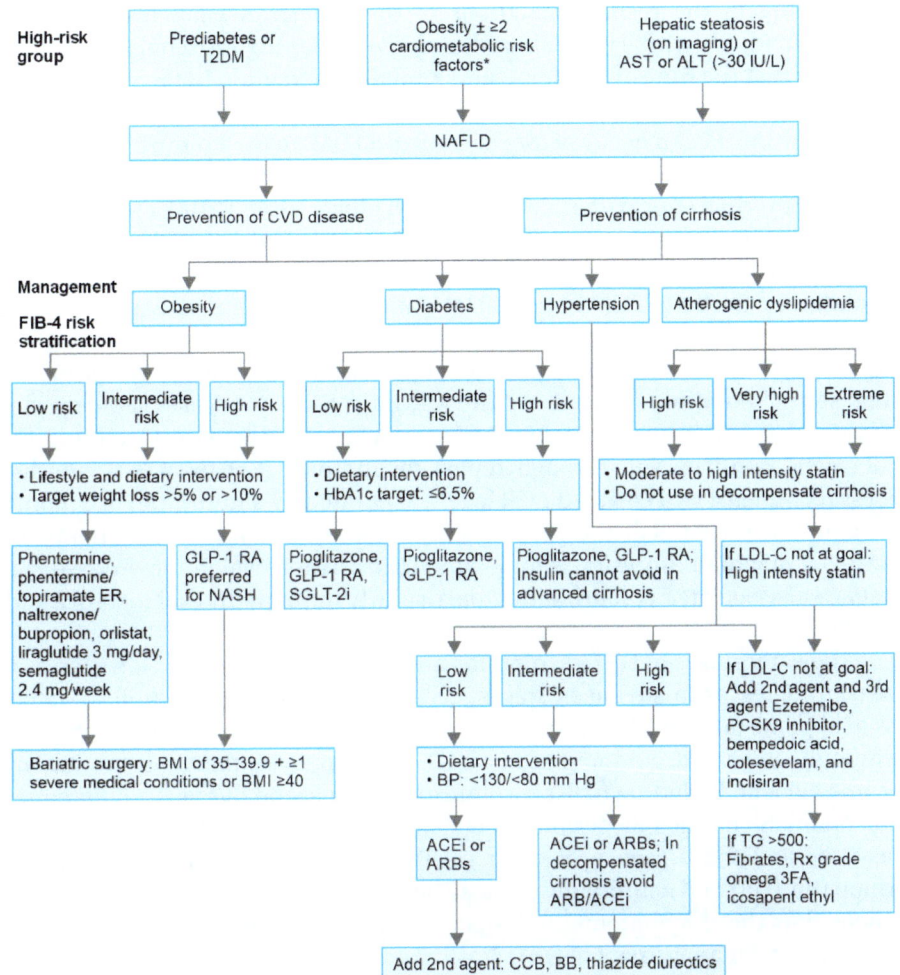

**Secondary causes of liver steatosis or elevated transaminases (AST or ALT) are excessive alcohol consumption (≥14 drinks/week for women or ≥21 drinks/week for men), hepatitis B, hepatitis C (genotype 3), Wilson's disease, alpha 1 antitrypsin deficiency, lipodystrophy, starvation, parenteral nutrition, abetalipoproteinemia, hemochromatosis, mass lesions, medications, and other causes.

Low Risk: FIB-4 <1.3 or LSM <8 kPa or ELF <7.7 (or if a liver biopsy was performed fibrosis stage is F0-F1).
Intermediate Risk: FIB-4 1.3–2.67 or LSM 8–12 kPa or ELF 7.7–9.8 (liver specialist to consider need for biopsy).
High Risk: FIB-4 >2.67 or LSM >12 kPa or ELF >9.8 (or if a liver biopsy was performed fibrosis stage is F2-F4).

FLOWCHART 1: Management algorithm for NAFLD based on recommendation by AACE practice guidelines 2022.52

Note: Cardiometabolic risk factors of the metabolic syndrome are waist circumference >40 inches men, 35 inches women, triglycerides ≥150 mg/dL HDL-c <40 mg/dL men, <50 mg/dL women, BP ≥130/≥85 mm Hg, fasting plasma glucose ≥100 mg/dL (NCEP ATP III).

(ACEIs: angiotensin converting enzyme inhibitors; ALT: alanine aminotransferase; ARBs: angiotensin II receptor blockers; AST: aspartate aminotransferase; BB: beta blockers; CCB: calcium channel blockers; CVD: cardiovascular disease; GLP-1 RA: glucagon-like peptide-1 receptor agonists; SGLT-2i: sodium-glucose cotransporter-2 inhibitor; T2DM: type 2 diabetes mellitus)

According to the recommendations of the American Diabetes Association (ADA), individuals with T2DM should undergo screening for renal function and albuminuria at the time of diagnosis and annually thereafter. In the case of T1DM, screening typically begins after 5 years of diagnosis. However, considering that microalbuminuria can occur before 5 years in T1DM, with a prevalence reaching 18%, it is advisable to initiate screening as early as 1 year after diagnosis. It is worth noting that approximately 7% of individuals with T2DM already exhibit microalbuminuria at the time of diabetes diagnosis. If the initial screening test does not indicate the presence of microalbuminuria, annual screening should still be conducted for both T1DM and T2DM patients. Albuminuria can be assessed using spot urine measurements, specifically the albumin-creatinine ratio (ACR), or through 24-hour urine collection. Renal function evaluation is recommended using serum creatinine based on the Chronic Kidney Disease Epidemiology Collaboration (CKD-EPI) equation. In cases where an increase in albuminuria is detected, confirmation through repeat testing over a span of 3-6 months is necessary. At least two elevated ACR levels, separated by a minimum of 3 months, are required to establish the presence of increased albuminuria. Patients with micro- or macroalbuminuria should undergo further evaluation to assess the presence of associated comorbidities, particularly retinopathy and macrovascular disease.[35]

In the early stages of DKD, symptoms are often absent or mild. However, as the disease progresses to advanced stages, certain symptoms may manifest. Fatigue, loss of appetite (anorexia), and swelling of the extremities are the main complaints commonly observed. In advanced DKD, clinical symptoms of uremia may become evident, including nausea, vomiting, hiccups, and dysgeusia (altered taste perception). Signs such as peripheral edema (swelling), hypertension (high blood pressure), and the presence of other microvascular complications like diabetic retinopathy (DR) and neuropathy can also be observed concurrently. It is important to note that these symptoms and signs indicate the need for further medical evaluation and management of DKD.[36]

Nephropathy Management

The management of DN involves two main goals—preserving renal function to reduce the risk of end-stage kidney disease (ESKD) and minimizing the risks of cardiovascular events and mortality. Additionally, individuals with DN are also at higher risk for other complications such as retinopathy, neuropathy, and foot ulcers, so increased attention and vigilance are important for the early detection and management of these issues. Various international and national organizations have developed treatment guidelines for DN, which provide recommendations and strategies for optimal management. For a summary of these guidelines, please refer to **Table 2**.[36-44] These guidelines serve as valuable resources in ensuring comprehensive and effective care for individuals with DN.

Evidence from Clinical Trials on Effect of Glycemic Control

The clinical benefits of intensive glycemic control [target glycated hemoglobin (HbA1c) <53 mmol/mol (<7%)] in terms of onset and progression of microalbuminuria are modest, but its effects on the progression to ESKD, death, and

TABLE 2: Summary of treatment goals for key therapeutic targets in international guidelines on diabetes and CKD.[36-44]

	KDIGO (2022, 2021, 2013)	EASD (2019)	ADA (2021)	NICE (2022, 2015, 2023)
Dietary sodium	<2 g/day (or <5 g/day salt)	-	<2,300 mg/day	-
Physical activity	>150 minutes/week moderate intensity	>150 minutes/week aerobic and resistance activity	>150 minutes/week aerobic activity	>150 minutes/week moderate intensity, aerobic activity
Weight loss	Achieve healthy weight (BMI 20–25 kg/m²)	Weight stabilization if BMI ≥25 kg/m²	>5% weight loss if BMI ≥25 kg/m²	Initial target 5–10% weight loss if BMI ≥25 kg/m²
Smoking cessation	Recommended	Obligatory	Advise against tobacco and e-cigarettes	Recommended
Blood pressure target	SBP <120 mm Hg <130/80 for adult kidney transplant recipients	SBP <130 mm Hg but not <120 DBP <80 mm Hg but not <70 If >65 years: SBP 139–130 mm Hg	<130/80 mm Hg if 10 year CV risk ≥15% <140/90 if lower risk	<130/80 mm Hg
RAASi	All patients with moderately-to-severely increased albuminuria*	First-line antihypertensive especially if albuminuria* or LVH present	First-line antihypertensive if albuminuria* present	First-line antihypertensive if albuminuria* present
HbA1c	<7% for most patients Higher target if risk of hypoglycemia, severe comorbidities, or limited life expectancy	<7% for most patients <6.5% for early stages of diabetes and younger patients <8% in elderly or those with severe multimorbidity	<7% for most patients <6.5% if low risk of hypoglycemia <8% if high risk of hypoglycemia of multimorbidity	<7.0% if risk of hypoglycemia <6.5% if low risk of hypoglycemia Relax target if: • High risk of hypoglycemia • Reduced life expectancy • Severe multimorbidity • Elderly or frail

Continued

Continued

	KDIGO (2022, 2021, 2013)	EASD (2019)		ADA (2021)	NICE (2022, 2015, 2023)
Lipid management	Statin therapy for all patients with diabetes and CKD	Statin therapy as first line		High-intensity statin for all patients aged 50–70 years with multiple CV risk factors	Statin therapy for all patients with diabetes and CKD
		Moderate CV risk: LDL-c <2.6 mmol/L (100 mg/dL)		Moderate intensity statin for patients aged 40–75 years without additional CV risk factors	
		High CV risk: LDL-c <1.8 mmol/L (70 mg/dL)			
		Very high CV risk: LDL-c <1.4 mmol/L (55 mg/dL)			
Nephrology referral criteria	• CKD stage 4 • CKD progression	–		• CKD stage 4 • Renal diagnosis uncertain • Rapid CKD progression	• CKD 4 • >25% reduction in GFR plus progression to the next CKD category • GFR reduction of >15 mL/minute/1.73 m² in 12 months

*Albuminuria is defined as urine albumin excretion >30 mg/day or equivalent (urine albumin-to-creatinine ratio >3 mg/mmol or >30 mg/g).

(ADA: American Diabetes Association; BMI: body mass index; CKD: chronic kidney disease; CV: cardiovascular; DBP: diastolic blood pressure; EASD: European Association for the Study of Diabetes; GFR: glomerular filtration rate; HBA1c: glycated hemoglobin; KDIGO: Kidney Disease Improving Global Outcomes; LDL-c: low density lipoprotein cholesterol; NICE: National Institute for Health and Care Excellence; RAASi: renin–angiotensin–aldosterone system inhibitor; SBP: systolic blood pressure) major cardiovascular events in individuals with DKD remain uncertain. In the Diabetes Control and Complications Trial (DCCT) and its long-term follow-up study, the Epidemiology of Diabetes Interventions and Complications (EDIC), intensive glycemic control demonstrated a slower decline in estimated glomerular filtration rate (eGFR) and development of albuminuria in people with T1DM. For individuals with T2DM, a meta-analysis conducted by Zoungas et al., which included patient-level data from four large trials (UKPDS, VADT, ACCORD, and ADVANCE), reported a 20% reduction in the risk (HR 0.80, 95% CI 0.72–0.88; $p < 0.0001$) of the composite outcome comprising macroalbuminuria, ESKD, and death with intensive glycemic control. Please note that the overall impact of intensive glycemic control on the progression of DKD, mortality, and major cardiovascular events in individuals with DKD requires further investigation and clarification.[45]

Treatment of Neuropathy in Different Comorbid Conditions

Hyperglycemia management: The management of hyperglycemia in diabetes requires a comprehensive approach that incorporates various factors, such as weight loss, exercise, dietary modifications, and medication. The initial focus should be on lifestyle changes and the use of metformin as first-line therapy. Analysis of data from large trials indicates that medications from different drug classes may have benefits in reducing the progression to DKD independent of their glucose-lowering effects. Specifically, GLP-1 RAs and dipeptidyl-peptidase-4 (DPP-4) inhibitors have shown promise in slowing the progression of albuminuria, while SGLT-2is have demonstrated effectiveness in reducing the rates of renal disease progression and the need for renal replacement therapy. Due to their inherent renal protective effects, GLP-1 agonists and SGLT-2is are recommended as second-line therapy for patients who fail to achieve their target HbA1c levels with lifestyle changes and metformin alone.[46]

Blood pressure control: To reduce the incidence of microvascular disease, including DKD, it is recommended to maintain SBP below 140 mm Hg and diastolic blood pressure below 90 mm Hg. Lower targets (130/80 mm Hg) may be appropriate for certain patients, such as those with established DKD or increased risk of atherosclerotic CVD, as long as achieving these targets does not impose significant treatment burden or adverse effects. Initial treatment of hypertension in patients with diabetes should primarily involve lifestyle management, including dietary sodium restriction (<2,300 mg/day), weight loss if overweight or obese, increased physical activity, and moderation of alcohol intake. A patient-specific treatment plan should be established at the time of diagnosis, and pharmacologic therapy should be considered to achieve the target blood pressure.[46]

Angiotensin-converting enzyme (ACE) inhibitors and angiotensin receptor blockers (ARBs) have been shown to delay and reduce the progression of DKD. A Cochrane review conducted in 2012 concluded that ACE inhibitors reduce the risk of new onset microalbuminuria or macroalbuminuria in individuals with diabetes, both with or without hypertension. The same review also found that ACE inhibitors reduce the risk of death in patients with diabetes compared to placebo. In a large randomized controlled trial in 2011, olmesartan (Benicar) was shown to delay the onset of microalbuminuria compared to placebo, even when both groups achieved blood pressure targets. A follow-up study in 2014 confirmed the sustained benefit of olmesartan over time. Combining ACE inhibitors and ARBs does not provide additional benefits but increases the risks of hyperkalemia, hypotension, and renal failure.[46]

Aldosterone antagonists, when used in combination with ACE inhibitors or ARBs, have therapeutic benefits. However, they carry a high risk of hyperkalemia and require careful monitoring when prescribed. Calcium channel blockers and thiazide diuretics have shown cardioprotective effects but do not appear to have the same level of benefit in preventing the progression of DKD.[46]

Lipid management: DKD has a significant impact on lipid metabolism, resulting in increased levels of LDL-c complexes and a higher risk of adverse outcomes related to atherosclerotic CVD. Although statin therapy does not have a substantial effect on slowing the progression of DKD, it has been shown to reduce the incidence of cardiac events and mortality in patients with renal disease who are not yet on dialysis, regardless of whether they have diabetes. It is important to note that many statins are metabolized by the kidneys, so dose adjustments may be necessary in patients with significantly reduced eGFR. However, atorvastatin (Lipitor) does not require dose adjustment in such cases.[46]

Dietary modification: Dietary modification holds potential for preventing the progression of DKD; however, the evidence regarding specific interventions is varied. The ADA recommends a protein-restricted diet (0.8 g/kg/day) for patients with DKD, as studies have shown that it can slow the decline of GFR and the progression to end-stage renal disease (ESRD). The Mediterranean diet and the Dietary Approaches to Stop Hypertension (DASH) diet have demonstrated beneficial outcomes. These diets emphasize whole-grain carbohydrates, fiber, fresh fruits and vegetables, omega-3 and omega-9 fats, and a daily sodium intake of <2,300 mg. It is important to avoid foods that are high in sugar, saturated fats, and processed carbohydrates. For patients with DKD, regular monitoring of phosphorus, potassium, and vitamin D levels can guide additional dietary modifications.[46]

METABOLIC DYSFUNCTION-ASSOCIATED STEATOTIC LIVER DISEASE

Nonalcoholic fatty liver disease (NAFLD) affects a significant portion of the global adult population, with approximately 25% being affected. The prevalence varies across regions, with lower rates observed in Africa (13%) and higher rates in Central and South America (nearly 40%). NAFLD is closely associated with obesity and T2DM, often considered as the hepatic manifestation of metabolic syndrome. The presence of multiple metabolic components in individuals with NAFLD is linked to an increased risk of mortality, underscoring the role of metabolic factors in the disease's progression.[47]

In recent years, there has been a growing understanding of the complex pathophysiology of this condition. As a result, a panel of international experts proposed a new term, metabolic dysfunction-associated fatty liver disease (MAFLD), to better encompass the underlying mechanisms involved. MAFLD encompasses a spectrum of liver conditions, ranging from simple steatosis (accumulation of fat) to nonalcoholic steatohepatitis (inflammation and liver cell damage), which can ultimately progress to cirrhosis. Obesity, T2DM, and metabolic syndrome are identified as the primary risk factors for MAFLD, emphasizing their significance in the development and progression of the disease.[47,48]

The proposed criteria for metabolic dysfunction-associated steatotic liver disease (MASLD) simplify the definition of NAFLD in both lean and non-lean patients by incorporating five components of metabolic syndrome, including central or overall obesity, while removing homeostatic model assessment for insulin resistance (HOMA-IR) and high-sensitivity C-reactive protein (hs-CRP). This change means that even a lean centrally obese nondiabetic individual with NAFLD would meet the MASLD criteria, whereas they would require an additional risk factor to satisfy the previously suggested MAFLD criteria. This shift in nomenclature makes MASLD and SLD more relevant for lean patients with NAFLD compared to the previous MAFLD terminology.[49]

Prevalence

Metabolic dysfunction-associated fatty liver disease has emerged as the most prevalent chronic liver disease worldwide over the past two decades. The global prevalence of MAFLD is estimated at 25.24%, with the highest rates observed in the Middle East (31.79%) and South America (30.45%), followed by Asia (27.37%), North America (24.13%), and Europe (23.71%). In contrast, Africa has a lower prevalence of MAFLD at 13.48%. In China, the prevalence of MAFLD has been steadily increasing, from 23.8% in 2001 to 32.9% in 2018, coinciding with the rise in metabolic syndrome, T2DM, CVD, and other metabolic disorders. Projections indicate that the number of MAFLD cases worldwide will reach approximately 314.58 million by 2030, highlighting the substantial impact of MAFLD in the coming decades.[48]

A recent meta-analysis and systematic review involving 10,739,607 individuals examined the prevalence, clinical characteristics, and associated factors of MAFLD. The analysis included a sensitivity analysis distinguishing between lean and nonobese MAFLD individuals. Among the pooled analysis of 3,320,108 individuals, the overall prevalence of MAFLD was found to be 38.77%. The highest prevalence of MAFLD was observed in Europe, with a rate of 55.33% (95% CI 36.20% to 73.00%). Asia had the second highest prevalence at 36.31% (95% CI 29.89% to 43.26%), while North America had the lowest prevalence at 35.99% (95% CI 30.68% to 41.66%). Specifically, 5.37% of lean individuals and 29.78% of nonobese individuals were diagnosed with MAFLD. The study also identified significant associations between lean and nonobese MAFLD and metabolic complications such as hypertension [odds ratio (OR) 2.63 and OR 2.03, respectively] and diabetes (OR 3.80 and OR 3.46, respectively), emphasizing the relevance of these factors in the development of MAFLD.[50]

Metabolic dysfunction-associated fatty liver disease patients exhibited several distinct characteristics compared to non-MAFLD controls. They were more likely to be males (OR 1.85, $p < 0.0001$) and significantly older [mean difference (MD) 2.17, $p < 0.0001$]. In terms of anthropometric measurements, MAFLD patients had higher BMI (MD 4.40, $p < 0.0001$) and waist circumference (MD 11.70, $p < 0.0001$). They also had higher SBP (MD 8.43, $p < 0.0001$) and diastolic blood pressure (MD 5.70, $p < 0.0001$).[50]

Furthermore, MAFLD patients had elevated levels of HbA1c (MD 0.33, $p < 0.0001$) and fasting blood glucose (MD 0.56, $p < 0.0001$) compared to non-MAFLD controls. In terms of lipid profile, MAFLD patients showed higher levels of triglycerides (MD 0.85, $p < 0.0001$) and low-density lipoprotein (LDL) cholesterol (MD 0.19, $p < 0.0001$), as well as lower levels of high-density lipoprotein (HDL) cholesterol (MD −0.22, $p < 0.0001$). Liver enzymes aspartate aminotransferase (AST) (MD 3.65, $p = 0.01$), alanine transaminase (ALT) (MD 10.96, $p < 0.0001$), and gamma-glutamyl transferase (GGT) (MD 22.51, $p < 0.0001$) were significantly higher in MAFLD patients.[50]

Additionally, MAFLD patients exhibited higher levels of uric acid (MD 53.51, 95% CI 39.11–67.92, $p < 0.0001$) and lower eGFR (MD −2.84, 95% CI −4.75 to −0.94, $p = 0.003$) compared to non-MAFLD controls. These findings highlight the distinct metabolic and biochemical characteristics associated with MAFLD.[50]

In Taiwan, the overall prevalence of MAFLD in the general population was estimated to be 11.4%. However, certain subpopulations showed even higher prevalence rates, such as the elderly with a prevalence of 50.1%, and taxi drivers who typically lead inactive lifestyles, with a prevalence of 66.4%. In Hong Kong, a community study that utilized proton-magnetic resonance spectroscopy (MRS) indicated a prevalence of 28.8% for MAFLD. Among the subjects, the prevalence was 19.3% in nonobese individuals and 60.5% among the obese. In the Far East region, the community prevalence of MAFLD was found to range from 23 to 26%. In Japan and Korea, abdominal ultrasonography during routine health screenings revealed a fatty liver prevalence of 27.3% in both countries. In rural India, which is characterized by traditional lifestyles and diets, the prevalence of MAFLD is remarkably low at around 9%. However, in urban populations, the prevalence rates align with those of other Asian countries, ranging from 16 to 32%.[51]

Diagnosis

The proposed criteria for a positive diagnosis of MAFLD involve evidence of hepatic steatosis (fat accumulation in the liver) based on histological, imaging, or blood biomarker findings, along with the presence of one of the following: overweight/obesity, T2DM, or evidence of metabolic dysregulation. Metabolic dysregulation is defined by the presence of at least two metabolic risk abnormalities:[52]

- Waist circumference ≥102/88 cm in Caucasian men and women or ≥90/80 cm in Asian men and women)
- Blood pressure ≥130/85 mm Hg or specific drug treatment
- Plasma triglycerides ≥150 mg/dL (≥1.70 mmol/L) or specific drug treatment
- Plasma HDL-c <40 mg/dL (<1.0 mmol/L) for men and <50 mg/dL (<1.3 mmol/L) for women or specific drug treatment.
- Prediabetes [i.e., fasting glucose levels 100–125 mg/dL (5.6 to 6.9 mmol/L), or 2-hour post-load glucose levels 140–199 mg/dL (7.8–11.0 mmol) or HbA1c 5.7–6.4% (39–47 mmol/mol)]
- Homeostasis model assessment of insulin resistance score ≥2.5
- Plasma high-sensitivity C-reactive protein level >2 mg/L.

Ultrasound is recommended as the first-line diagnostic modality for detecting steatosis, although it has limitations in sensitivity, particularly for detecting steatosis below 20%, and its performance may be suboptimal in individuals with a BMI over 40 kg/m². CT or MRI can be used for diagnosing moderate and severe steatosis if available, while MRS provides a quantitative estimation of liver fat but has limitations in terms of cost, availability, and software requirements.[52]

In the future, noninvasive tests that capture both disease activity and fibrosis stage should aim to categorize the disease effectively. Liver biopsy should be reserved for complex cases where it may be necessary to rule out other liver diseases or further characterize the disease process, as the pathology score reflects not only the amount of fat but also factors such as location and parenchymal alterations, including vascular changes.[52]

Management of Metabolic Dysfunction-associated Steatotic Liver Disease

Once MAFLD has been diagnosed and its severity and associated complications assessed, the treatment goals align with those established for NAFLD. This includes implementing lifestyle changes such as caloric restriction and increased physical activity to achieve weight loss. In suitable individuals with obesity, bariatric surgery may be considered. It is also crucial to control cardiometabolic risk factors and prevent the development and progression of liver and non-liver complications. Medications commonly used for cardiovascular risk reduction and renoprotection in T2DM, such as statins and renin-angiotensin system blocking drugs, may have additional anti-fibrotic properties.[53,54]

While interventions such as vitamin E, prebiotics, probiotics, synbiotics, and polyunsaturated fatty acids (PUFA) have been suggested as potential modifiers for MAFLD, the evidence regarding their effects remains uncertain. Recent reviews have highlighted the lack of conclusive data on their impact on clinical outcomes, and there are concerns that PUFA supplementation may increase adverse events. Therefore, further research is needed to better understand the efficacy and safety of these interventions in the context of MAFLD.[53,55]

When considering blood glucose-lowering medications for the treatment of diabetes, it has been observed that pioglitazone can improve liver histology in individuals with biopsy-proven nonalcoholic steatohepatitis (NASH). Pioglitazone is also included in guidelines for the management of NAFLD. However, the effects of pioglitazone on fibrosis have shown inconsistent results. In more recent clinical trials, the use of GLP-1 RA and SGLT-2is has demonstrated favorable effects on reducing hepatic fat content. These medications have shown promising outcomes in addressing the specific issue of hepatic fat accumulation. Tirzepatide, a dual GIP agonist and GLP-1 RA, is an innovative therapy used for the treatment of T2DM. It is also currently being studied as a potential treatment for NASH in individuals with or without diabetes. The unique mechanism of action of tirzepatide, targeting both GIP, and GLP-1 receptors, makes it a promising candidate for addressing NASH, a condition characterized by liver inflammation and fat accumulation. Ongoing research aims to evaluate the effectiveness of tirzepatide in managing NASH and its associated complications.[53-55]

A wide range of novel agents are currently being developed for the treatment of NAFLD/MAFLD, and several of them are also being studied in the context of T2DM. Among the most promising agents are:[54]

- *Obeticholic acid*: This is a semisynthetic derivative of chenodeoxycholic acid found in bile. In a Phase 2 trial, obeticholic acid demonstrated improvements in biochemical markers of fibrosis in individuals with T2DM.
- *Lanifibranor:* This agent is a pan-peroxisome proliferator-activated receptor activator with antifibrotic properties. It is currently being evaluated in a Phase 2 trial for the treatment of NAFLD in individuals with T2DM, with changes in surrogate indices of fibrosis (plasma biomarkers and imaging) as an endpoint.
- *Resmetirom:* This is a liver-directed thyroid hormone receptor-β agonist. In a study involving 125 participants with NASH, nearly 40% of whom had diabetes, resmetirom demonstrated a significant reduction in hepatic fat.

These agents represent promising advancements in the development of therapeutic options for NAFLD/MAFLD, and their evaluation in individuals with T2DM highlights the potential for managing both conditions simultaneously. Ongoing research will further elucidate their efficacy and safety profiles.[54]

OSTEOARTHRITIS

The prevalence of overweight and obesity has significantly increased worldwide since 1980, with nearly one-third of the global population now classified as overweight or obese. This has become a major public health concern, as obesity has detrimental effects on various physiological functions of the body. It significantly raises the risk of developing several diseases, including DM, CVD, various types of cancers, musculoskeletal disorders, and mental health issues. These conditions not only reduce the quality of life but also impact work productivity and healthcare costs.[56]

Among the musculoskeletal disorders associated with obesity, both degenerative and inflammatory conditions are prevalent.[57] Osteoarthritis (OA) is a particularly common condition, with knee OA being highly prevalent, especially with increasing age. In 2010, the global prevalence of symptomatic knee OA confirmed through radiographic examination was estimated to be 3.8%. It was higher in females (mean 4.8%) compared to males (mean 2.8%), and its prevalence peaked around the age of 50. The Asia Pacific high-income region had the highest prevalence, followed by Oceania and North Africa/Middle East, while South and Southeast Asia had the lowest prevalence.[58]

According to pooled data, the global prevalence of knee OA is estimated to be 16.0% in individuals aged 15 and over. When focusing on individuals aged 40 and over, the prevalence increases to 22.9%. Based on these figures, it is estimated that there are approximately 654.1 million individuals worldwide aged 40 and older living with knee OA in 2020. The prevalence of knee OA varies across different regions. In Asia, the prevalence is reported to be 19.2%. In Europe, it is 13.4%, while in North America, it is 15.8%. South America has a prevalence of 4.1%, Oceania has 3.1%, and Africa has the highest prevalence at 21.0%.[4] The risk of both prevalence and incidence of knee OA increases with age, reaching its peak at advanced ages.

The prevalence risk curve demonstrates this trend showing a gradual increase with age. Similarly, the incidence risk curve peaks between the ages of 70 and 79. Furthermore, females have a higher risk compared to males. The prevalence risk for females is 1.69 times higher ($p < 0.00$) than males, while the incidence risk is 1.39 times higher ($p < 0.00$). This indicates that females are more susceptible to both the prevalence and incidence of knee OA.[59]

Globally, hip and knee OA ranked as the 11th highest contributor to global disability in terms of YLDs in 2010, among the 291 conditions studied. The YLDs associated with hip and knee OA increased from 10.5 million in 1990 to 17.1 million in 2010. In 1990, OA accounted for 1.8% of total YLDs, which rose to 2.2% in 2010. Additionally, the overall DALYs for hip and knee OA increased from 0.42% of total DALYs in 1990 to 0.69% in 2010.[58]

These statistics highlight the significant impact of obesity and its association with musculoskeletal disorders, particularly knee OA. The increasing burden of these conditions underscores the need for effective prevention and management strategies to address the global public health challenge posed by obesity-related musculoskeletal disorders.

Pathophysiology of Metabolic Osteoarthritis

The pathophysiology of obesity-related OA is likely to be multifactorial, involving both mechanical and metabolic factors. Structural joint damage occurs due to increased forces around the joint, decreased muscle strength, altered biomechanics during everyday activities, and metabolic factors **(Fig. 5)**. It is important to note that obesity can increase the risk of OA even in non-weight-bearing joints such as the hands.[57,60]

One of the major mechanical contributions is the increased loading of weight-bearing joints, particularly the knee. The knee adduction moment, which represents the inward force on the knee joint, is an important mechanical variable associated with the development of knee OA. Individuals with obesity experience higher knee adduction moments due to their increased body mass and may adopt compensatory gait patterns such as slower walking velocity and increased toe-out angle.[57]

Adipokines, which are signaling molecules secreted by adipose tissue, also play a significant role in the pathogenesis and progression of obesity-induced OA. These adipokines can directly induce or inhibit catabolic or apoptotic pathways and affect bone metabolism. Some adipokines, such as leptin, chemerin, resistin, visfatin, and lipocalin-2, are believed to have detrimental effects on joint tissue. However, others such as progranulin, vaspin, and omentin-1 have been reported to maintain cartilage integrity and reduce osteophyte formation. Adipokines have emerged as potential targets for disease-modifying OA drugs, especially in obese patients.[60]

Dyslipidemia, characterized by abnormal lipid levels, also contributes to OA development and progression. LDL, triglycerides (TAG), free fatty acids (FFA), and ROS, along with low levels of HDL, contribute to OA through various mechanisms. These mechanisms include increased cytokine production, synovial inflammation,

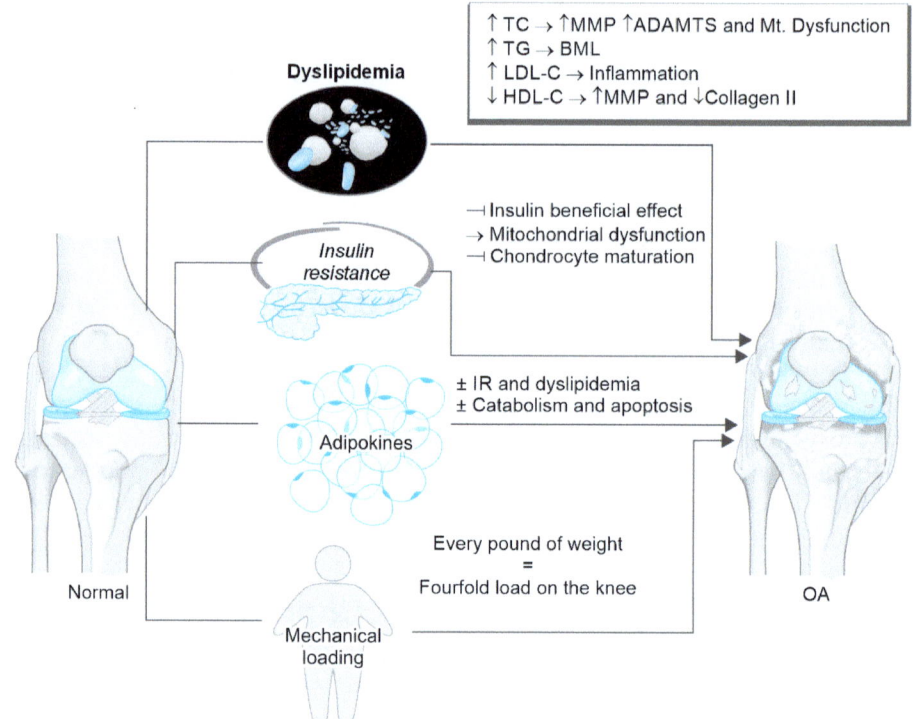

FIG. 5: Multi-factorial interplay between obesity and OA. Dyslipidemia, insulin resistance, adipokines, and mechanical loading are the four aspects by which obesity affects normal knee and induces OA. The arrows represent a summary of how each aspect leads to OA development.

(ADAMTS: a disintegrin and metalloproteinase with thrombospondin motifs; BML: bone marrow lesions; HDL-c: high-density lipoprotein cholesterol; IR: insulin resistance; LDL-c: low-density lipoprotein cholesterol; MMP: matrix metalloproteinases; Mt. dysfunction: mitochondrial dysfunction; OA: osteoarthritis; TAG: triglycerides; TC: total cholesterol)

ectopic bone formation, cholesterol oxidation products, mitochondrial-oxidative stress, and increased matrix metalloproteinase (MMP) production. Dyslipidemia is also associated with the occurrence of bone marrow lesions, which contribute to pain in OA.[60]

Insulin resistance (IR) plays a role in the degenerative process of OA. During IR, insulin receptors in chondrocytes and synovium become less responsive to insulin's beneficial effects, leading to the overproduction of cytokines. FFA accumulation in the joints results in mitochondrial dysfunction, cytokine release, and apoptosis. Hyperinsulinemia, a consequence of IR, hinders the formation of mature chondrocytes and disrupts the balance of thyroid hormones, further contributing to OA progression.[60]

Overall, the interplay of mechanical factors, metabolic factors, adipokines, dyslipidemia, and insulin resistance contributes to the development and progression of obesity-related OA. Understanding these underlying mechanisms can help guide therapeutic interventions and management strategies for individuals with OA, particularly those affected by obesity.

Diagnosis

The primary symptom of OA is joint pain, which typically worsens with activity and improves with rest. This pain is often accompanied by morning stiffness, but unlike rheumatoid arthritis, the stiffness in OA lasts for <30 minutes. Patients may also experience joint locking or instability, leading to a loss of function, and limitations in daily activities.[61]

Osteoarthritis commonly affects joints such as the hands, knees, hips, and spine, although it can involve almost any joint in the body. The condition often manifests asymmetrically, meaning that one joint may be severely affected while the opposite joint retains relatively normal function.[61]

To confirm the diagnosis and rule out other conditions, plain radiography (X-rays) can be useful. Advanced imaging techniques such as computed tomography (CT) or magnetic resonance imaging (MRI) are rarely necessary unless there is uncertainty in the diagnosis or suspicion of an alternative cause, such as a meniscal injury.[61]

Therapeutic Strategies for Obesity-related Osteoarthritis

A consensus from Malaysia (2021), focused on managing knee osteoarthritis (OA), provides nine recommendations for the management of patients with knee OA. These recommendations advocate an algorithmic approach to guide healthcare providers in their management strategies **(refer to Flowchart 2)**.[62]

The consensus emphasizes a multimodal intervention strategy as the primary approach to managing knee OA. The choice of interventions, whether single or multimodal, may vary depending on the stage and progression of the disease. It is recommended that all patients receive a nonpharmacological core treatment set consisting of patient education, weight loss (if applicable), and exercise. These interventions form the foundation of OA management for all patients.[62]

When pharmacotherapy is necessary, the use of symptomatic slow-acting drugs for OA is recommended during the early stages of the disease. These drugs can be combined with physical therapy as a background treatment to provide relief and manage symptoms. If patients do not respond sufficiently to the background treatment, advanced pharmacotherapy options can be considered. This may include the use of NSAIDs, intraarticular injections, and short-term weak opioids. The selection of advanced pharmacotherapy should be tailored to the individual patient's needs and preferences.[62]

For patients with severe symptomatic knee OA, knee replacement surgery should be considered as a treatment option. The consensus advises that management should prioritize specific treatments with the least systemic exposure or toxicity. The choice of treatment should be made through shared decision-making between patients and their healthcare providers.[62]

In summary, the Malaysian consensus on knee OA management recommends a multimodal approach that includes nonpharmacological interventions, such as patient education, weight loss, and exercise, as well as pharmacotherapy when necessary. The choice of treatment should be personalized, taking into account the individual patient's needs and preferences, and a shared decision-making approach should be adopted between patients and healthcare providers.[62]

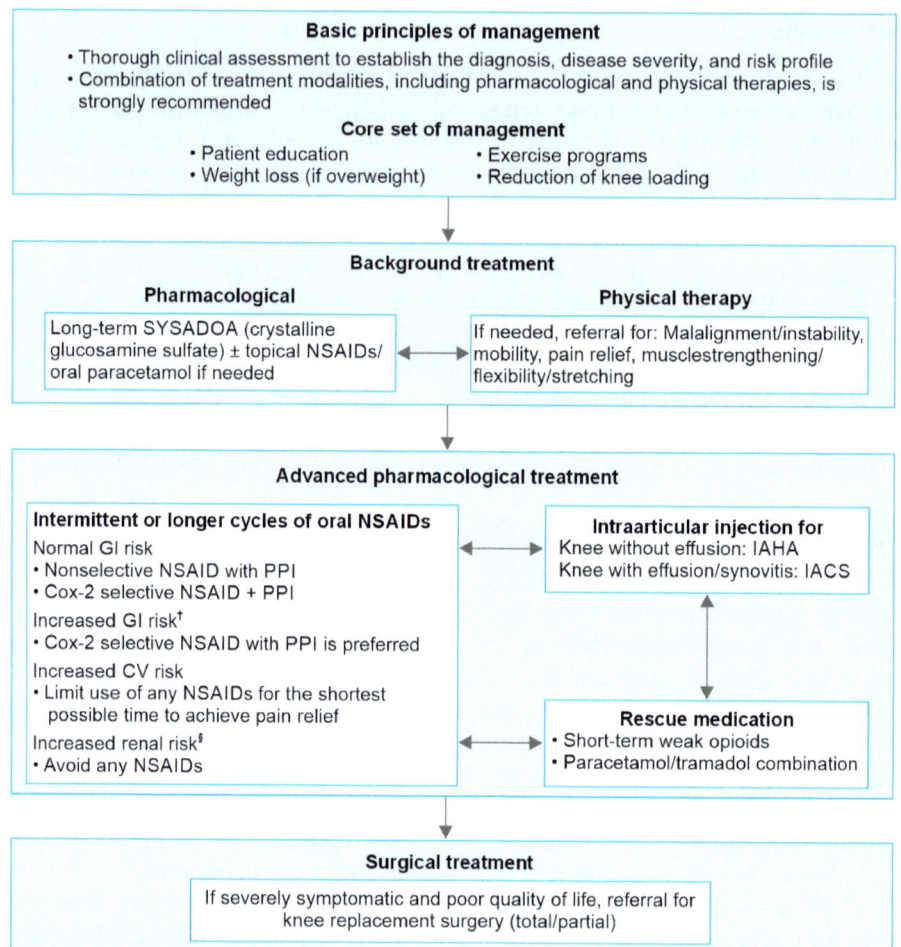

† Including use of low-dose aspirin.

§ With glomerular filtration rate <30 mL/min (caution in other cases).

FLOWCHART 2: Malaysian consensus on the management of knee OA (2021): Recommended algorithm.

(IACS: intraarticular corticosteroid; IAHA: intraarticular hyaluronate; NSAID: nonsteroidal anti-inflammatory drugs; PPI: proton pump inhibitor; SYSADOA: symptomatic slow-acting drugs of osteoarthritis)

OBSTRUCTIVE SLEEP APNEA

Prevalence

Obstructive sleep apnea (OSA) is a clinical condition characterized by repeated instances of complete or partial obstruction of the upper airway during sleep. This obstruction leads to negative intrathoracic pressure, fragmented sleep, and intermittent episodes of reduced oxygen levels (hypoxia). Recent research has shown that approximately one-third of sleep studies reveal some degree of OSA, defined as an apnea-hypopnea index (AHI) of five or more events per hour of sleep.[63]

Among adults aged 30–70, around 13% of men and 6% of women have moderate to severe forms of OSA, with an AHI of 15 or more events per hour of sleep. These estimates represent a significant increase compared to data from two decades ago and can largely be attributed to the ongoing obesity epidemic. It is estimated that 50–60% of individuals who are obese or have metabolic syndrome also have OSA. The prevalence of OSA is even higher in obese individuals with diabetes mellitus and morbid obesity. Despite this strong association, OSA often goes unrecognized in a majority of these patients, despite having a high probability of having the condition.[63]

A literature-based analysis conducted by Benjafield et al. used the 2012 scoring criteria of the American Academy of Sleep Medicine and defined OSA as an AHI threshold of five or more events per hour and 15 or more events per hour. The global estimate suggests that approximately 936 million adults aged 30–69 have mild to severe OSA, and 425 million adults in the same age group have moderate to severe OSA. Among affected individuals, the highest numbers were found in China (176 million and 66 million for the two thresholds), followed by the USA (54 million and 24 million), Brazil (49 million and 25 million), and India (52 million and 29 million).[64]

Pathogenesis

Numerous studies have consistently demonstrated a strong and positive link between obesity and OSA. The relationship between obesity and OSA is multifaceted, and several potential mechanisms have been proposed to explain their association (see Fig. 6).[65]

Traditionally, it has been suggested that the increased mass of adipose tissue mechanically restricts the airflow, leading to airway obstruction during sleep. This is particularly relevant in the tongue and pharyngeal areas, where excess fat deposits create a physical weight that hinders normal breathing, resulting in apnea or hypopnea. Furthermore, obesity affects the mechanics of the lungs, reducing their functional capacity and tidal volume, which further contributes to respiratory disturbances.[65]

However, emerging hypotheses indicate that physiological factors related to obesity play a significant role in the development of OSA. Factors such as glycemic control, insulin action, and leptin signaling are currently being investigated for their potential impact on OSA. Obese individuals may experience greater reductions in muscle tone in the pharyngeal dilator muscles, making them more susceptible to airway blockages during sleep. This reduction in muscle tone could be influenced by chronically increased muscle activity, autonomic responses, or inflammatory pathways that lead to histological changes in the muscle tissue. Additionally, the physiological characteristics associated with obesity may contribute to disordered breathing and central sleep apnea through a decreased sensitivity to chemical stimuli.[65]

These evolving hypotheses suggest that the relationship between obesity and OSA extends beyond the mechanical effects of excess fat mass. Physiological factors, including metabolic and hormonal dysregulation, likely play significant roles in the development and progression of OSA. Further research is necessary to fully

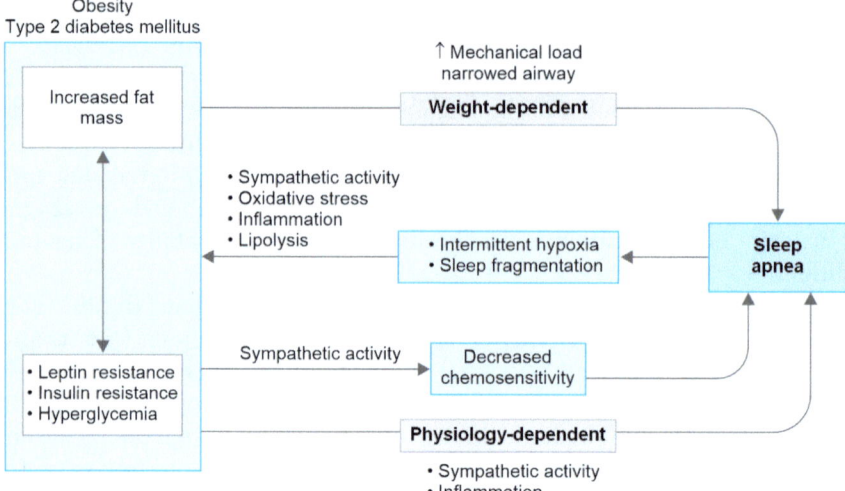

FIG. 6: The bidirectional relationship between obstructive sleep apnea and metabolic disease. Sleep apnea results in intermittent hypoxia and sleep fragmentation which lead to and exacerbate obesity and type 2 diabetes mellitus by increasing sympathetic activity, oxidative stress, inflammation, and lipolysis. Moreover, metabolic disease can lead to, or exacerbate, sleep apnea through weight-dependent and physiology-dependent mechanisms. While weight-dependent mechanisms are a function of the physical increase in body mass or fat mass (e.g., increased mechanical load, narrowed airway), physiology-dependent mechanisms are physiological changes coincident with obesity or diabetes which go on to influence chemosensitivity and sleep apnea either directly or via action on sympathetic activity, inflammation, or other mechanisms.

understand the complex interplay between obesity and OSA and to develop targeted interventions for this common sleep disorder.

Diagnosis

The diagnosis of OSA begins with a comprehensive evaluation of the patient's medical history and a thorough physical examination to identify the characteristic signs and symptoms of the condition. Patients commonly report symptoms such as snoring, disrupted sleep, daytime sleepiness, decreased libido, and may also have a history of hypertension, CVD, and diabetes. However, relying solely on a clinician's subjective analysis for OSA diagnosis may lead to inaccuracies due to the nonspecific and variable nature of the disorder.[66]

To improve the accuracy of OSA diagnosis, several outpatient screening questionnaires have been developed. These questionnaires, including the Epworth Sleepiness Scale (ESS), Berlin Questionnaire, STOP-BANG questionnaire, Sleep Apnea of Sleep Disorder Questionnaire (SA-SDQ), OSA50 questionnaire, and others, can assist in identifying individuals who may be at risk for OSA. These screening tools provide additional objective measures to supplement the clinician's assessment and aid in the identification of potential OSA patients.[66]

Overnight polysomnography is considered the gold standard for diagnosing OSA. To identify patients at high risk and in urgent need of polysomnography and/or further treatment, a screening tool is necessary to stratify individuals based on their clinical symptoms, physical examinations, and risk factors.[66]

Diagnostic polysomnography involves using a computerized polysomnographic system to monitor various physiological parameters during sleep. This includes electroencephalogram (EEG), submental and anterior tibial electromyogram (EMG), oxygen saturation (SaO_2), electrocardiogram (ECG), inductance plethysmography of the chest walls and abdomen, nasal pressure sensor, and oronasal thermistor. The polysomnographic recording is manually scored by a sleep specialist, following the guidelines outlined in the American Academy of Sleep Medicine (AASM) Manual for the Scoring of Sleep and Associated Events. The total obstructive AHI is calculated by determining the number of obstructive apneas and hypopneas per hour of total sleep time (TST). A threshold of AHI ≥5 is used to diagnose OSA. The severity of OSA is then classified based on specific cut-off levels of AHI, which are determined using standardized criteria.[66]

Management of Obstructive Sleep Apnea

Effective treatments for OSA encompass various approaches, including behavioral measures, medical devices, and surgery. Behavioral measures involve lifestyle modifications such as abstaining from alcohol, avoiding the supine sleep position, engaging in regular aerobic exercise, and weight loss. Weight loss, in particular, is recommended for all patients with overweight or obesity in conjunction with other therapies, as it has shown to improve OSA severity. Lifestyle interventions, bariatric surgery, and weight loss medication have been associated with improved OSA severity **(Flowchart 3)**.[66,67]

In the Sleep AHEAD study, which focused on patients with overweight or obesity, T2DM, and OSA, participants were randomized to undergo a lifestyle intervention involving weight loss through diet and exercise, or a diabetes education control. At the 1-year follow-up, the lifestyle intervention group exhibited a significantly greater reduction in weight (10.2 kg) and a greater reduction in the AHI by 9.7 events/hour.[68]

Exercise has shown potential in improving OSA independent of weight loss. There is a dose-dependent association between exercise and a lower prevalence of OSA. Individuals engaging in vigorous exercise demonstrated reduced odds ratios for moderate to severe OSA, with ratios of 0.62 for 1–2 hours of exercise per week, 0.39 for 3–6 hours/week, and 0.31 for at least 7 hours/week, after adjusting for factors such as age, sex, body habitus, and daytime sleepiness.[69]

Positive airway pressure (PAP) is considered the primary therapy for individuals with symptomatic OSA of any severity. PAP devices deliver pressurized air to the airway through a mask worn over the nose or nose and mouth, acting as a splint to prevent airway collapse during inspiration. PAP therapy has been shown to normalize the AHI in over 90% of patients while wearing the device.[67]

Positive airway pressure is widely regarded as the first-line treatment for most patients with OSA due to its effectiveness, cost-effectiveness, and noninvasive nature. It directly counteracts the collapse of the oropharynx by delivering pressure through a nasal or oronasal mask during sleep. PAP can be delivered in different modes—continuous positive airway pressure (CPAP), where a fixed pressure is applied; bilevel positive airway pressure (BiPAP), where different pressures are applied during inhalation and exhalation; and autotitrating positive airway

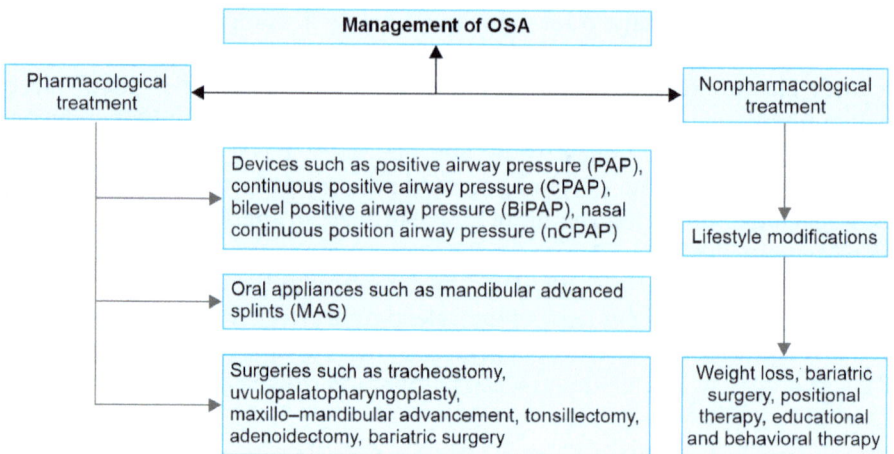

FLOWCHART 3: Treatment algorithm of obstructive sleep apnea (OSA).

pressure (APAP), where the delivered pressure varies based on machine feedback. To determine the ideal pressure needed to prevent airway collapse, patients may undergo further attended in-lab polysomnography.[70]

The benefits of PAP therapy depend on adherence to the treatment, with greater hours of nightly use associated with improved symptom relief and reduction in blood pressure. A 2019 report involving over 2.6 million patients who initiated PAP therapy revealed that 75% of patients achieved adequate adherence within the first 90 days of treatment. Overall, PAP was used on 93% of nights, with a mean duration of 6.0 (2.0) hours/night. Approximately 65% to 80% of patients continue using PAP therapy after 4 years.[67]

Factors that enhance adherence to PAP therapy include education about the risks of OSA and the expected benefits of treatment, monitoring of PAP use with reinforcement and support for technical issues, and behavioral interventions such as cognitive-behavioral therapy and motivational enhancement therapy. These interventions can increase PAP adherence by >30 minutes/night, with behavioral interventions having a mean effect size of up to 80 minutes/night.[67]

Oral appliances, specifically mandibular repositioning devices (MADs), are effective treatment options, particularly for individuals with mild to moderate OSA. MADs are an alternative to PAP therapy for OSA. A MAD works by positioning the mandible (lower jaw) in a protruded position during sleep, which increases the airway's caliber and activates stretch receptors, reducing upper airway collapsibility.[67,70]

A large multicenter study involving over 400 patients treated with a MAD found significant improvements in OSA outcomes. Specifically, 37% of patients achieved complete resolution of their OSA (AHI <5), 52% experienced a reduction in AHI to <10, and 64% had their AHI more than halved.[71] Furthermore, a meta-analysis demonstrated that MADs can reduce blood pressure similarly to PAP therapy. Compared to an inactive control group, MADs were associated with a reduction in SBP of 2.1 mm Hg ($p = 0.002$) and a reduction in diastolic blood pressure (DBP) of 1.9 mm Hg ($p = 0.008$).[72] Another meta-analysis of 34 randomized clinical trials showed that MADs were associated with a mean reduction in AHI of 13.6 events/hour.[67]

Surgical treatment of OSA may be considered for appropriate candidates who have obstructing anatomy or are unable to tolerate PAP therapy. The surgical procedures aim to alleviate areas of airway obstruction during sleep and can be categorized based on their intended anatomical targets. Nasal procedures such as septoplasty (correction of a deviated nasal septum) and nasal valve surgery focus on addressing nasal airway blockages. Oral/palatal procedures, such as uvulopalatoplasty (removal or modification of the uvula and/or soft palate) and tonsillectomy (removal of the tonsils), target obstructions in the oral and palatal regions. Hypopharyngeal procedures, such as radiofrequency ablation of the tongue, aim to address obstructions in the base of the tongue area. Other surgical options include maxillomandibular advancement (MMA), which involves repositioning the upper and lower jaws, and tracheostomy, which creates a bypass for airflow by surgically opening the trachea.[73]

A recent systematic review indicated that tracheostomy had the most evidence supporting reduced cardiovascular outcomes. However, tracheostomy is generally considered an antiquated and highly invasive procedure for the treatment of OSA. Pharyngeal surgery, including uvulopalatopharyngoplasty (UPPP), showed mixed improvements in cardiovascular endpoints. MMA demonstrated some evidence for improved hypertension.[74]

Hypoglossal nerve stimulation is a newer surgical procedure used to increase the tone of the pharyngeal dilator muscles during sleep. The US Food and Drug Administration has approved a specific device for this procedure, which involves the unilateral placement of an electrode on the medial branch of the hypoglossal nerve. The electrode enhances tongue protrusion, while a pressure sensor is positioned between the internal and external intercostal muscles to detect inspiratory effort. Additionally, a small neurostimulator is implanted in the chest wall, which triggers the hypoglossal electrode in response to respiratory effort. In the Stimulation Therapy for Apnea Reduction (STAR) trial, this hypoglossal nerve stimulation device was evaluated. The trial demonstrated that the treatment significantly reduced the median AHI from 29.3 to 9.0 events/hour. The median change in AHI was -17.3 events/hour, with sustained benefits observed even after 5 years of therapy.[75,76]

These findings highlight the importance of behavioral interventions and lifestyle modifications in the management of OSA. Incorporating these measures along with medical devices and surgical options as appropriate, can contribute to improved OSA outcomes and overall patient well-being.

MALIGNANCIES

Obesity is associated with a significant increase in the risk of various cancer types, estimated to be around 20%. This elevated cancer risk is influenced by factors such as diet, weight fluctuations, body fat distribution, and physical activity. Strong evidence from organizations such as the International Agency for Research into Cancer and the World Cancer Research Fund links obesity to several specific cancer types, including endometrial, esophageal adenocarcinoma, colorectal, postmenopausal breast, prostate, and renal cancers. Less common malignancies, such as leukemia, non-Hodgkin's lymphoma, multiple myeloma, malignant melanoma, and thyroid tumors, are also affected. Studies consistently show that as BMI increases from normal to overweight to obese categories, the risk of cancer rises in a dose-response manner. However, successful and sustained weight loss has been shown to reduce this future cancer risk.[77]

Leukemia, non-Hodgkin's lymphoma, and myeloma are among the cancers associated with obesity, as supported by large cohort studies and meta-analyses. The mechanisms underlying this association could involve changes in metabolism, endocrine function, immunity, inflammation, and DNA regulation. Obesity may increase cell mutation rates, disrupt gene function, hinder DNA repair, or induce epigenetic changes that favor the development of cancer. Alternatively, obesity may create an environment that allows dormant cancer cells to become active. The link between obesity and cancer risk is primarily attributed to anthropometric factors such as BMI, weight gain, and the amount of body fat, particularly visceral fat. Lifestyle factors, including sedentary behavior and diet quality (especially a high-calorie and low-quality diet), also play a significant role. Biological mechanisms mediating the adverse effects of these factors include hyperinsulinemia, insulin resistance, insulin-like growth factors (IGFs), sex hormones, inflammation, adipokine and vascular growth factor production, oxidative stress, endocrine disruptors, and immune function alterations.[77,78]

Data from the American Cancer Society indicate that overweight and obesity are associated with higher death rates from liver, pancreatic, myeloma, and non-Hodgkin's lymphoma cancers. Over the past few decades, it has become evident that obesity is a causative factor in approximately 20% of cancer-related deaths in women and around 14% in men, making it the second leading preventable cause of cancer after smoking. Abdominal obesity, in particular, has been linked to a 24% increase in cancer mortality. Epidemiological studies further highlight the contribution of obesity to both the incidence and mortality of colon, endometrial, kidney, and postmenopausal breast cancers. In the European Union, preventing overweight and obesity could potentially reduce the annual incidence of colon cancer by up to 21,000 cases and breast cancer by up to 13,000 cases. Additionally, obesity's impact on cancer potency and progression likely contributes to lower survival rates among individuals with cancer.[78]

REFERENCES

1. World Health Organization. (2021). Obesity and overweight. [online] Available from https://www.who.int/news-room/fact-sheets/detail/obesity-and-overweight [Last accessed October, 2023].
2. Pati S, Irfan W, Jameel A, Ahmed S, Shahid RK. Obesity and Cancer: A Current overview of epidemiology, pathogenesis, outcomes, and management. Cancers (Basel). 2023;15(2):485.
3. Chong B, Jayabaskaran J, Kong G, Chan YH, Chin YH, Goh R, et al. Trends and predictions of malnutrition and obesity in 204 countries and territories: an analysis of the Global Burden of Disease Study 2019. EClinicalMedicine. 2023;57:101850.
4. Malnick SDH, Knobler H. The medical complications of obesity. QJM. 2006;99:565-79.
5. Medscape. (2013). Obesity's Toll: 1 in 5 deaths linked to excess weight. [online] Available from http://www.medscape.com/viewarticle/809516. [Last accessed October, 2023].
6. Maggs FG. Problem based review: the morbidly obese patient. Acute Med. 2012;11:107-12.

7. GBD 2013 Mortality and Causes of Death Collaborators. Global, regional, and national age–sex specific all-cause and cause-specific mortality for 240 causes of death, 1990–2013: a systematic analysis for the Global Burden of Disease Study 2013. Lancet. 2015;385(9963):117-71.
8. Roglic G, Unwin N. Mortality attributable to diabetes: estimates for the year 2010. Diabetes Res Clin Pract. 2010;87(1):15-9.
9. International Diabetes Federation. (2021). IDF Diabetes Atlas. 10th edition. [online] Available from http://www.diabetesatlas.org/. [Last accessed October, 2023].
10. Vos T, Barber RM, Bell B, Bertozzi-Villa A, Biryukov S, Bolliger I, et al. Global, regional, and national incidence, prevalence, and years lived with disability for 301 acute and chronic diseases and injuries in 188 countries, 1990–2013: a systematic analysis for the Global Burden of Disease Study 2013. Lancet. 2015;386(9995):743-800.
11. Forouzanfar MH, Afshin A, Alexander LT, Anderson HR, Bhutta ZA, Biryukov S, et al. Global, regional, and national comparative risk assessment of 79 behavioural, environmental and occupational, and metabolic risks or clusters of risks, 1990–2015: a systematic analysis for the Global Burden of Disease Study 2015. Lancet. 2016;388(10053):1659-724.
12. Litwak L, Goh SY, Hussein Z, Malek R, Prusty V, Khamseh ME. Prevalence of diabetes complications in people with type 2 diabetes mellitus and its association with baseline characteristics in the multinational A1chieve study. Diabetol Metab Syndr. 2013;5(1):57.
13. Gregg EW, Sattar N, Ali MK. The changing face of diabetes complications. Lancet Diabetes Endocrinol. 2016;4(6):537-47.
14. Zimmet PZ, Magliano DJ, Herman WH, Shaw JE. Diabetes: a 21st century challenge. Lancet Diabetes Endocrinol. 2014;2(1):56-64.
15. Zhuo X, Zhang P, Hoerger TJ. Lifetime direct medical costs of treating type 2 diabetes and diabetic complications. Am J Prev Med. 2013;45(3):253-61.
16. Reusch JEB, Manson JE. Management of type 2 diabetes in 2017: Getting to goal. JAMA. 2017;317(10):1015-6.
17. Harding JL, Pavkov ME, Magliano DJ, Shaw JE, Gregg EW. Global trends in diabetes complications: a review of current evidence. Diabetologia. 2019;62(1):3-16.
18. Zheng Y, Ley SH, Hu FB. Global aetiology and epidemiology of type 2 diabetes mellitus and its complications. Nat Rev Endocrinol. 2018;14(2):88-98.
19. Polovina M, Lund LH, Đikić D, Petrović-Đorđević I, Krljanac G, Milinković I, et al. Type 2 diabetes increases the long-term risk of heart failure and mortality in patients with atrial fibrillation. Eur J Heart Fail. 2020;22(1):113-25.
20. Kozakova M, Morizzo C, Fraser AG, Palombo C. Impact of glycemic control on aortic stiffness, left ventricular mass and diastolic longitudinal function in type 2 diabetes mellitus. Cardiovasc Diabetol. 2017;16(1):78.
21. Grubić Rotkvić P, Planinić Z, Liberati Pršo AM, Šikić J, Galić E, Rotkvić L. The mystery of diabetic cardiomyopathy: from early concepts and underlying mechanisms to novel therapeutic possibilities. Int J Mol Sci. 2021;22(11):5973.
22. Jia G, Whaley-Connell A, Sowers JR. Diabetic cardiomyopathy: a hyperglycaemia- and insulin-resistance-induced heart disease. Diabetologia. 2018;61(1):21-8.
23. Li Y, Liu Y, Liu S, Gao M, Wang W, Chen K, et al. Diabetic vascular diseases: molecular mechanisms and therapeutic strategies. Signal Transduct Target Ther. 2023;8(1):152.
24. Sarma S, Sockalingam S, Dash S. Obesity as a multisystem disease: trends in obesity rates and obesity-related complications. Diabetes Obes Metab. 2021;23 Suppl 1:3-16.
25. Ren J, Wu NN, Wang S, Sowers JR, Zhang Y. Obesity cardiomyopathy: evidence, mechanisms, and therapeutic implications. Physiol Rev. 2021;101(4):1745-807.
26. Lopez-Jimenez F, Almahmeed W, Bays H, Cuevas A, Di Angelantonio E, le Roux CW, et al. Obesity and cardiovascular disease: mechanistic insights and management strategies. A joint position paper by the World Heart Federation and World Obesity Federation. Eur J Prev Cardiol. 2022;29(17):2218-37.
27. Zhang Y, Lazzarini PA, McPhail SM, van Netten JJ, Armstrong DG, Pacella RE. Global disability burdens of diabetes-related lower-extremity complications in 1990 and 2016. Diabetes Care. 2020;43(5):964-74.
28. Yang H, Sloan G, Ye Y, Wang S, Duan B, Tesfaye S, et al. New Perspective in Diabetic Neuropathy: From the Periphery to the Brain, a Call for Early Detection, and Precision Medicine. Front Endocrinol (Lausanne). 2020;10:929.
29. Sandireddy R, Yerra VG, Areti A, Komirishetty P, Kumar A. Neuroinflammation and oxidative stress in diabetic neuropathy: futuristic strategies based on these targets. Int J Endocrinol. 2014;2014:674987.

30. Rosenberger DC, Blechschmidt V, Timmerman H, Wolff A, Treede RD. Challenges of neuropathic pain: focus on diabetic neuropathy. J Neural Transm (Vienna). 2020;127(4):589-624.
31. Khdour MR. Treatment of diabetic peripheral neuropathy: a review. J Pharm Pharmacol. 2020;72(7):863-72.
32. Chen J, Liu Q, He J, Li Y. Immune responses in diabetic nephropathy: Pathogenic mechanisms and therapeutic target. Front Immunol. 2022;13:958790.
33. Gross JL, de Azevedo MJ, Silveiro SP, Canani LH, Caramori ML, Zelmanovitz T. Diabetic nephropathy: diagnosis, prevention, and treatment. Diabetes Care. 2005;28(1):164-76.
34. Deng Y, Li N, Wu Y, Wang M, Yang S, Zheng Y, et al. Global, Regional, and National Burden of Diabetes-Related Chronic Kidney Disease From 1990 to 2019. Front Endocrinol (Lausanne). 2021;12:672350.
35. Samsu N. Diabetic Nephropathy: Challenges in pathogenesis, diagnosis, and treatment. Biomed Res Int. 2021;2021:1497449.
36. Kidney Disease: Improving Global Outcomes (KDIGO) Diabetes Work Group. KDIGO 2022 Clinical Practice Guideline for Diabetes Management in Chronic Kidney Disease. Kidney Int. 2022;102(5S):S1-S127.
37. Kidney Disease: Improving Global Outcomes (KDIGO) Blood Pressure Work Group. KDIGO 2021 Clinical Practice Guideline for the Management of Blood Pressure in Chronic Kidney Disease. Kidney Int. 2021;99(3S):S1-S87.
38. Wanner C, Tonelli M; Kidney Disease: Improving Global Outcomes Lipid Guideline Development Work Group Members. KDIGO Clinical Practice Guideline for Lipid Management in CKD: summary of recommendation statements and clinical approach to the patient. Kidney Int. 2014;85(6):1303-9.
39. Task Force on diabetes, pre-diabetes, and cardiovascular diseases of the European Society of Cardiology (ESC); European Association for the Study of Diabetes (EASD), Rydén L, Grant PJ, Anker SD, Berne C, et al. ESC guidelines on diabetes, pre-diabetes, and cardiovascular diseases developed in collaboration with the EASD - summary. Diab Vasc Dis Res. 2014;11(3):133-73.
40. American Diabetes Association. 11. Microvascular Complications and Foot Care: Standards of Medical Care in Diabetes-2021 [published correction appears in Diabetes Care. 2021 Sep;44(9):2186-2187]. Diabetes Care. 2021;44(Suppl 1):S151-67.
41. Type 2 diabetes in adults: management. London: National Institute for Health and Care Excellence (NICE); 2022. [online] Available from https://www.ncbi.nlm.nih.gov/books/NBK553486/ [Last accessed October, 2023].
42. Chronic kidney disease in adults: assessment and management. London: National Institute for Health and Care Excellence (NICE); 2015.
43. Cardiovascular disease: risk assessment and reduction, including lipid modification. London: National Institute for Health and Care Excellence (NICE); 2023. [online] Available from https://www.ncbi.nlm.nih.gov/books/NBK554923/ [Last accessed October, 2023].
44. Hypertension in adults: diagnosis and management. London: National Institute for Health and Care Excellence (NICE); 2022. Available from: https://www.ncbi.nlm.nih.gov/books/NBK547161/ [Last accessed October, 2023].
45. Crasto W, Patel V, Davies MJ, Khunti K. Prevention of microvascular complications of diabetes. Endocrinol Metab Clin North Am. 2021;50(3):431-55.
46. McGrath K, Edi R. Diabetic kidney disease: diagnosis, treatment, and prevention. Am Fam Physician. 2019;99(12):751-9.
47. Nguyen VH, Le MH, Cheung RC, Nguyen MH. Differential clinical characteristics and mortality outcomes in persons with NAFLD and/or MAFLD. Clin Gastroenterol Hepatol. 2021;19(10):2172-81.e6.
48. Yuan Q, Wang H, Gao P, Chen W, Lv M, Bai S, et al. Prevalence and risk factors of metabolic-associated fatty liver disease among 73,566 individuals in Beijing, China. Int J Environ Res Public Health. 2022;19(4):2096.
49. De A, Bhagat N, Mehta M, Taneja S, Duseja A. Metabolic dysfunction-associated steatotic liver disease (MASLD) definition is better than MAFLD criteria for lean patients with non-alcoholic fatty liver disease (NAFLD) [published online ahead of print, 2023]. J Hepatol. 2023;S0168-8278(23)05044-4.
50. Chan KE, Koh TJL, Tang ASP, Quek J, Yong JN, Tay PWL, et al. Global prevalence and clinical characteristics of metabolic-associated fatty liver disease: a meta-analysis and systematic review of 10,739,607 individuals. J Clin Endocrinol Metab. 2022;107(9):2691-700.
51. Eslam M, Sarin SK, Wong VW, Fan JG, Kawaguchi T, Ahn SH, et al. The Asian Pacific Association for the Study of the Liver clinical practice guidelines for the diagnosis and management of metabolic associated fatty liver disease. Hepatol Int. 2020;14(6):889-919.
52. Eslam M, Newsome PN, Sarin SK, Anstee QM, Targher G, Romero-Gomez M, et al. A new definition for metabolic dysfunction-associated fatty liver disease: An international expert consensus statement. J Hepatol. 2020;73(1):202-9.

53. Cusi K, Isaacs S, Barb D, Basu R, Caprio S, Garvey WT, et al. American Association of Clinical Endocrinology Clinical Practice Guideline for the Diagnosis and Management of Nonalcoholic Fatty Liver Disease in Primary Care and Endocrinology Clinical Settings: Co-Sponsored by the American Association for the Study of Liver Diseases (AASLD). Endocr Pract. 2022;28(5):528-62.
54. Davis TME. Diabetes and metabolic dysfunction-associated fatty liver disease. Metabolism. 2021;123:154868.
55. Venkatesan K, Haroon NN. Management of metabolic-associated fatty liver disease. Endocrinol Metab Clin North Am. 2023 Sep;52(3):547-57.
56. Chooi YC, Ding C, Magkos F. The epidemiology of obesity. Metabolism. 2019;92:6-10.
57. King LK, March L, Anandacoomarasamy A. Obesity & osteoarthritis. Indian J Med Res. 2013;138(2):185-93.
58. Cross M, Smith E, Hoy D, Nolte S, Ackerman I, Fransen M, et al. The global burden of hip and knee osteoarthritis: estimates from the global burden of disease 2010 study. Ann Rheum Dis. 2014;73(7):1323-30.
59. Cui A, Li H, Wang D, Zhong J, Chen Y, Lu H. Global, regional prevalence, incidence and risk factors of knee osteoarthritis in population-based studies. EClinicalMedicine. 2020;29-30:100587.
60. Sobieh BH, El-Mesallamy HO, Kassem DH. Beyond mechanical loading: The metabolic contribution of obesity in osteoarthritis unveils novel therapeutic targets. Heliyon. 2023;9(5):e15700.
61. Sinusas K. Osteoarthritis: diagnosis and treatment [published correction appears in Am Fam Physician. 2012 Nov 15;86(10):893]. Am Fam Physician. 2012;85(1):49-56.
62. Yeap SS, Abu Amin SR, Baharuddin H, Koh KC, Lee JK, Lee VKM, et al. A Malaysian Delphi consensus on managing knee osteoarthritis. BMC Musculoskelet Disord. 2021;22(1):514.
63. Drager LF, Togeiro SM, Polotsky VY, Lorenzi-Filho G. Obstructive sleep apnea: a cardiometabolic risk in obesity and the metabolic syndrome. J Am Coll Cardiol. 2013;62(7):569-76.
64. Benjafield AV, Ayas NT, Eastwood PR, Heinzer R, Ip MSM, Morrell MJ, et al. Estimation of the global prevalence and burden of obstructive sleep apnoea: a literature-based analysis. Lancet Respir Med. 2019;7(8):687-98.
65. Framnes SN, Arble DM. The Bidirectional Relationship Between Obstructive Sleep Apnea and Metabolic Disease. Front Endocrinol (Lausanne). 2018;9:440.
66. Jyothi I, Renuka Prasad K, Rajalakshmi R, Satish Kumar R, Ramphanindra T, Vijayakumar T, et al. Obstructive Sleep Apnea: A Pathophysiology and Pharmacotherapy Approach [Internet]. Noninvasive Ventilation in Medicine - Recent Updates. IntechOpen; 2019. [online] Available from: http://dx.doi.org/10.5772/intechopen.77981 [Last accessed October, 2023].
67. Gottlieb DJ, Punjabi NM. Diagnosis and management of obstructive sleep apnea: a review. JAMA. 2020;323(14):1389-1400.
68. Foster GD, Borradaile KE, Sanders MH, Millman R, Zammit G, Newman AB, et al. A randomized study on the effect of weight loss on obstructive sleep apnea among obese patients with type 2 diabetes: the Sleep AHEAD study. Arch Intern Med. 2009;169(17):1619-26.
69. Peppard PE, Young T. Exercise and sleep-disordered breathing: an association independent of body habitus. Sleep. 2004;27(3):480-4.
70. Lee JJ, Sundar KM. Evaluation and management of adults with obstructive sleep apnea syndrome. Lung. 2021;199(2):87-101.
71. Sutherland K, Takaya H, Qian J, Petocz P, Ng AT, Cistulli PA. Oral Appliance Treatment Response and Polysomnographic Phenotypes of Obstructive Sleep Apnea. J Clin Sleep Med. 2015;11(8):861-68.
72. Bratton DJ, Gaisl T, Wons AM, Kohler M. CPAP vs mandibular advancement devices and blood pressure in patients with obstructive sleep apnea: a systematic review and meta-analysis. JAMA. 2015;314(21):2280-93.
73. Smith DF, Cohen AP, Ishman SL. Surgical management of OSA in adults. Chest. 2015;147(6):1681-90.
74. Halle TR, Oh MS, Collop NA, Quyyumi AA, Bliwise DL, Dedhia RC. Surgical treatment of OSA on cardiovascular outcomes: a systematic review. Chest. 2017;152(6):1214-29.
75. Strollo PJ Jr, Soose RJ, Maurer JT, de Vries N, Cornelius J, Froymovich O, et al. Upper-airway stimulation for obstructive sleep apnea. N Engl J Med. 2014;370(2):139-49.
76. Woodson BT, Strohl KP, Soose RJ, Gillespie MB, Maurer JT, de Vries N, et al. Upper Airway Stimulation for Obstructive Sleep Apnea: 5-Year Outcomes. Otolaryngol Head Neck Surg. 2018;159(1):194-202.
77. Lichtman MA. Obesity and the risk for a hematological malignancy: leukemia, lymphoma, or myeloma. Oncologist. 2010;15(10):1083-1101.
78. De Pergola G, Silvestris F. Obesity as a major risk factor for cancer. J Obes. 2013;2013:291546.

CHAPTER 9

Special Populations and Issues

Key Highlights

- *Children and adolescents*: Multidisciplinary approach, careful insulin dosing, dietary education, and promoting physical activity.
- *Older adults*: Individualized treatment plans, regular monitoring, and medication adjustments as needed.
- *Pregnant women and gestational diabetes*: Tight glycemic control, regular prenatal check-ups, and close monitoring of blood sugar levels. Lifestyle modifications as first-line treatment, insulin or other medications if necessary.
- Weight management in special populations requires tailored approaches to address unique challenges, such as menopausal hormonal changes, polycystic ovarian syndrome (PCOS)-related insulin resistance, and aging-related body composition changes.
- Lifestyle modifications, including balanced diets, regular exercise (both aerobic and resistance training), and behavioral therapy, are essential components of weight management in special populations.
- Medications approved by the Food and Drug Administration (FDA), such as orlistat, phentermine/topiramate, naltrexone/bupropion, and liraglutide 3 mg, may be considered for long-term use in managing obesity.

PEDIATRIC AND ADOLESCENT OBESITY AND DIABETES

Pediatric and Adolescent Obesity

Amidst the global health crisis caused by the escalating issue of excess weight in children, the member states of the World Health Organization (WHO) have taken action by endorsing the goal of "no increase in childhood overweight by 2025." This objective is part of the "Comprehensive Implementation Plan for Maternal, Infant, and Young Child Nutrition," aligning with the aim set for obesity and diabetes from 2010 to 2025 in the "WHO Global Action Plan for the Prevention and Control of Noncommunicable Diseases 2013–2020".[1]

The obesity epidemic has the potential to undermine the remarkable strides made in improving life expectancy worldwide. Despite emerging as a concern several decades ago, the issue of excess weight during childhood and adolescence continues to be a pressing matter in global health. In 2014, an estimated 41 million children under the age of 5 years were affected by overweight or obesity, defined as weight-for-height Z-score values exceeding 2 and 3 standard deviations (SDs), respectively, from the WHO growth standard median.[2]

The situation in Africa is particularly alarming, as the number of overweight or obese children has nearly doubled since 1990, increasing from 5.4 to 10.3 million. In 2014, 48% of children under age of 5 years who were overweight resided in Asia, and 25% were in Africa. Surprisingly, more overweight and obese children are found in low- and middle-income countries than in high-income countries (HICs) when considering prevalence in absolute numbers.[2]

Examining the period between 1975 and 2016, for the age group of 5–19 years, the global prevalence of obesity [body mass index (BMI) >2 SD above the median of the WHO growth reference] has soared to 5.6% in girls and 7.8% in boys, showing an approximately eight-fold increase. While HICs have reached a plateau in obesity rates, other regions, notably parts of Asia, have experienced an acceleration in obesity rates. Analyzing the age group of 2–4 years between 1980 and 2015, the prevalence of obesity [International Obesity Task Force (IOTF) definition, equivalent to an adult BMI of ≥30 kg/m^2] has risen from 3.9 to 7.2% in boys and from 3.7 to 6.4% in girls.[1,3]

The future health risks associated with pediatric obesity in adulthood are well-documented. For instance, a data linkage prospective study in Israel with 2.3 million participants revealed that individuals with obesity (≥95th percentile BMI for age) had a substantially higher risk of death from coronary heart disease, stroke, and sudden death compared to those with BMI falling between the 5th and 24th percentiles at age of 17 years. The study revealed that individuals with obesity had a heightened risk of death from coronary heart disease, with a hazard ratio (HR) of 4.9, also faced a higher risk of stroke, with an HR of 2.6, and had an increased risk of sudden death, with an HR of 2.1. The gravity of the excess weight crisis in children demands urgent and concerted efforts from governments, healthcare organizations, and society as a whole to address and reverse this alarming trend.[4]

According to a systematic review conducted in 2019, children and adolescents affected by obesity face significantly higher risks of various health conditions compared to those with a healthy weight. Specifically, the findings showed that individuals with obesity were 1.4 times more likely to have prediabetes, 1.7 times more likely to have asthma, 4.4 times more likely to have high blood pressure, and a staggering 26.1 times more likely to have fatty liver disease.[5]

Considering these alarming statistics, projections have been made regarding the potential impact of childhood obesity on global health. By the year 2025, it is estimated that there could be approximately 12 million children aged 5–17 years with glucose intolerance, 4 million with type 2 diabetes mellitus (T2DM), 27 million with hypertension, and 38 million with fatty liver disease worldwide.[6] These high prevalence rates of obesity-related health conditions carry significant implications for both pediatric and adult health services.

Pediatric and Adolescent Obesity: Management

The Expert Committee recommendations propose a shift in the approach to addressing obesity, advocating for a move from merely identifying cases of obesity to universal assessment, preventive health messages, and early intervention. To combat the childhood obesity epidemic effectively, primary care providers should assess obesity risk for all patients and offer guidance on healthy behaviors to minimize those risks. The recommendations provided by the expert committee and writing groups cover all stages of care, from normal-weight, low-risk children to severely obese children **(Flowchart 1)**.[7]

Body mass index serves as the initial screening tool at each well-child visit and forms the basis for categorizing health risks. Children in the healthy-weight category (BMI between the 5th and 84th percentile) generally have lower risks and efforts should focus on maintaining or adopting healthy lifestyle behaviors through preventive measures. As BMI increases to the 85th to 94th percentile (overweight category), children may require prevention counseling and if health risks, others might need more active intervention rises.[7] Children with a BMI above the 95th percentile (obese) are highly likely to face obesity-related health risks, necessitating a focus on weight control practices as per the staged approach **(Flowchart 1)**.[7]

Obesity is further classified into three distinct classes:[8]
- *Class I obesity*: BMI at least 95th percentile—BMI <120% of the 95th percentile or BMI <35 kg/m², whichever is lower.
- *Class II obesity*: BMI at least 120% of the 95th percentile or a BMI at least 35 kg/m², whichever is lower—BMI <140% of the 95th percentile.
- *Class III obesity*: BMI at least 140% of the 95th percentile or a BMI at least 40 kg/m², whichever is lower.

Severe obesity encompasses classes II and III obesity. It is important to track weight status over time using a specific BMI-for-age chart. Interventions for obesity are tailored based on severity, clinical capacity, and family motivation, involving a multidisciplinary team of experts including pediatrician, dietitian, mental health counselor, coordinator, exercise specialist, and, when necessary, a bariatric surgeon.[8] These approaches aim to enhance obesity management by facilitating early assessment, personalized intervention, and appropriate tracking for better health outcomes in children and adolescents.

Lifestyle Intervention

Nutrition: The recommendations for adolescents involve consuming five or more servings of fruits and vegetables daily, minimizing sugar-sweetened beverages, eating breakfast, limiting meals outside the home, portion control, and promoting balanced macronutrient intake. At stage 2, a structured eating plan based on dietary reference intake (DRI) recommendations is used. For stage 3 and 4, focusing on weight loss, very low-energy diets (VLED) with ≤800 kcal/day using

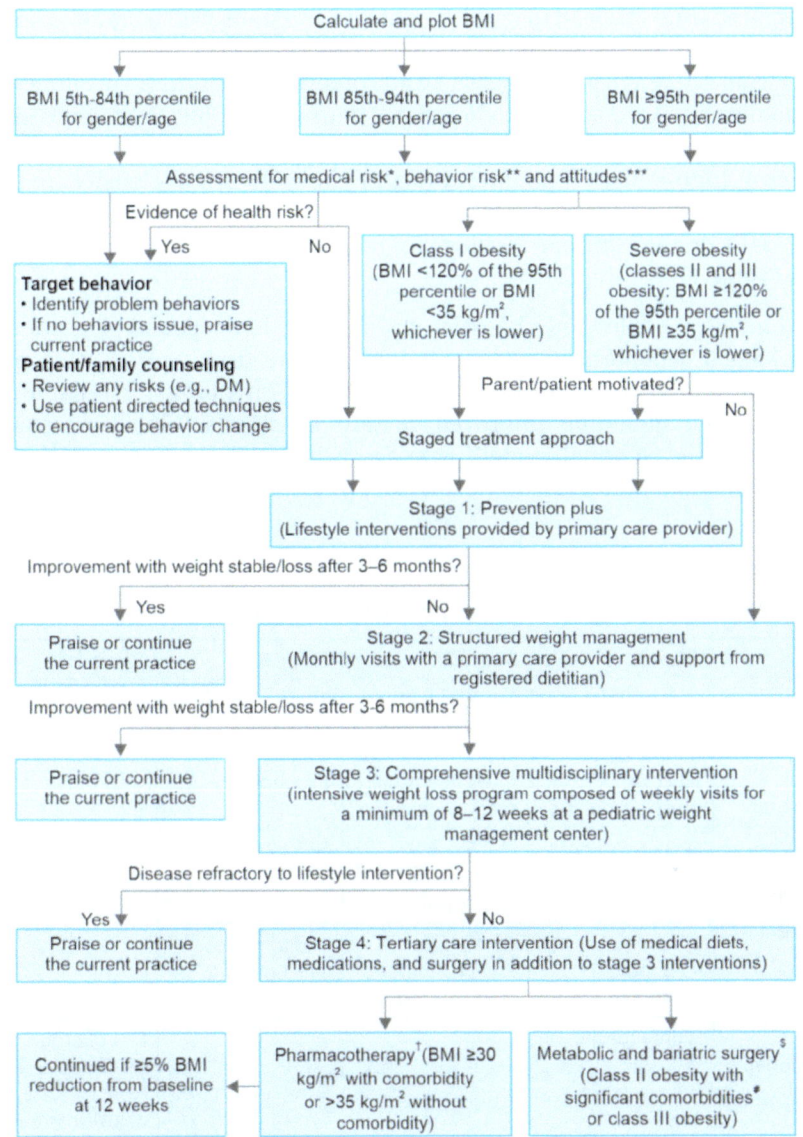

*Child history and examination, child growth, parental obesity, family history, and laboratory as needed when to screen for common conditions associated with obesity including dyslipidemia, type 2 diabetes mellitus (T2DM), and nonalcoholic fatty liver disease (NAFLD).
**Sedentary time, eating, and physical activity.
***Family and patient concern and motivation.
[†]Two Food and Drug Administration (FDA)-approved antiobesity medications (AOMs) for use in the adolescent population: Orlistat and phentermine.
[#]Including severe obstructive sleep apnea, T2DM, idiopathic intracranial hypertension, nonalcoholic steatohepatitis, Blount's disease, slipped capital femoral epiphysis (SCFE), gastroesophageal reflux disease (GERD), or hypertension.
[$]Options available including laparoscopic adjustable gastric band (LAGB), vertical sleeve gastrectomy (VSG), Roux-en-Y gastric bypass (RYGB), and biliopancreatic diversion (BPD) with or without duodenal switch.

FLOWCHART 1: Suggested approach to management of adolescent obesity based on Expert Committee Recommendations and Johnson et al.[7,8]

(BMI: body mass index; DM: diabetes mellitus)

meal replacements can lead to rapid weight loss and improved metabolic markers.[8] A 2019 meta-analysis showed VLED programs resulted in average weight loss ranging from 4.1 kg at 8 weeks to 30.4 kg at 5 months for children and adolescents.[9] Additionally, VLED also have shown to improve various metabolic markers including insulin sensitivity, glucose levels, glycated hemoglobin (HbA1c), total cholesterol, high-density lipoprotein (HDL) cholesterol, low-density lipoprotein (LDL) cholesterol, and triglycerides. The use of revised protein-sparing modified fast (rPSMF) or intermittent fasting has recently been studied in tertiary care centers **(Table 1)**.[8]

Physical activity: Adolescent obesity is closely linked to reduced physical activity and prolonged sedentary behavior. Studies indicate that incorporating physical activity, particularly within family-based therapy for obesity, brings numerous health benefits, including improved insulin sensitivity, blood pressure, and cholesterol levels. National guidelines suggest that adolescents engage in at least 60 minutes of moderate-to-vigorous intensity physical activity daily.[8,10]

TABLE 1: Staging and blood glucose monitoring in T1DM patients.

	Stage 1	Stage 2	Stage 3	Remark
Definition	Multiple islet autoantibodies, normal blood glucose, presymptomatic	Multiple islet autoantibodies, abnormal glucose tolerance, usually presymptomatic	Blood glucose above ADA diagnostic thresholds	NA
Oral glucose tolerance test (OGTT)	FPG <5.6 mmol/L (<100 mg/dL)	FPG 5.6–6.9 mmol/L (100–125 mg/dL)	FPG ≥7.0 mmol/L (≥126 mg/dL)	The gold standard for staging children
	2-hour glucose <7.8 mmol/L (<140 mg/dL)	2-hour glucose 7.8–11.1 mmol/L (140–199 mg/dL)	2-hour glucose ≥11.1 mmol/L (≥200 mg/dL)	
Glycated hemoglobin (HbA1c)	Highly specific			Risk of progression to "clinical disease": HbA1c >5.7%, or 10% rise over 3–12 months
Continuous glucose monitoring	Provides real-time data and may be useful in identifying children with increased glucose variability			Further validation is needed, especially in very young children
Random venous glucose	A simple and low-cost measurement with comparable predictive characteristics to that of OGTT-derived 2-hour glucose value			Relatively poor sensitivity and a specificity
Self-monitoring of blood glucose	Simple use at home but little evidence exists for the accuracy			Immediate result

(ADA: American Diabetes Association; T1DM: type 1 diabetes mellitus)

For toddlers, 60–90 minutes of moderate-to-vigorous-intensity physical activity, such as running, is recommended during an 8-hour day, while preschoolers are advised to have 90–120 minutes of such activity. Limiting "screen time" (excluding homework) to <2 hours per day is recommended for children older than 2 years, and for those younger than 2 years, no screen time is recommended. Adolescents should aim to spend no >2 hours daily on noneducational media activities. Encouraging regular physical activity and reducing sedentary behavior are vital aspects of obesity prevention and management in adolescents.[8,10]

Behavior interventions: Family-based intervention (FBT) is considered the primary treatment for childhood obesity, targeting both children and parents/caregivers. FBT involves modifying dietary and energy expenditure behaviors through goal setting, self-monitoring, reward systems, and stimulus control. Studies have demonstrated that FBT leads to clinically significant weight loss in children, with approximately 80–85% experiencing BMI Z-score changes ≥0.5 at 6 months and 67% maintaining these changes at 10 years.[8]

Motivational interviewing (MV), an extension of FBT, offers an alternative approach for obesity treatment and prevention, utilizing a directive person-centered method to explore ambivalence and stimulate motivation for change.[8]

However, it is important to note that behavioral interventions for treating overweight and obesity in children show a low-to-moderate treatment effect, with reported weight loss and BMI reductions being modest (ranging from 1 to 3 kg/m² of BMI). Additionally, dropout rates tend to be relatively high in these interventions. Despite these challenges, FBT and MV remain important strategies in the fight against childhood obesity.[8,10]

Sleep management: Shorter sleep duration is linked to an increased likelihood of obesity, with up to an 80% higher risk. National guidelines recommend that adolescents should aim for 8–10 hours of sleep per night for optimal health.[8]

Pharmacotherapy

Pharmacotherapy plays a crucial role in treating severe adolescent obesity in tertiary care centers, as a significant percentage of adolescents with severe obesity do not respond well to intensive lifestyle interventions. Antiobesity medications (AOMs) are necessary in such cases, and two Food and Drug Administration (FDA)-approved options for adolescents are orlistat and phentermine.[8,10]

Orlistat, approved for adolescents aged 12 years or older, functions as a lipase inhibitor, blocking the absorption of approximately one-third of fat from meals. The recommended dose is 120 mg three times a day with meals, and it is also available over-the-counter at a lower dose of 60 mg three times a day. Orlistat's efficacy is modest, with a 1-year placebo-subtracted change in BMI being <1 kg/m².[8,10]

Phentermine, indicated for ages 16 years or older with a BMI ≥30 or ≥27 with comorbidities, suppresses appetite as a sympathomimetic amine. A 12-week trial demonstrated that phentermine was well-tolerated in the pediatric population, showing no changes in baseline systolic or diastolic blood pressure. However, there is currently no long-term safety data available for phentermine's use in this population.[8]

Bariatric Surgery

It is reserved as a treatment option for severe obesity in adolescents, and the number of surgeries performed is increasing annually. Surgical options include gastric sleeve resection, Roux-en-Y gastric bypass, and laparoscopic adjustable gastric banding, all conducted in experienced surgical centers.[11]

Current recommendations for adolescent bariatric surgery include a BMI >35 kg/m² with moderate-to-severe comorbidities, or a BMI >40 kg/m² with skeletal and sexual maturity (typically around age 14 for girls and 15 for boys). To prepare for surgery, adolescents should participate in a weight loss program led by a multidisciplinary team, including pediatric surgery, nutrition, psychology, and pediatric specialists. Females receive counseling on increased fertility, and all adolescents provide informed consent. However, significant psychiatric disease is considered an exclusion criterion.[11]

Limited data on outcomes are available, but a 3-year study showed promising results, with a mean percent weight loss of 27%, 74% achieving normalized blood pressure, 66% normalizing lipid levels, and over 50% experiencing remission of T2DM after surgery. Bariatric surgery can be an effective treatment option for severely obese adolescents, but careful patient selection and a comprehensive approach are essential to achieve successful outcomes.[11]

Pediatric and Adolescent Diabetes

According to the International Diabetes Federation (IDF) Diabetes Atlas 2022 report, there were approximately 8.75 million individuals worldwide living with type 1 diabetes mellitus (T1DM) in 2022, with 1.9 million of them residing in low-income and lower-middle-income countries. Among the total T1DM population, 1.52 million (17.0%) were aged below 20 years, 5.56 million (64.0%) were between 20 and 59 years old, and 1.67 million (19.9%) were aged 60 years or older. The increase in the estimate of 1.52 million individuals aged below 20 years from the 2021 Atlas is due to improved methodology considering incidence data for countries lacking recent data and accounting for population growth. In 2022, there were 530,000 new cases of T1DM diagnosed across all age groups, with 201,000 of these cases occurring in individuals below 20 years old. In 2022, there were an estimated 182,000 deaths attributed to T1DM worldwide. The distribution of these deaths by region was as follows in high- to low-Southeast Asia region: 42,000 deaths, Africa: 38,000 deaths, Europe: 34,000 deaths, North America and Caribbean: 20,000 deaths, Middle East and North Africa: 20,000 deaths, Western Pacific (WP): 14,000 deaths, and South and Central America (SACA): 13,000 deaths.[12]

The Lancet study by Ward et al. in 2022 estimates that, in 2021, there were a total of 355,900 new cases of T1DM globally among children and adolescents. Among these cases, only 56% (200,400 cases) were diagnosed at the time. The underdiagnosis rates vary significantly across regions, with over 95% of new T1DM cases being diagnosed in regions such as Australia, New Zealand, western and northern Europe, and North America. However, in regions like west Africa, south and southeastern Asia, and Melanesia, <35% of new T1DM cases were diagnosed.

The research further projects that the total number of incident childhood cases of T1DM is expected to increase to 476,700 by the year 2050.[13]

The findings reveal that the global incidence of childhood and adolescent T1DM is larger than previously estimated, with nearly half of the children currently undiagnosed. To address this concerning trend, policymakers are urged to plan for sufficient diagnostic and medical capacity to enhance timely detection and treatment of T1DM, especially as the incidence is projected to rise worldwide, with the highest numbers of new cases expected in Africa. Early detection and intervention are crucial in managing T1DM and reducing its impact on the health of children and adolescents.[13]

In 2021, there were an estimated 41,600 newly clinically diagnosed cases of T2DM among children and adolescents worldwide. The top three countries with the highest number of incident cases are China: 7,300 cases, India: 4,000 cases, and the United States of America: 2,900 cases. Together, these three countries contribute to approximately 34% of the worldwide total estimated incident cases of T2DM in children and adolescents.[14]

Among the seven regions defined by the IDF, the WP region has the largest estimated number of new T2DM cases in children and adolescents, with 12,300 cases, accounting for almost 30% of the global total incident cases. The Africa (AFR) region follows with 6,700 estimated new cases. The distribution of incident cases is largest in the upper-middle-income countries (UMIC) group, contributing to about 41% of the worldwide total incident cases, while the low-income countries (LICs) group has the smallest contribution, accounting for approximately 10% of the global total.[14]

These data highlight the significant impact of diabetes on children and adolescents globally and emphasize the need for improved detection and treatment to address this growing health concern, especially in regions like Africa where the incidence is projected to increase substantially.

Pediatric and Adolescent Diabetes: Management

Type 1 diabetes mellitus is characterized by four stages, with individuals progressing from increased genetic risk to immune activation and the development of islet autoimmunity (stage 1), followed by preclinical dysglycemia (stage 2). Those who develop stage 3 T1DM may or may not show symptoms, and established T1DM is considered stage 4.[15]

Debate exists regarding the most effective screening strategy for T1DM, whether it should be population-wide or limited to first-degree family members. Evidence suggests that disease progression rates are not significantly different between individuals with a family history of T1DM compared to the general population. Screening strategies include population-wide islet autoantibody screening and genetic risk-stratified islet autoantibody screening. Advancements in islet autoantibody assays enable minimally invasive testing, such as using capillary samples or dried bloodspots, making it more convenient for home or community collection. Genetic risk factors can help identify children with an increased risk of T1DM who would benefit from islet autoantibody screening, particularly for prevention trials.[15]

For staging children for clinical trials, an oral glucose tolerance test (OGTT) is recommended as the gold standard. In cases where OGTT is not feasible, alternative approaches like HbA1c and postprandial or random glucose measurements can be used, depending on risk stratification. More frequent monitoring is offered to children at high risk of progression. Continuous glucose monitoring (CGM) can be added if dysglycemia is identified, providing valuable information for counseling and education. Self-monitoring of blood glucose (SMBG) measurements is helpful for real-time data, allowing early detection of hyperglycemia and prevention of diabetic ketoacidosis (DKA). Overall, screening strategies and monitoring play vital roles in identifying and managing T1DM in its early stages to improve outcomes for affected individuals.[15]

The presentation of youth-onset T2DM can vary, ranging from asymptomatic hyperglycemia, which is detected through screening during routine physical examinations, to DKA occurring in up to 25% of patients.

The diagnosis of T2DM involves two steps: first, confirming the presence of diabetes, and then determining the type of diabetes. Hyperglycemic symptoms, including polyuria (excessive urination), polydipsia (excessive thirst), nocturia (frequent urination at night), unexplained weight loss, and general fatigue, may be present. In cases where hyperglycemic symptoms are not clearly evident, laboratory testing is required to confirm the diagnosis. To establish a definitive diagnosis, the hyperglycemia should be confirmed using a different test from the same sample or on a different day to rule out transient hyperglycemia and ensure accurate results. The criteria for the diagnosis of T2DM in children and adolescents include symptoms of hyperglycemia, one of the following laboratory values and negative islet autoantibodies:[16]

- Fasting plasma glucose (FPG) ≥126 mg/dL (7.0 mmol/L)
- 2-hour plasma glucose on an OGTT ≥200 mg/dL (11.1 mmoL/L). OGTT: 1.75 g/kg (maximum 75 g) anhydrous glucose dissolved in water
- Random plasma glucose ≥200 mg/dL (11.1 mmol/L)
- HbA1c ≥6.5% (48 mmol/mol) by a NGSP-certified device, standardized to the DCCT (Diabetes Control and Complications Trial) assay.

For children and adolescents with T1DM and their families, it is crucial to have access to a multidisciplinary team of healthcare professionals trained in pediatric diabetes management. This team should be sensitive to the unique challenges that children and adolescents with T1DM face and the impact it has on their families. The diabetes-specific care provided by this multidisciplinary team should include diabetes self-management education and support, medical nutrition therapy, and psychosocial support. These components should be offered at the time of diagnosis and regularly thereafter, presented in a developmentally appropriate format that takes into account the child's prior knowledge and experiences. The healthcare professionals comprising the diabetes team should be well-versed in the biological, educational, nutritional, behavioral, and emotional needs of growing children and their families. They should be adept at addressing the psychosocial aspects of living with T1DM and take into consideration the developmental stage of the child when providing guidance and support.[17]

Nutrition management for youth with T1DM should be highly personalized, taking into account various factors such as family habits, food preferences, religious or cultural needs, financial constraints, schedules, physical activity levels, and the youth's and family's abilities in numeracy, literacy, and self-management. Visits with a registered dietitian nutritionist are essential and should involve a comprehensive assessment. This assessment should consider changes in food preferences over time, access to food, growth and development, weight status, cardiovascular risk, and the potential for disordered eating.[17]

It is recommended that youth engage in 60 minutes of daily physical activity, which should include a combination of moderate-intensity activities such as brisk walking and dancing, as well as vigorous-intensity activities like running and jumping rope. This routine can also incorporate resistance training and flexibility exercises. However, intense physical activity should be postponed if the individual has marked hyperglycemia (glucose levels ≥350 mg/dL or 19.4 mmol/L), moderate to large urine ketones, and/or a beta-hydroxybutyrate (β-OHB) level higher than 1.5 mmol/L. Caution should be exercised when β-OHB levels are equal to or exceed 0.6 mmol/L. To prevent and manage hypoglycemia associated with physical activity, individuals can take the following steps:[17]

- *Adjusting prandial insulin*: Before engaging in exercise, they can reduce the insulin dose for the meal or snack preceding the activity to avoid a drop in blood sugar levels.
- *Increasing food intake*: Consuming additional carbohydrates before or during exercise can help prevent low blood sugar levels.
- *Modifying insulin pump settings*: For those using insulin pumps, they can lower basal insulin rates by 10–50% or suspend insulin delivery for 1–2 hours during exercise to prevent excessive insulin action.

Given that a significant part of a youth's day is spent at school or day care, it is crucial to train school or day care personnel to provide care according to the child's individualized diabetes medical management plan. This training is vital for ensuring optimal diabetes management and safe participation in all school or day care-sponsored activities. By equipping school and day care staff with the necessary knowledge and skills, we can create a supportive environment that allows children with diabetes to access educational and developmental opportunities while managing their condition effectively and safely.[17]

Automated insulin delivery systems should be made available for youth with T1DM who can safely use the device, either independently or with the help of caregivers. The decision on which device to use should be based on the unique circumstances, preferences, and requirements of the individual and their family. For those on multiple daily injections (MDIs) with T1DM who can safely manage an insulin pump, it should also be offered as a viable option for diabetes management. Like with automated systems, the choice of device should consider the specific needs and preferences of the individual and their family. In both cases, providing access to appropriate diabetes management technologies can help improve glucose control and enhance the overall quality of life for youth with T1DM. The individual's ability to safely and effectively use the device is a critical consideration in the decision-making process.[17]

The treatment approach for youth-onset T2DM should include three main components: (1) lifestyle management, (2) diabetes self-management education and support, and (3) pharmacologic treatment. Initial treatment of youth with obesity and diabetes should consider that the specific diabetes type may be uncertain during the first few weeks of treatment due to overlapping clinical presentations. Additionally, a significant percentage of youth with T2DM may present with clinically significant ketoacidosis. Therefore, the primary focus of initial therapy should be on addressing hyperglycemia and associated metabolic abnormalities, regardless of the ultimate diabetes type. Once metabolic compensation has been achieved and additional information, such as islet autoantibody results, becomes available, adjustments to therapy can be made accordingly.[17]

Flowchart 2 provides a step-by-step approach to the initial treatment of new-onset diabetes in youth with overweight or obesity who are clinically suspected of having T2DM, guiding healthcare providers in managing the condition effectively.[16-18]

WEIGHT MANAGEMENT OF GESTATIONAL DIABETES AND PREGNANCY MANAGEMENT

Weight Management of Gestational Diabetes

The documented prevalence of gestational diabetes mellitus (GDM) varies widely worldwide, with rates ranging from 1 to over 30%. This variability is due to the lack of consensus and uniformity in screening standards and diagnostic criteria for GDM, making it challenging to compare prevalence across countries and regions.

A review of global GDM prevalence based on studies conducted between 2005 and 2015 found that the Middle East and North Africa had the highest prevalence of GDM, with a median estimate of 12.9%. It was followed by Southeast Asia, Western Pacific, SACA, Africa, and North America and the Caribbean, with median prevalence rates of 11.7, 11.7, 11.2, 8.9, and 7%, respectively. In contrast, Europe had the lowest median prevalence of 5.8%.[19,20]

Within the Western Pacific region, GDM prevalence estimates showed a wide range, varying from 4.5% in Japan to 25.1% in Singapore due to different GDM diagnosis criteria being applied. Similarly, European countries exhibited significant variations in estimates, with Norway having the highest prevalence (median 22.3%) and Ireland the lowest prevalence at 1.8%. In the North America and Caribbean region, there was relatively less variability, with GDM prevalence ranging from 6.5% in Canada to 11.9% in Barbados. In the Middle East and North Africa region, which had the highest average prevalence of GDM, estimates ranged from 8.4% in Iran to 24.5% in the United Arab Emirates. Qatar, Bahrain, and Israel had intermediate estimates of 16.3, 12.9, and 8.8%, respectively. In Southeast Asia, Malaysia had the highest GDM prevalence of 18.3%, followed by India (13.6%), Bangladesh (9.7%), and Sri Lanka (8.1%). For SACA, GDM data were available in only two countries, with Cuba and Brazil reporting prevalence rates of 16.6 and 5.7%, respectively. Likewise, only two countries in Africa had qualified and available data, with Nigeria reporting 8.2% and Tanzania 9.5% prevalence of GDM.[20]

CHAPTER 9: Special Populations and Issues

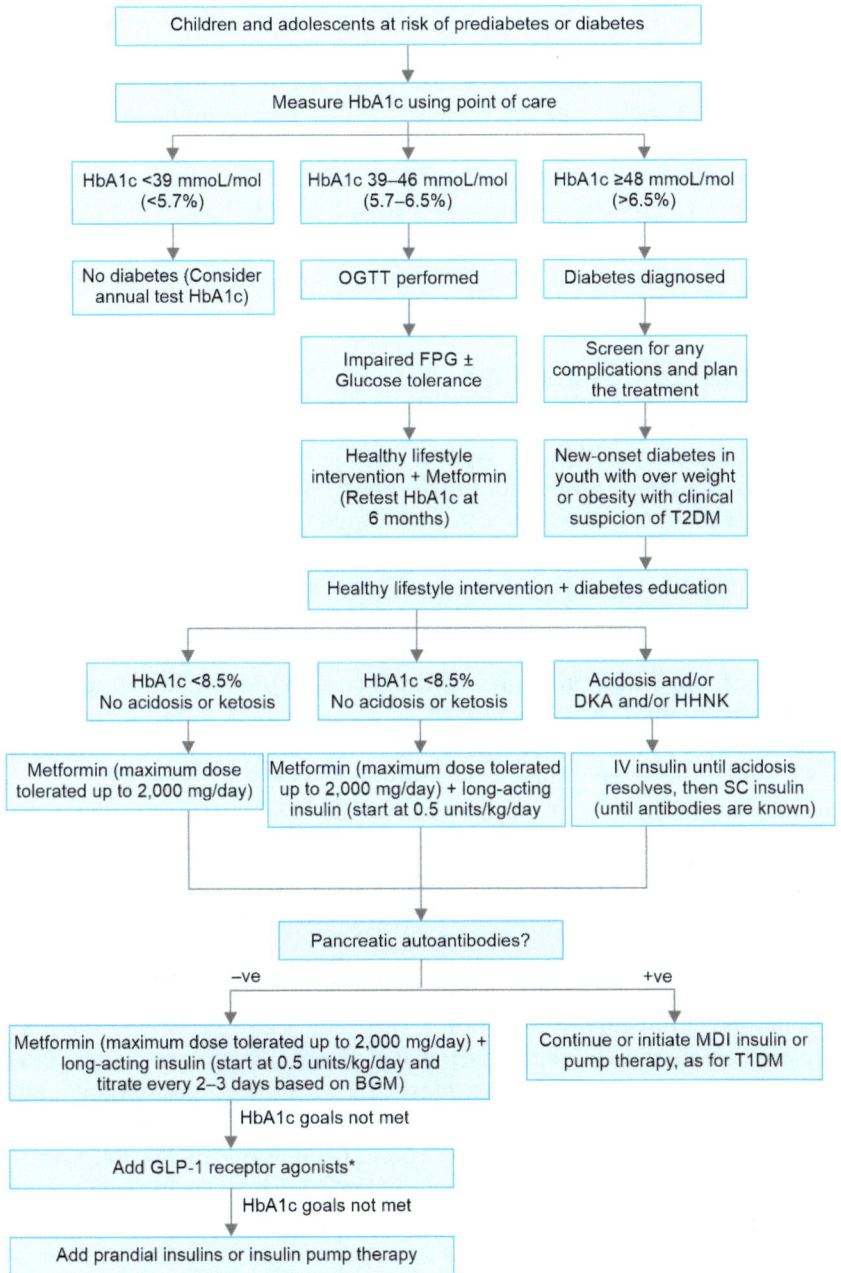

*Children 10 years of age or older if they have no past medical history or family history of medullary thyroid carcinoma or multiple endocrine neoplasia type 2.

FLOWCHART 2: Recommended approach to management of T2DM based on Australasian Paediatric Endocrine Group guidelines 2020, American Diabetes Association (ADA) 2023, and ISPAD Clinical Practice Consensus Guidelines 2022.[16-18]

(BGM; blood glucose monitoring; DKA: diabetic ketoacidosis; FPG: fasting plasma glucose; GLP1: glucagon-like peptide 1; HbA1c: glycated hemoglobin; HHNK: hyperosmotic hyperglycemic nonketotic state; IV: intravenous; MDI: multiple daily injection; OGTT: oral glucose tolerance test; SC: subcutaneous; T2DM: type 2 diabetes mellitus)

Subsequent updates on GDM prevalence between August 2015 and December 2018 revealed that the Middle East and some North African countries continued to have the highest prevalence of GDM, with a median of 15.2%. Southeast Asia followed with a median of 15.0%, while the Western Pacific, SACA, sub-Saharan Africa, and North America and the Caribbean had median prevalence rates of 10.3, 11.2, 10.8, and 7.0%, respectively. The region with the lowest GDM prevalence and the widest variation was Europe, with a median prevalence of 6.1%. Even within each region, there remained significant variation in GDM prevalence, both within countries and between them. For instance, in the Western Pacific region, prevalence ranged from 4.5% in Japan to 18.0% in Singapore.[19]

Risk of Metabolic Syndrome

The most significant risk factor for GDM is being overweight or obese before pregnancy, defined by a BMI ≥25 kg/m². There is suggestive evidence linking low plasma levels of vitamin D and vitamin C in early pregnancy, along with increased dietary fat intake during pregnancy, to an elevated risk of developing GDM.[19]

Observational studies on prepregnancy diets have identified several dietary factors that may independently increase GDM risk, regardless of body adiposity and physical activity. These factors include higher consumption of sugar-sweetened beverages, potatoes, fried foods, heme iron, animal fat, and protein. Moreover, a diet low in carbohydrates but high in animal fat and protein, as well as an overall "western" dietary pattern characterized by a high intake of red meat, processed meat, refined grain products, sweets, French fries, and pizza, are associated with an increased risk of GDM. Collectively, findings from observational studies suggest that around 45% of GDM cases may be preventable by adopting a healthy diet before pregnancy, maintaining a BMI below 25 kg/m², engaging in at least 30 minutes of daily exercise, and avoiding cigarette smoking. These lifestyle modifications can play a crucial role in reducing the risk of developing GDM during pregnancy.[19]

Long-term Consequences on Maternal and Offspring

Mild hyperglycemia during pregnancy can have adverse effects on maternal health, increasing the risk of hypertensive disorders, preterm labor, cesarean delivery, and later metabolic disorders. GDM during pregnancy can also predispose women to later cardiovascular disease. Studies have shown that GDM significantly increases a woman's risk of developing T2DM up to seven-fold over her lifetime. The increased risks associated with GDM include gestational hypertension (threefold increase), cardiovascular disease (1.7-fold increase), metabolic syndrome (2.5-fold increase), preterm birth (2.1-fold increase), and cesarean delivery (2.2-fold increase).[21]

Moreover, exposure to hyperglycemia during pregnancy can significantly impact the long-term health of the child as well. Newborns exposed to high glucose levels during pregnancy may face lifelong risks of glucose intolerance and obesity, even after birth when they are no longer exposed to a high glucose environment. Children born to mothers with GDM have nearly double the risk of developing childhood obesity and/or metabolic syndrome compared to children born to nondiabetic mothers (**Fig. 1**).[21,22]

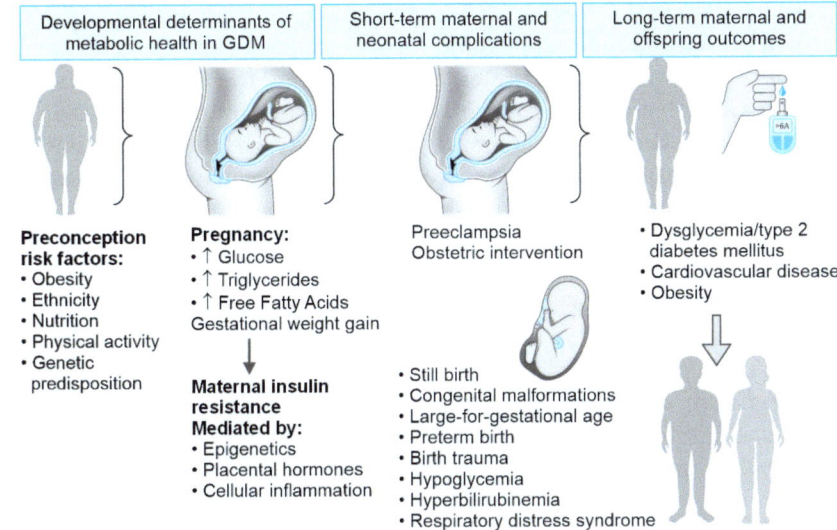

FIG. 1: Short-term and long-term maternal and neonatal complications in gestational diabetes mellitus (GDM).

These findings highlight the importance of managing and controlling hyperglycemia during pregnancy to safeguard both maternal and child health in the short-term and long-term. Early detection and appropriate management of GDM can help reduce the associated risks and promote better health outcomes for both mother and child.

Weight Management in Gestational Diabetes Mellitus

Diagnosis

The landmark Hyperglycemia and Adverse Pregnancy Outcome (HAPO) study, published in 2008, aimed to establish evidence-based guidelines for GDM risk assessment. This extensive international prospective observational study involved over 25,000 pregnant women and examined the relationship between glucose levels from the 75-g 2-hour OGTT performed at 24–32 weeks of gestation (mean 27.8 weeks) and primary outcomes such as birthweight above the 90th percentile for gestational age, primary cesarean section delivery, neonatal hypoglycemia, and cord blood serum C-peptide above the 90th centile. The results revealed a continuous positive linear relationship between maternal fasting, 1-, and 2-hour plasma glucose levels obtained during the OGTT, even below the diagnostic thresholds for diabetes outside of pregnancy.[22]

Following the HAPO study, various screening and testing approaches for the diagnosis of GDM have been adopted worldwide. The International Association of Diabetes and Pregnancy Study Groups (IADPSG) and WHO recommend universal testing of all pregnant women between 24 and 28 weeks of gestation using the 75-g 2-hour OGTT. These revised recommendations have received significant support from various organizations including the American Diabetes Association (ADA), Endocrine Society, International Federation of Gynecology and Obstetrics,

Australasian Diabetes in Pregnancy Association, Japan Diabetes Society, Ministry of Health of China, and the European Board of Gynecology and Obstetrics.[22]

However, the National Institutes of Health and the American College of Obstetricians and Gynecologists (ACOG) continue to recommend a two-step testing approach. This involves initial screening using the glucose challenge test (GCT) for all pregnant women, and those who screen positive proceed to the diagnostic 100-g 3-hour OGTT. This approach is also endorsed by the ADA.[22]

After a diagnosis of GDM, treatment typically begins with medical nutrition therapy, physical activity, and weight management, tailored to the pregestational weight of the individual. Glucose monitoring is essential, aiming to achieve specific targets recommended by the Fifth International Workshop-Conference on Gestational Diabetes Mellitus:[23]

- *Fasting glucose*: <95 mg/dL (5.3 mmol/L)
- *1-hour postprandial glucose*: <140 mg/dL (7.8 mmol/L)
- *2-hour postprandial glucose*: <120 mg/dL (6.7 mmol/L)

Management

In many cases, GDM can be effectively managed with lifestyle interventions alone in approximately 80–90% of women, depending on the specific diagnostic criteria used. The ADA does not provide specific dietary recommendations for GDM but refers to the DRI for pregnant women, suggesting a minimum intake of 175 g of carbohydrates, 71 g of protein, and 28 g of fiber. On the other hand, the Endocrine Society offers more specific dietary guidance, suggesting limiting carbohydrate intake to 35–45% of total calories, distributed across three small-to-moderate-sized meals and 2–4 snacks, including an evening snack.[23,24]

Self-monitoring of blood glucose is important and should be performed at least four times daily including fasting and 1–2 hours after meals. For women whose GDM is well controlled with diet alone, the frequency of SMBG may be reduced but should generally still be performed at least twice a day. HbA1c may be used as a secondary measure for glycemic control, with a target of <6–6.5% if not contraindicated due to underlying hemoglobinopathy. Pharmacologic therapy may be considered in cases of significant initial hyperglycemia or if SMBG consistently shows glucose values above the recommended targets during pregnancy.[24]

Pharmacologic therapy is recommended for cases of significant initial hyperglycemia or when SMBG consistently shows glucose values above the targeted levels during pregnancy. Two large randomized studies, as reviewed by the US Preventive Services Task Force, have demonstrated that treatment of GDM with lifestyle modifications and insulin can improve perinatal outcomes.[23,24]

In the United States, insulin is the first-line agent for the pharmacologic treatment of GDM. It can be administered as a single bedtime injection, MDIs, or via continuous subcutaneous insulin infusion (CSII) **(Flowchart 3)**. Although limited evidence supports the efficacy of metformin and glyburide in reducing glucose levels for GDM treatment, they are not recommended as the first-line treatment due to their ability to cross the placenta, raising concerns about long-term safety for the offspring. Additionally, separate studies have shown that glyburide and metformin may not provide adequate glycemic outcomes in a significant percentage

CHAPTER 9: Special Populations and Issues

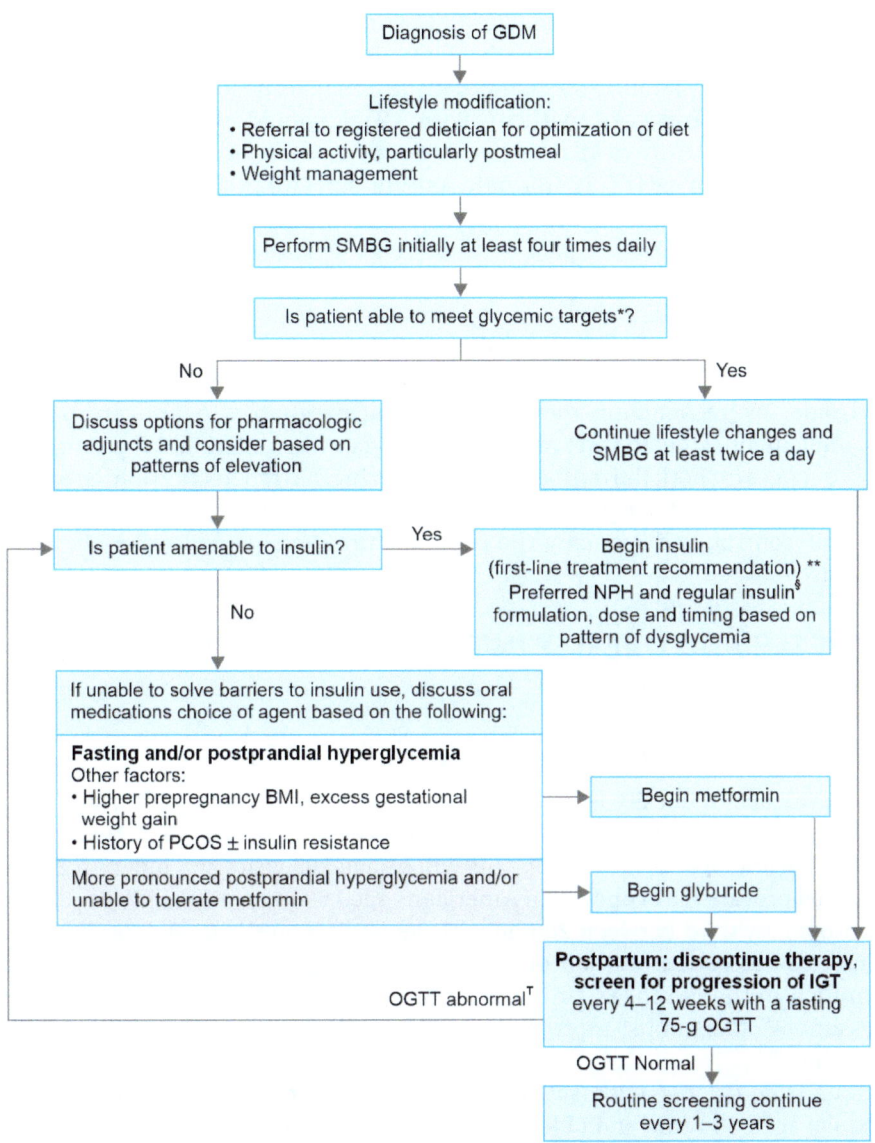

*Glycemic targets (mg/dL): Fasting <95; 1-hour postprandial <140; 2-hour postprandial <120.

**If consistent fasting and postprandial hyperglycemia is present, basal/bolus regimens using up to 0.7–1.0 units/kg may be required in a ratio of approximately 50% long- or intermediate-acting and 50% short- or rapid-acting.

§Insulins assigned a pregnancy category B include regular insulin (U-100 and U-500), insulin aspart, insulin lispro (U-100 and U-200), NPH, and insulin detemir. Pregnancy category C designation has been assigned to insulin glulisine, insulin degludec, and inhaled human insulin. Insulin glargine (U-100 and U-300) has no pregnancy category.

†If fasting plasma glucose (≥126 mg/dL) and 2-hour plasma glucose (≥200 mg/dL) are abnormal in a single-screening test.

FLOWCHART 3: Comprehensive management GDM.[23,24]

(BMI: body mass index; GDM: gestational diabetes mellitus; IGT: impaired glucose tolerance; OGTT: oral glucose tolerance test; PCOS: polycystic ovarian syndrome; SMBG: selfmonitoring of blood glucose) of participants with GDM (23 and 25–28%, respectively). However, metformin can be considered a reasonable alternative for patients who decline insulin therapy or are unable to safely administer or afford insulin, according to ACOG guidelines.[23,24]

Following delivery, all patients with GDM should undergo an OGTT at 4–12 weeks postpartum to identify persistent glucose intolerance or overt diabetes. If the postpartum OGTT is normal, routine screening should continue every 1–3 years, and for subsequent pregnancies, early screening for recurrent GDM is recommended. Persistent glucose intolerance is found in up to 20% of women during postpartum follow-up, and their subsequent risk of developing T2DM is significantly increased.[23,24]

Indeed, with the increasing prevalence of obesity and T2DM, GDM represents a crucial opportunity to identify women at risk for developing T2DM and metabolic syndrome. By recognizing these risks during pregnancy, healthcare providers can implement targeted interventions to mitigate the potential long-term health consequences for both the mother and her offspring. Early detection and appropriate management of GDM can pave the way for promoting healthier lifestyles, optimizing glycemic control, and reducing the risk of future metabolic disorders in affected women.

DIABETES AND OBESITY IN THE ELDERLY AND GERIATRIC PATIENTS

Obesity in the Elderly and Geriatric Patients

The prevalence of obesity is on the rise worldwide, even among older age groups. By the year 2030–2035, it is estimated that over 20% of the adult United States population and over 25% of Europeans will be aged 65 years and older. In 2010, the predicted prevalence of obesity in Americans aged 60 years and older was 37%, and in Europe, it varied between 20 and 30% depending on the model used, resulting in approximately 20.9 million obese individuals aged 60+ years in the USA and 32 million in the European Union in 2015.[25] Japan and Taiwan had lower obesity rates among older adults, approximately 20% in 2012, with 30.5% in men and 21.3% in women.[26]

Data from the Behavioral Risk Factor Surveillance System showed that 20.3% of adults aged 65 years and older in the US were classified as obese, with a higher prevalence (25%) in the 65- to 74-year age group compared to the 75- to 84-year age group (16.6%) and the ≥85-year age group (9.9%). In France, the Obepi survey between 1997 and 2006 found that obesity prevalence was 17.9% in those aged 65 years or older, with similar rates in both sexes, and severe obesity (BMI ≥40 kg/m^2) was present in 1.1%. In Spain, 35% of individuals aged 65 years or older were obese, with higher rates in females (38.3%) compared to males (30.6%). The prevalence of obesity in the Netherlands was 18% in men and 20% in women aged 60 years or older, while increased waist circumference was more common, affecting 40% of men and 56% of women.[25]

In Malaysia, the prevalence of obesity in adults aged >18 years was 17.7% in 2016, and among older adults aged ≥60 years, it increased from 14% in 2006 to 20.5% in 2015, with higher rates in females.[26] Indian studies demonstrated that

34% of men and 40.3% of women aged 65–74 years were overweight and obese, and this prevalence decreased to nearly half (20.9%) in those aged 85 years and above. Among Indian females, 42.1% of the elderly were obese/overweight, compared to 20.9% of males. These findings highlight the concerning trend of obesity in older populations and its potential impact on health outcomes and public health efforts to mitigate the associated risks.[27,28]

Consequences of Obesity

As individuals age, significant changes occur in body composition and metabolism. Between the ages of 20 and 70 years, there is a gradual decline in fat-free mass, primarily muscle mass, by approximately 40%, while fat mass increases. Age-related changes also impact fat distribution, leading to a greater accumulation of visceral fat, particularly in women. Additionally, fat tends to be deposited within skeletal muscles and the liver.[29]

The increase in visceral fat is a major contributing factor to impaired glucose tolerance in older adults. Intramuscular and intrahepatic fat accumulation further exacerbates the problem by releasing adipokines and free fatty acids, which impair insulin action locally. Furthermore, increased pancreatic fat is associated with declining β-cell function, contributing to the development of insulin resistance and impaired glucose regulation in aging individuals. These changes in body composition and fat distribution play a significant role in the age-related decline in metabolic health and may increase the risk of metabolic disorders, including T2DM, in the elderly population.[29]

As individuals age, not only does fat mass increase, but its distribution also changes, with a greater accumulation of fat in the abdominal and subscapular regions. This shift in fat distribution is associated with increased risks of metabolic syndrome and other cardiovascular risk factors. Interestingly, in females, peripheral adiposity or fat accumulation in the typical female distribution may have a protective effect. Over recent years, the general adiposity of the elderly population has risen due to social changes and differences in dietary and lifestyle habits. However, it is important to note that the level of adiposity associated with increased health risks may be higher in the elderly compared to younger age groups. In addition to the increased fat deposition in traditional fat depots, elderly individuals with obesity may experience ectopic fat deposition. This means fat may accumulate in organs like the liver, leading to nonalcoholic fatty liver disease (NAFLD), and within muscle tissue, leading to insulin resistance. These changes further contribute to the increased risk of metabolic disorders, particularly T2DM, in the elderly population.[30]

Management

Obesity-related complications, such as diabetes, hyperlipidemia, and hypertension, should be treated in the elderly population. The treatment approach should be adapted to suit the specific age-related considerations. Various therapeutic tools are available for weight management in the elderly and these tools include:[25,29]

- Lifestyle intervention involving diet, physical activity, and behavioral modification

- Pharmacotherapy
- Endoscopic interventions
- Surgery

Lifestyle Intervention Involving Diet, Physical Activity, and Behavioral Modification

A lifestyle intervention for weight management in older individuals should include a calorie-deficit diet of about 500 kcal (2.1 MJ)/day, although the deficit can range from 500 to 1,000 kcal (2.1–4.2 MJ)/day **(Flowchart 4)**. The diet should provide sufficient high-quality protein at a rate of 1 g/kg of body weight. Adequate supplementation of calcium (1,000 mg/day), vitamin D (10–20 μg/day), multivitamins, and minerals is also important. The intervention should be combined with regular exercise and behavioral therapy. While increased physical activity and exercise are not mandatory for initial weight loss, they play a crucial role in preserving lean body

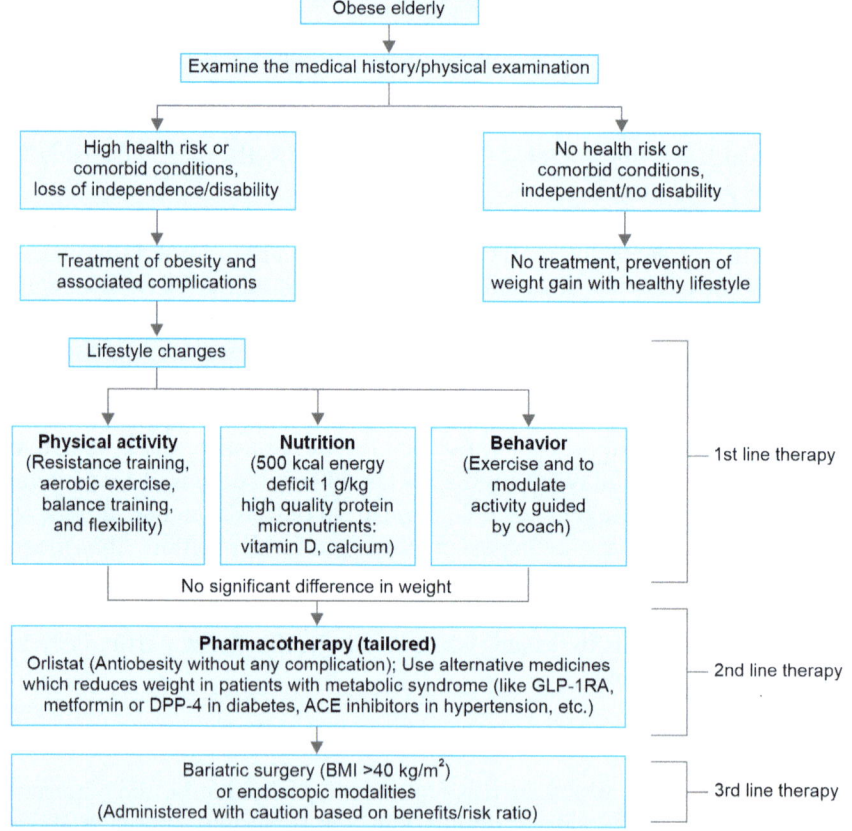

FLOWCHART 4: Simplified treatment algorithm for obese elderly individuals suggested by Mathus-Vliegen et al.[25]

(ACE: angiotensin-converting enzyme; BMI: body mass index; DPP-4: dipeptidyl peptidase-4; GLP-1RA: glucagon-like peptide-1 receptor agonist)

mass, maintaining weight loss, and preventing weight regain. A well-rounded exercise program may include elements of aerobic exercise, resistance training, balance, and flexibility training, particularly beneficial for older individuals as it improves physical function and helps counter frailty. Behavioral therapy components such as self-monitoring, goal setting, social support, stimulus control, and relapse prevention are vital for long-term success.[25,29]

This combined approach of a moderate energy-deficit diet, increased physical activity, and behavioral modification typically results in moderate weight loss, ranging from 0.4 to 0.9 kg/week, or approximately 8–10% of body weight after 6 months. The intervention is effective in improving obesity-related medical complications and physical dysfunction, with only a small risk of treatment-associated complications.[25,29]

The Diabetes Prevention Program (DPP) conducted a study that included obese men and women up to the age of 84 years. Participants followed a program that involved moderate physical activity of at least 2.5 hours per week, a reduction in total dietary fat to <25% of total energy intake and counseling sessions with a lifestyle counselor. The results of the study showed that every kilogram of weight loss achieved through diet and exercise reduced the incidence of T2DM by 16% over a period of 3.2 years. In the 60- to 85-year age group, the incidence of diabetes was 3.3 cases per 100 patient-years, which was half of the incidence observed in the younger age group of 25–44 years.[31] Systematic review of weight loss interventions in people aged over 60 years have demonstrated significant positive outcomes. These interventions led to improved glucose tolerance and physical functioning, a reduced incidence of newly developed diabetes, and significant benefits for those with osteoarthritis, diabetes, and coronary heart disease.[32]

Medical nutrition therapy: In the treatment of individuals with sarcopenic obesity or those at risk of it, the energy deficit should be more moderate, ranging from 200 to 750 kcal (840–3,150 kJ). There should be a strong emphasis on increasing protein intake to support muscle health and prevent muscle protein breakdown. Protein intake can be increased to up to 1.5 g/kg of high biological quality protein. Maintaining or increasing protein intake is essential when restricting energy intake, as dietary protein and amino acids are effective in slowing or preventing muscle protein breakdown. Additionally, protein supplementation has the added benefit of increasing satiety, which can help reduce hunger and adherence to an energy-deficient diet. It is important to avoid excessive protein intake, especially in individuals with renal function disturbances, to prevent potential complications.[25,29]

Another strategy to enhance protein synthesis is the supplementation of essential amino acids. Mixtures of arginine and glutamine or arginine and lysine have been studied for this purpose. Leucine, found in foods like legumes (soybeans) and animal products (fish and beef), is particularly beneficial for muscle protein synthesis. Adding leucine to a mixed nutrient meal in older individuals resulted in a significant increase in muscle protein synthesis.[25,29]

In addition to protein, specific micronutrients should be addressed to support overall health. Vitamin D is essential for protein synthesis and muscle health, while magnesium is associated with insulin resistance. Vitamin B6, vitamin B12, and selenium are also important for preventing functional decline.[25,29]

Physical activity: The American College of Sports Medicine recommends a comprehensive multicomponent training exercise program, including strength, endurance, balance, and flexibility exercises, to improve and maintain physical function in older adults. Resistance training has been studied as a potential approach to counteract sarcopenia in older adults by stimulating protein synthesis and promoting muscle hypertrophy, leading to increased muscle mass, strength, and improved physical functioning. Endurance training, on the other hand, focuses on improving aerobic capacity. Most studies have utilized a multicomponent exercise program with three 90-minute sessions per week. These sessions typically include 15 minutes of balance training, 15 minutes of flexibility exercises, 30 minutes of aerobic exercise, and 30 minutes of high-intensity resistance training.[25,29]

A specific study conducted by Davidson et al. examined the impact of different exercise modalities on obese subjects aged 60–80 years. The subjects were randomized into four groups: a control group, a group undergoing progressive resistance training, a group performing aerobic exercise, and a group combining progressive resistance training with aerobic exercise. After 6 months, the study showed that body weight decreased by 0.6 kg in the resistance training group, 2.8 kg in the aerobic exercise group, and 2.3 kg in the combined exercise group. Abdominal fat and visceral fat also decreased in the aerobic and combined exercise groups. Moreover, endurance capacity improved significantly in the aerobic and combined exercise groups. Interestingly, skeletal mass increased in the resistance training and combined exercise groups, and muscle strength improved in these groups as well. Additionally, insulin resistance improved by 31% in the aerobic exercise group and by 45% in the combined exercise group, while it remained unchanged in the resistance training group.[33]

Why Add Exercise to a Diet?

Adding exercise to a diet has been shown to offer various benefits in different populations:[25,34]

- In individuals with added exercise, higher basal and stimulated lipolysis was observed in the abdominal and gluteal regions. This suggests that exercise can help promote fat breakdown and mobilization in specific areas.
- In frail older adults, it reduces the loss of fat-free mass and lean tissue mass while increasing muscle strength. This indicates an improvement in muscle quality and preservation of muscle mass with exercise.
- Also associated with improvements in endurance capacity, muscle strength, plasma triglycerides, LDL cholesterol, and diastolic blood pressure.
- Shown positive effects on intrahepatic fat content and insulin sensitivity. This can lead to a reduction in the risk of insulin resistance and related metabolic complications.

Several systematic reviews of interventions in the elderly population have also demonstrated the positive outcomes of adding physical activity to dietary advice. One review in obese older individuals (aged 60 years or older, BMI >30 kg/m^2) showed that combined dietary advice and physical activity achieved the highest weight loss and a greater decrease in serum total cholesterol, contributing to improved cardiovascular health. Another review combined the effects of energy restriction and exercise on fat-free mass in middle-aged and older adults, which is crucial for addressing sarcopenic obesity. The addition of exercise to energy restriction significantly attenuated the loss of fat-free mass from 24 to 11%, reducing the negative impact on muscle health.[35,36]

Pharmacotherapy

The exclusion of older subjects from most clinical trials of pharmacological agents for weight loss is a common issue, as the average age of participants in these trials typically ranges from 34 to 54 years. One pharmacological agent that has been approved for long-term treatment in patients with obesity is orlistat. Orlistat is a lipase inhibitor that blocks the digestion and absorption of up to one-third of ingested fat, leading to an energy deficit of approximately 300 kcal/day (1,260 kJ).[29]

Studies have shown that adding orlistat to a diet and lifestyle intervention results in additional weight loss of 2–3 kg compared to adding a placebo. Moreover, orlistat has been found to improve glucose tolerance and blood pressure, which is dependent on the rate of weight loss. Interestingly, orlistat also has weight loss-independent beneficial effects on dyslipidemia and insulin resistance.[29]

In a study by Jain et al., orlistat was evaluated in obese patients. Compared to placebo, orlistat caused significant reductions ($p < 0.05$) in weight (4.65 kg vs. 2.5 kg; orlistat vs. placebo, respectively), BMI (1.91 kg/m^2 vs. 0.64 kg/m^2), and waist circumference (4.84 cm vs. 2 cm). Orlistat also resulted in reductions in cholesterol levels (10.68 mg vs. 6.18 mg) and LDL levels (5.87 mg vs. 2.33 mg). The study also noted gastrointestinal side effects, such as loose stools, oily stools/spotting, abdominal pain, and fecal urgency in the orlistat group. Overall, orlistat was deemed to be an effective and well-tolerated antiobesity drug, and it can be used in combination with therapeutic lifestyle changes to achieve and maintain optimal weight.[37]

Regarding the management of diabetes, certain medications, such as acarbose (α-glucosidase inhibitor), metformin, and gliptins [dipeptidyl peptidase-4 (DPP-4) inhibitors] are considered weight neutral. On the other hand, glucagon-like peptide-1 (GLP-1) receptor agonists have been shown to lead to a moderate reduction in body weight. A meta-analysis of 25 studies demonstrated that GLP-1 receptor agonists lead to a 2.9% reduction in body weight. In patients without diabetes (3 trials), weight losses were 3.2 kg (95% confidence interval, 2.1–4.3 kg), and in patients with diabetes, weight losses were 2.8 kg (95% confidence interval, 2.3–3.4 kg).[29]

Endoscopic Interventions and Bariatric Surgery

The use of antiobesity drugs and surgical options may be limited for patients with a BMI between 30 and 40 kg/m^2. In this context, endoscopic treatments have emerged as potential alternatives. One such option is the intragastric balloon, which has been used in thousands of obese subjects, but most of the data are from patients between 31 and 43.3 years of age. Another endoscopic treatment is the EndoBarrier, which is an endoscopically delivered duodeno-jejunal bypass device. It has shown promise in ameliorating the symptoms of T2DM soon after its positioning. However, there is a lack of extensive clinical studies specifically focusing on elderly obese patients, and the available data may not show significant differences in this population.[25]

The absence of a clear patient-tailored stepwise treatment plan for individuals with a BMI between 30 and 40 kg/m² highlights the need for more research and options in this category. As the field of endoscopic treatments continues to evolve, further studies and data collection in elderly obese patients will be essential to determine the effectiveness and safety of these approaches in this specific population.

Bariatric surgery is recommended for patients with severe obesity, typically those with a BMI ≥40 kg/m² or a BMI ≥35 kg/m² with obesity-related comorbidities, such as diabetes, cardiorespiratory disease, sleep apnea, and severe osteoarthritis. These comorbidities are expected to improve with surgically-induced weight loss. More recent guidelines, such as those from the International Federation of Diabetes, suggest that a lower BMI threshold (>30 kg/m²) should be considered for individuals with T2DM.[25,29]

In elderly patients, bariatric surgery has shown positive outcomes, with clinically significant weight loss and improvements in obesity-related comorbidities. The weight loss achieved through surgery has been associated with reduced medication requirements and an overall enhancement in health. It is important to note that overall mortality after bariatric surgery is low, and the risk-to-benefit ratio is considered acceptable. Therefore, the elderly population should not be denied bariatric surgery solely based on age grounds. The decision to undergo bariatric surgery should be made on an individual basis, considering the patient's health status, comorbidities, and overall goals for weight management and health improvement.[25,29]

SARCOPENIC OBESITY

Recently, the concept of sarcopenic obesity has evolved to consider not only muscle mass but also muscle strength in relation to waist circumference, leading to the introduction of dynapenic abdominal obesity (DAO). Muscle and fat are interconnected pathogenically, as they share common pathways of damage and communication.

As individuals age, there is a gradual decline in fat-free mass, resulting in reduced total energy expenditure, often linked to decreased physical activity. This decline in energy expenditure may contribute to weight gain, particularly an increase in visceral abdominal fat. Both muscle and fat have been recognized as endocrine organs capable of producing peptides called myokines, which play roles in autocrine and paracrine signaling. Physical exercise induces the production of myokines, such as irisin, which may have positive effects on fat metabolism. For instance, irisin produced by myocytes during exercise can promote browning of white fat, potentially controlling fat gain. Therefore, a decrease in physical activity with aging may lead to reduced production of irisin by muscles, resulting in an increase in fat mass and potentially contributing to sarcopenic obesity. This highlights the intricate relationship between muscle, fat, and physical activity in the context of aging and its impact on body composition and metabolic health **(Flowchart 5)**.[38,39]

The accurate prevalence rates for sarcopenic obesity face a challenge due to the lack of a consistent definition for either sarcopenia or obesity. Several different definitions have been used, leading to significant variations in reported rates. For

CHAPTER 9: Special Populations and Issues

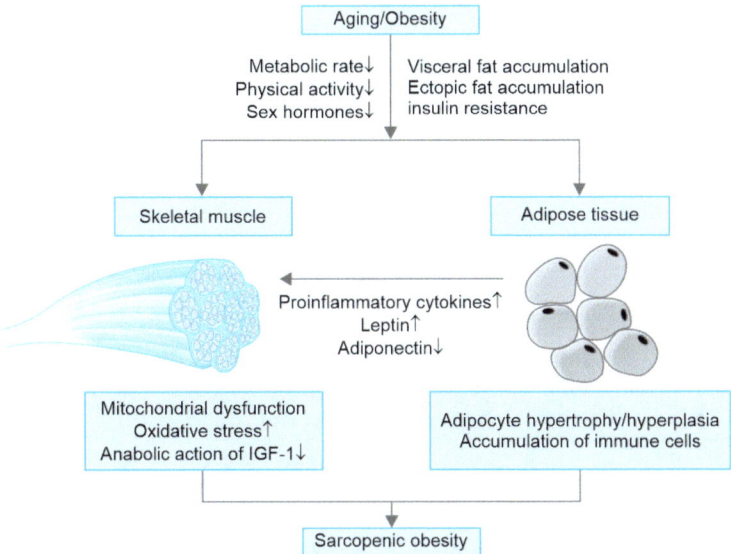

FLOWCHART 5: Schematic biological pathways that lead to sarcopenic obesity with age. Aging accompanies with reduced metabolic rate, decreased physical activity, and sex-specific hormonal changes. These changes contribute to aging-related decrease in muscle mass and strength as well as increase in body fat and unfavorable changes in body fat composition, such as a loss of subcutaneous fat, an accumulation of visceral fat, and ectopic fat deposition. Obesity in aged individuals stimulates ectopic fat accumulation in skeletal muscles, which leads to marked impairment of mitochondria fatty acid oxidation, increased oxidative stress, and insulin resistance, resulting in decline in muscle mass and strength. Moreover, obesity-associated adipose tissue inflammation can affect skeletal muscle mass and function by the increased production of proinflammatory cytokines and adipokine leptin, and decreased action of adiponectin and insulin-like growth factor 1 (IGF-1). Aging-associated sarcopenic obesity is correlated to multiple adverse cardiometabolic effects and contributes to poor health outcomes.

instance, a review of eight definitions for sarcopenic obesity revealed a 19- to 26-fold variation in sex-specific rates. Similarly, when bioelectrical impedance was used to define sarcopenia and percentage of body fat to define obesity, rates of sarcopenic obesity showed an increasing trend with age. In another study, individuals with a BMI ≥35 kg/m² were evaluated for sarcopenic obesity using dual X-ray absorptiometry (DXA)-defined body fat. The reported rates varied widely, ranging from 0 to 84.5% in women and 0 to 100% in men, depending on the specific definition applied. A population-based cohort study using National Health and Nutrition Examination Survey (NHANES) data applied the criteria of the Foundation for the National Institutes of Health (FNIH) for appendicular lean mass. The study found that rates of sarcopenic obesity were 12.6% in men and 33.5% in women. As age increased, the rates of sarcopenic obesity also increased significantly, reaching 48.0% in females and 27.5% in males among those aged over 80 years.[40]

Management of Sarcopenic Obesity

Screening and Diagnosis

The European Society for Clinical Nutrition and Metabolism (ESPEN) and the European Association for the Study of Obesity (EASO) have collaborated to develop

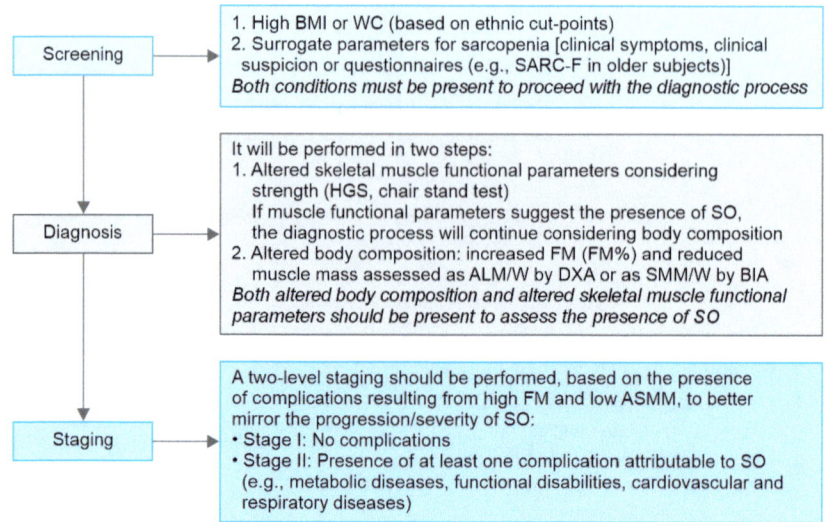

FLOWCHART 6: Diagnostic procedure for the assessment of sarcopenic obesity.

(ALM/W: appendicular lean mass adjusted to body weight; ASMM: absolute skeletal muscle mass; BIA: bioelectrical impedance analysis; BMI: body mass index; DXA: dual X-ray absorptiometry; FM: fat mass; HGS: handgrip strength; SARC-F: strength, assistance with walking, rising from a chair, climbing stairs, and falls; SMM/W: total skeletal muscle mass adjusted by weight; SO: sarcopenic obesity; WC: waist circumference)

a definition and diagnostic procedures for sarcopenic obesity. Their approach involves screening and diagnosis, allowing for staging the disease on two levels **(Flowchart 6)**.[40]

Screening for sarcopenic obesity entails assessing individuals for the simultaneous presence of an elevated BMI or waist circumference using ethnicity-specific cut points. In addition, surrogate indicators of sarcopenia, such as clinical symptoms or validated questionnaires like SARC-F (strength, assistance with walking, rising from a chair, climbing stairs, and falls) for older subjects, are considered. The recommended cut points for BMI are those provided by the WHO, while references by the National Institutes of Health and Misra et al. are suggested for waist circumference in Caucasian and Asian populations, respectively. Once a positive screening result is obtained, a diagnostic evaluation is conducted to confirm or reject the presence of sarcopenic obesity. This evaluation includes body composition measurements using appropriate techniques and devices when available. Upon establishing the sarcopenic obesity diagnosis, a two-level staging process is performed, taking into account the presence of complications. The aim is to stratify patients based on the severity of sarcopenic obesity. This staging process helps in understanding the disease's impact and guiding appropriate management strategies for affected individuals.[41]

Treatment

The most effective and evidence-based therapeutic approach for sarcopenic obesity is lifestyle modification, which includes a combination of regular aerobic and resistance exercise along with diet modifications. The goal of this approach is

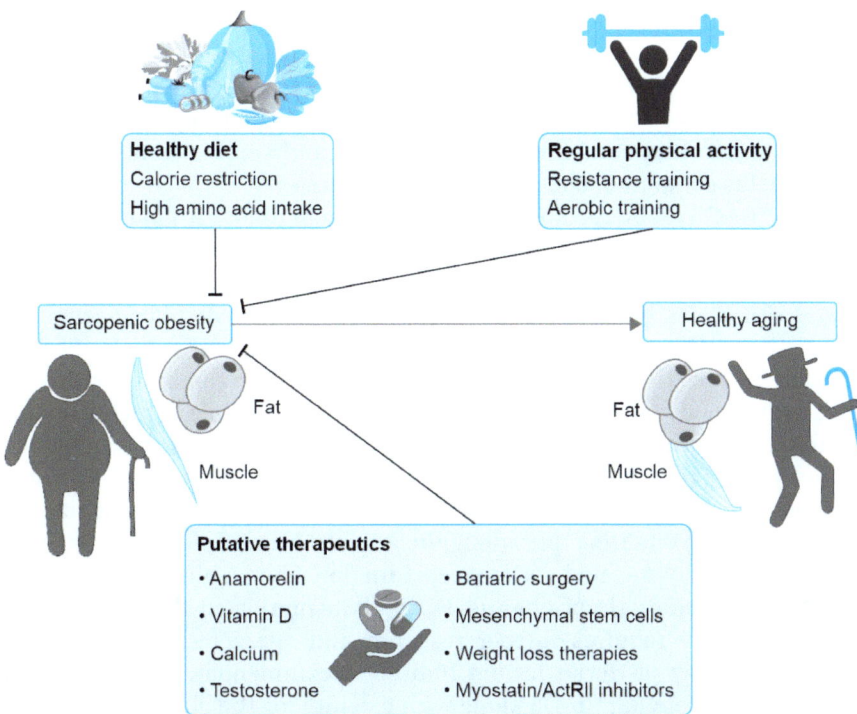

FIG. 2: Therapeutic strategies to counter-act sarcopenic development. Various therapeutic approaches are proposed against sarcopenic obesity. Caloric restriction could be considered cautiously, especially in elderly subjects associated with high-quality protein intake. Physical activity is a cornerstone in the management of sarcopenic obesity and should combine aerobic and resistance exercises. Various pharmacological treatments are considered and include myostatin inhibitors, anamorelin, vitamin D, testosterone and selective androgen receptor modulators, and weight loss therapies.

(ActRII: activin type II receptor)

to reduce fat mass and increase muscle mass and function, ultimately leading to improved quality of life and reduced mortality **(Fig. 2)**.[42,43]

Caloric restriction is a key component of lifestyle modification, but the precise quantity of calorie reduction per day has not been universally defined. However, it is generally recommended to consume fewer than 750 kcal/day than the usual intake. Additionally, a high-quality protein intake of 1–1.2 g/kg/day is recommended, especially with sources that contain leucine, which is essential for muscle protein synthesis. However, caution is necessary while consuming high-protein diets to avoid potential impairment of renal function.[42,43]

Physical exercise plays a crucial role in countering various pathophysiological aspects of both sarcopenia and obesity. Regular exercise promotes mitochondrial biogenesis, reduces low-grade inflammation, decreases insulin resistance, and helps prevent skeletal muscle cell apoptosis. Aerobic and resistance exercises are considered safe even for individuals at risk of falling. Aerobic exercise and various sporting activities, such as walking, running, swimming, cycling, and rowing, offer significant benefits for individuals with sarcopenic obesity and older people in general. These exercises improve cardiovascular function, reduce insulin resistance, enhance skeletal muscle capacity, and contribute to reducing mortality in older individuals. However, resistance exercise is considered the most effective form of physical training for older people with sarcopenic obesity. It helps induce muscle hypertrophy, enhance muscle function, and promote weight loss. An individualized exercise program that combines both resistance and aerobic activities may offer greater benefits compared to either intervention alone.[40,42]

The PROT-AGE group recommends a daily protein intake of 1.0–1.1 g/kg of body weight, divided into multiple doses. This recommendation takes into account the complex physiological changes that occur during the aging process. A protein intake of 25.0–30.0 g per meal, containing 2.5–2.8 g of leucine, has been found to have beneficial effects in slowing down frailty in older individuals. Early pilot studies have shown that meals enriched with protein, when combined with a weight loss intervention, can improve physical function. For example, a high-protein diet in combination with resistance training has been shown to preserve appendicular lean mass during weight loss.[40]

Supplementation with calcium and vitamin D is also crucial in managing sarcopenic obesity. Vitamin D plays a significant role in muscle function, as it triggers gene transcription associated with muscle function when it binds to the vitamin D receptor. The specific role of vitamin D supplementation in the management of sarcopenic obesity requires further research and characterization. As per the American Academy of Geriatrics, an indirect recommendation suggests a daily intake of 1,000 IU of vitamin D3 along with calcium for the older nonhospitalized population aged 65 years and above. This recommendation aims to maintain serum vitamin D levels at 30 ng/mL.[42]

Despite ongoing research on various pharmacological interventions for sarcopenic obesity, there are currently no approved drugs specifically designed for this condition. Several potential treatments, such as testosterone supplements, selective androgen receptor modulators, and myostatin inhibitors, are under investigation, but their efficacy and safety need further evaluation before they can be used as standard treatments.[40,42]

Weight-loss therapies, such as those utilizing GLP-1 receptor agonists, have shown promise in preclinical studies for sarcopenic obesity. However, more specific and targeted studies are needed to assess their effectiveness in improving muscle mass and function in individuals with sarcopenic obesity. Bariatric surgery, which induces weight loss through restrictive or malabsorptive mechanisms, has a consistent impact on reducing adipose tissue mass. However, its benefits for skeletal muscle and sarcopenic obesity require further investigation and evaluation. Whole-body vibration therapy, which stimulates muscle contraction, has been suggested as a potential treatment for sarcopenic obesity. However, its routine use in management requires additional assessment due to limited available evidence, especially regarding its impact on sarcopenic obesity. Anamorelin, an oral ghrelin receptor agonist known for its potential to improve lean mass and counteract cancer cachexia, is being considered for sarcopenic obesity due to its anabolic and anti-inflammatory properties. While it has demonstrated positive effects on lean mass in cancer cachexia, its impact on muscle function and sarcopenic obesity requires further investigation.[40,42]

Overall, more research is needed to identify effective pharmacological interventions for sarcopenic obesity and to better understand their potential benefits and risks. As of now, lifestyle modifications, including dietary changes and physical exercise, remain the cornerstone of management for sarcopenic obesity.

POLYCYSTIC OVARY SYNDROME

Polycystic ovary syndrome (PCOS) is a complex endocrine and metabolic disorder that affects females at various stages of life, including puberty, childbearing years, and perimenopause. The exact cause of PCOS is not fully understood, but it is believed to result from a combination of genetic and environmental factors. Obesity is recognized as one of the environmental factors that can contribute to the development and exacerbation of PCOS. Unhealthy dietary habits and an imbalance between food intake and energy expenditure can lead to obesity, which can further impact hormonal and metabolic functions in individuals with PCOS. In addition to obesity, exposure to certain environmental chemicals that disrupt endocrine functions during critical stages of growth and development may also play a role in the pathogenesis of PCOS. These chemicals, known as endocrine disruptors, can interfere with the body's hormonal regulation and contribute to the development of PCOS symptoms. The interplay between genetic predisposition and environmental factors in the development of PCOS highlights the importance of a comprehensive approach to managing this condition.[44]

Globally, the estimated prevalence of PCOS ranges between 5 and 15%. Compelling evidence suggests that women with PCOS have significantly higher risks of obesity, dyslipidemia, impaired glucose tolerance, and long-term complications, such as diabetes, endometrial cancer, and cardiovascular disease. Globally, women of reproductive age accounted for 1.55 million incident cases of PCOS and 0.43 million associated disability-adjusted life-years (DALYs). The global age-standardized PCOS incidence rate among women of reproductive age increased to 82.44 per 100,000 population in 2017, representing an increase of 1.45% from 2007 to 2017. The rate of age-standardized DALYs increased to 21.96 per 100,000 population in 2017, representing an increase of 1.91% from 2007 to 2017. Over the study period, the greatest increase in the age-standardized PCOS incidence and DALYs rates were observed in the middle- and high-middle socio-demographic index (SDI) regions, respectively. At the Global Burden of Disease (GBD) regional level, the largest increases in the age-standardized incidence rates from 2007 to 2017 were observed in Tropical Latin America (4.29%), East Asia (3.70%), and Eastern Sub-Saharan Africa (2.76%). Tropical Latin America (4.58%), East Asia (3.62%), and Eastern Sub-Saharan Africa (2.77%) had the steepest increases in the age-standardized DALYs rates from 2007 to 2017, whereas only North Africa and the Middle East exhibited a downward trend during this period (−1.05%). At the national level, Ecuador, Peru, Bolivia, Japan, and Bermuda had the highest age-standardized incidence rates and DALYs rates in both 2007 and 2017. The highest increases in both the age-standardized incidence rates and DALYs rates from 2007 to 2017 were observed in Ethiopia, Brazil, and China.[45]

Diagnosis

Polycystic ovary syndrome is diagnosed based on three main criteria: (1) hyperandrogenism, (2) ovulatory dysfunction, and (3) the presence of polycystic ovaries [polycystic ovarian morphology (PCOM)]. Hyperandrogenism is assessed both clinically by evaluating hirsutism using a visual scoring system like the modified Ferriman–Gallwey (mFG) method and biochemically by measuring circulating androgen levels. Ovulatory dysfunction is typically identified through a history of irregular menstrual cycles (polymenorrhea or oligo-amenorrhea) or by assessing ovulation using luteal phase progesterone levels in hirsute women with otherwise regular periods. PCOM is identified through ovarian ultrasonography. Additionally, related or mimicking disorders like hyperprolactinemia and thyroid dysfunction, which can cause ovulatory problems, should be excluded during the evaluation process.[46]

Weight Management in Polycystic Ovary Syndrome

The treatment of PCOS should be personalized to each individual patient and often involves multiple approaches. Lifestyle interventions are typically the first-line treatment, and even small changes in lifestyle habits can have significant positive effects on metabolic dysfunction, ovulation, fertility, and mood. Other treatment options aim to address specific aspects of PCOS, such as metabolic dysfunction, hyperandrogenism, reproductive issues, and emotional well-being.[46]

It has been observed that about half of overweight women with PCOS do not engage in sufficient physical activity to promote weight loss. To address obesity in PCOS patients, various methods can be utilized. These may include implementing diet and lifestyle modifications, using medications like insulin sensitizers, and considering bariatric surgery in some cases. By tailoring the treatment plan to the unique needs of each patient, better outcomes can be achieved in managing PCOS and its associated symptoms **(Fig. 3)**.[46,47]

Lifestyle modification: Lifestyle changes are a sensible and effective approach to managing obesity in patients with PCOS, especially when pregnancy is not a primary concern. Exercise alone may not be sufficient, and a combination of exercise, dietary modifications, caloric restriction, and behavioral interventions is often necessary. Paying attention to the quality and quantity of fats and making appropriate carbohydrate modifications can be beneficial, although further research is needed to fully understand the role of dietary glycemic index in PCOS.[47]

Recent meta-analyses have shown that lifestyle interventions lead to improvements in biochemical and endocrinological parameters, such as body composition, insulin resistance, and hyperandrogenism, although they may not have a significant effect on glucose tolerance and lipid profile. While physical exercise can contribute to reducing body weight, studies indicate that weight loss in women with PCOS may be modest or absent, even with more intensive exercise programs. Nonetheless, physical exercise has been found to improve insulin resistance, alter fat distribution, and reduce cardiovascular risk in women with PCOS. To be effective, exercise should be performed for at least 30 minutes a day, at least 5 days a week.[46,47]

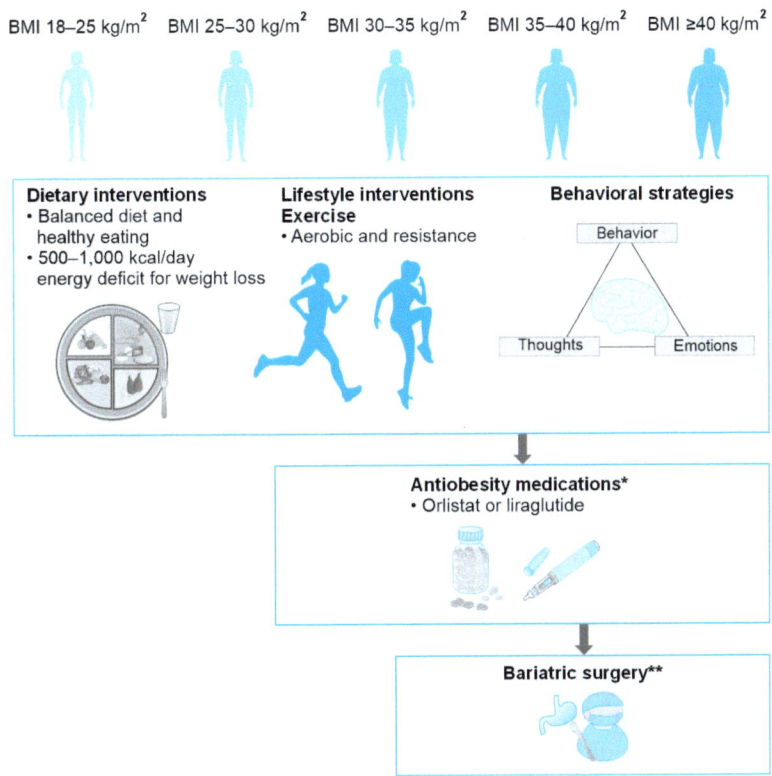

*Orlistat or liraglutide is suitable for patients with BMI >30 kg/m² and for patients with BMI >27 kg/m² with comorbidities as per the prescribing information.
**Bariatric surgery is suitable for patients with BMI >40 kg/m² and for patients with BMI >35 kg/m² with comorbidities.[46]

FIG. 3: Recommended weight management strategies for women with PCOS based on body mass index based on references 46 and 47.

(BMI: body mass index; PCOS: polycystic ovarian syndrome)

A comprehensive lifestyle program for PCOS management should include psychological support, social support, and the avoidance of toxic substances, such as smoking, alcohol, and drugs. By incorporating these various elements into the treatment plan, individuals with PCOS can experience positive changes in their health and well-being.[46]

Bariatric surgery: It has become an established and effective treatment option for obesity, especially for women with PCOS who struggle to control their weight through diet alone. It is typically recommended for women with severe obesity (BMI >40 kg/m²) or moderate obesity (BMI >35 kg/m²) who also have additional health issues. While its use in PCOS is limited, it is increasingly being applied to these patients with positive outcomes.[46]

A meta-analysis of 13 primary studies showed that bariatric surgery led to a significant reduction in PCOS symptoms, with the incidence decreasing from 45.6 to 7.1%. Additionally, the procedure resulted in a mean weight loss of 57.2%. In a prospective randomized evaluation, bariatric surgery led to substantial weight loss and improvement in PCOS-related factors including reduced serum androgens, improved insulin resistance, and restoration of ovulation and normal menstruation within 6 months.[48,49]

Medical treatment: When lifestyle modifications fail to effectively manage metabolic dysfunction and dyslipidemia in women with PCOS, pharmacological interventions can be considered. Many of these medications may also indirectly improve hyperandrogenism and ovulatory dysfunction in the disorder.

One of the most commonly used insulin-sensitizing drugs for PCOS is metformin. Studies have shown that metformin treatment may lead to body weight reduction, especially when combined with lifestyle interventions, particularly in PCOS women with a BMI >39 kg/m^2. However, in lean patients or those with a BMI of <30 kg/m^2, metformin does not appear to have a significant effect on body weight. Thiazolidinediones, which are peroxisome proliferator-activated receptor agonists or activators, are more effective than metformin in lowering fasting insulin levels and improving insulin resistance in PCOS. Other insulin sensitizers, such as troglitazone, rosiglitazone, and pioglitazone either increase body weight or have no substantial effect, and their usefulness in PCOS has not been fully assessed.[47]

Orlistat, a lipase inhibitor, has been found to be beneficial for obese PCOS patients. Its use results in improvements in insulin resistance, hyperandrogenemia, and cardiovascular risk factors. When combined with lifestyle modifications, such as diet, exercise, and behavioral changes, orlistat has been shown to be effective in addressing the endocrine and metabolic issues in obese patients with PCOS. Orlistat may also increase serum antimüllerian hormone (AMH) levels in obese PCOS patients. Studies have indicated that orlistat and metformin have similar effects in reducing BMI, insulin resistance markers, and serum testosterone levels in obese women with PCOS. Additionally, orlistat has been shown to induce ovulation and achieve similar ovulation rates as metformin in obese PCOS patients, with the advantage of minimal side effects and better tolerability compared to metformin.[50]

MENOPAUSE

Menopause is the stage in a woman's life when menstrual periods permanently cease, marking the end of the menopausal transition, also known as perimenopause. The perimenopause is a phase characterized by irregular menstrual cycles and hormonal fluctuations, often leading to unpleasant and uncomfortable symptoms. To diagnose menopause, a woman's menses must have stopped completely for 12 consecutive months, with no other physiological or pathological cause explaining the cessation. The diagnosis is primarily clinical, relying on the absence of menstruation. Additionally, elevated levels of serum follicle-stimulating hormone (FSH) may be indicative of menopause. FSH levels tend to increase as a woman's ovaries produce less estrogen during menopause. This hormonal change can be measured through a blood test and may aid in confirming the menopausal status.[51]

During the menopausal transition, the follicular ovarian pool continuously depletes, resulting in reduced estrogen production and relatively increased androgen levels. This hormonal imbalance disrupts energy homeostasis and the regulation of hunger and satiety signals. Estrogen normally inhibits hunger signals, preventing excessive calorie consumption. However, due to fluctuating estrogen levels during the menopausal transition, its ability to modulate hunger hormones is diminished. As a consequence, menopausal women experience intensified hunger signals, leading to increased food intake and promoting weight gain. Furthermore, the hormonal imbalance during menopause contributes to the accumulation of fat in the abdominal region. The combination of low estrogen levels and high androgen levels causes fat to shift from the gluteal and femoral regions to the abdomen, favoring the development of abdominal obesity.[52]

Diagnosis

According to the National Institute for Health and Care Excellence (NICE) guidelines from 2016, laboratory tests, specifically FSH measurements, are not necessary for diagnosing menopause in otherwise healthy women aged over 45 years with menopausal symptoms. The following diagnoses can be made without the need for FSH testing:[53]
- *Perimenopause*: This can be diagnosed based on the presence of vasomotor symptoms (such as hot flashes) and irregular periods in women over 45 years of age.
- *Menopause*: Women who have not had a period for at least 12 consecutive months and are not using hormonal contraception can be diagnosed with menopause based on their symptoms alone.
- *Menopause in women without a uterus*: In women without a uterus, menopause can be diagnosed based on the presence of menopausal symptoms.

However, in certain situations, considering an FSH test for diagnosing menopause is recommended:[53]
- Women aged 40-45 years with menopausal symptoms, including changes in their menstrual cycle, may benefit from an FSH test to confirm the diagnosis.
- In women under 40 years of age in whom menopause is suspected, an FSH test can be used to help establish the diagnosis.

Overall, for symptomatic women, the diagnosis of menopause should primarily rely on age and menstrual cyclicity (or lack of it) in the specified age groups, while FSH testing may be considered in specific cases as mentioned above.[53]

The Stages of Reproductive Aging Workshop (STRAW) introduced the STRAW+10 staging system, which is considered the gold standard for menopause staging. This system is primarily based on the characteristics of the menstrual cycle and divides menopausal status into three stages:[51]
1. *Reproductive stage*: In this stage, the menstrual cycle is regular, indicating that the woman is still in her reproductive years and is capable of conceiving.
2. *Menopause transition (perimenopause)*: This stage is characterized by variations in the duration of the menstrual cycle. Women in this stage may experience irregular periods and hormonal fluctuations as they approach menopause.
3. *Postmenopause*: In this stage, the menstrual cycle has ceased for at least 12 consecutive months, indicating the permanent cessation of menstruation. Women in the postmenopausal stage are no longer capable of conceiving naturally.

The STRAW+10 staging system provides a standardized classification of menopausal status, which is beneficial for researchers in conducting studies related to menopause.

Weight Management in Menopausal Women

Management strategies for weight reduction in obese individuals encompass various approaches including physical activity, calorie-controlled diet, pharmacotherapy, or bariatric surgery. Complementary and alternative treatments, such as acupuncture, yoga, and herbal supplements, may also complement weight loss efforts. These strategies can be used alone or in combination for enhanced efficacy.[54]

Dietary management involves creating a caloric deficit while improving the overall diet quality. Achieving a deficit of 500-750 kcal from the current caloric intake, considering caloric expenditure, baseline BMI, and comorbidities, is recommended. In general, a daily intake of 1,200-1,000 kcal is suggested. The proportion of protein (20-25%), fat (<30%), and carbohydrates (40-50%) with respect to total calories is determined accordingly. The diet should be rich in fiber, antioxidants from fruits, and vegetables to reduce oxidative stress that may impact ovarian follicles. Adequate water intake (at least 2 L/day), limitations on salt, sugar, and processed foods are essential. Corrective eating behaviors, such as 5-6 small and frequent meals, portion control, balanced meals, healthy snacking, and addressing emotional eating, should be incorporated.[52]

Physical activity, including both aerobic and resistance training, is vital for weight maintenance. Adults should engage in at least 150-300 minutes of moderate-intensity or 75-150 minutes of vigorous-intensity aerobic activity per week, along with full-body muscle-strengthening activities on two or more days a week. For patients with obesity, higher doses of exercise are recommended due to metabolic and cardiopulmonary benefits, as well as mitigating lean mass loss often observed with caloric reduction.[55,56]

Behavioral therapy employs various strategies, such as goal setting, problem-solving, addressing emotional eating, stimulus control, and relapse prevention, to enhance patient compliance with recommended dietary and exercise regimens. Sessions should be initiated after assessing the patient's readiness for behavior change and setting specific weight loss targets. Understanding the patient's knowledge, attitudes, and practices related to obesity can aid in providing personalized advice. Identifying primary behaviors linked to weight gain is crucial before counseling on necessary behavioral modification techniques.[52]

In addition to these lifestyle interventions, pharmacotherapy can be considered for long-term use in the treatment of obesity. The FDA has approved four medications for long-term use in the treatment of obesity: (1) orlistat, (2) phentermine/topiramate, (3) naltrexone/bupropion, and (3) liraglutide 3 mg. Among these, phentermine was the first medication approved for obesity in the United States and is commonly prescribed for short-term use. Additionally, phentermine is approved as a combination medication with topiramate-extended release (ER) (phentermine/topiramate ER) for chronic obesity treatment. Orlistat is another approved medication that reduces intestinal fat absorption, while bupropion sustained release/naltrexone combines a dopamine/norepinephrine reuptake inhibitor with an opioid receptor antagonist. Liraglutide 3 mg, a GLP-1 receptor agonist, has emerged as a promising pharmacologic treatment for obesity. Its potential to reduce insulin resistance could be particularly effective for managing obesity in postmenopausal women. These medications offer various mechanisms to help individuals with obesity achieve weight loss and improve overall health. It is important for healthcare providers to consider individual patient profiles and needs when selecting the most appropriate medication for long-term obesity management.[55]

Overall, a comprehensive approach that combines lifestyle modifications, behavioral therapy, and, when necessary, pharmacotherapy can contribute to effective weight reduction and improved overall health.

REFERENCES

1. Di Cesare M, Sorić M, Bovet P, Miranda JJ, Bhutta Z, Stevens GA, et al. The epidemiological burden of obesity in childhood: a worldwide epidemic requiring urgent action. BMC Med. 2019;17(1):212.
2. World Health Organization. Report of the Commission on Ending Childhood Obesity. Geneva: WHO; 2015.
3. NCD Risk Factor Collaboration (NCD-RisC). Worldwide trends in body-mass index, underweight, overweight, and obesity from 1975 to 2016: a pooled analysis of 2416 population-based measurement studies in 128·9 million children, adolescents, and adults. Lancet. 2017;390(10113):2627-42.
4. Twig G, Yaniv G, Levine H, Leiba A, Goldberger N, Derazne E, et al. Body-Mass Index in 2.3 Million Adolescents and Cardiovascular Death in Adulthood. N Engl J Med. 2016;374(25):2430-40.
5. Sharma V, Coleman S, Nixon J, Sharples L, Hamilton-Shield J, Rutter H, et al. A systematic review and meta-analysis estimating the population prevalence of comorbidities in children and adolescents aged 5 to 18 years. Obes Rev. 2019;20(10):1341-49.
6. Lobstein T, Jackson-Leach R. Planning for the worst: estimates of obesity and comorbidities in school-age children in 2025. Pediatr Obes. 2016;11(5):321-5.
7. Barlow SE; Expert Committee. Expert committee recommendations regarding the prevention, assessment, and treatment of child and adolescent overweight and obesity: summary report. Pediatrics. 2007;120 Suppl 4:S164-92.
8. Johnson VR, Cao M, Czepiel KS, Mushannen T, Nolen L, Stanford FC. Strategies in the Management of Adolescent Obesity. Curr Pediatr Rep. 2020;8(2):56-65.
9. Andela S, Burrows TL, Baur LA, Coyle DH, Collins CE, Gow ML. Efficacy of very low-energy diet programs for weight loss: A systematic review with meta-analysis of intervention studies in children and adolescents with obesity. Obes Rev. 2019;20(6):871-82.
10. Kumar S, Kelly AS. Review of Childhood Obesity: From Epidemiology, Etiology, and Comorbidities to Clinical Assessment and Treatment. Mayo Clin Proc. 2017;92(2):251-65.
11. Cuda SE, Censani M. Pediatric Obesity Algorithm: A Practical Approach to Obesity Diagnosis and Management. Front Pediatr. 2019;6:431.
12. International Diabetes Federation. (2022). IDF Atlas Reports: Type 1 diabetes numbers in children and adults. [online] Available from https://diabetesatlas.org/idfawp/resource-files/2022/12/IDF-T1D-Index-Report.pdf. [Last accessed October, 2023].
13. Ward ZJ, Yeh JM, Reddy CL, Gomber A, Ross C, Rittiphairoj T, et al. Estimating the total incidence of type 1 diabetes in children and adolescents aged 0-19 years from 1990 to 2050: a global simulation-based analysis. Lancet Diabetes Endocrinol. 2022;10(12):848-58.
14. Wu H, Patterson CC, Zhang X, Ghani RBA, Magliano DJ, Boyko EJ, et al. Worldwide estimates of incidence of type 2 diabetes in children and adolescents in 2021. Diabetes Res Clin Pract. 2022;185:109785.
15. Besser REJ, Bell KJ, Couper JJ, Ziegler AG, Wherrett DK, Knip M, et al. ISPAD Clinical Practice Consensus Guidelines 2022: Stages of type 1 diabetes in children and adolescents. Pediatr Diabetes. 2022;23(8):1175-87.
16. Shah AS, Zeitler PS, Wong J, Pena AS, Wicklow B, Arslanian S, et al. ISPAD Clinical Practice Consensus Guidelines 2022: Type 2 diabetes in children and adolescents. Pediatr Diabetes. 2022;23(7):872-902.
17. ElSayed NA, Aleppo G, Aroda VR, Bannuru RR, Brown FM, Bruemmer D, et al. 14. Children and Adolescents: Standards of Care in Diabetes-2023. Diabetes Care. 2023;46(Suppl 1):S230-53.

18. Peña AS, Curran JA, Fuery M, George C, Jefferies CA, Lobley K, et al. Screening, assessment and management of type 2 diabetes mellitus in children and adolescents: Australasian Paediatric Endocrine Group guidelines. Med J Aust. 2020;213(1):30-43.
19. McIntyre HD, Catalano P, Zhang C, Desoye G, Mathiesen ER, Damm P. Gestational diabetes mellitus. Nat Rev Dis Primers. 2019;5(1):47.
20. Zhu Y, Zhang C. Prevalence of Gestational Diabetes and Risk of Progression to Type 2 Diabetes: a Global Perspective. Curr Diab Rep. 2016;16(1):7.
21. Reece EA. The fetal and maternal consequences of gestational diabetes mellitus. J Matern Fetal Neonatal Med. 2010;23(3):199-203.
22. Sweeting A, Wong J, Murphy HR, Ross GP. A Clinical Update on Gestational Diabetes Mellitus. Endocr Rev. 2022;43(5):763-93.
23. ElSayed NA, Aleppo G, Aroda VR, Bannuru RR, Brown FM, Bruemmer D, et al. 15. Management of Diabetes in Pregnancy: Standards of Care in Diabetes-2023. Diabetes Care. 2023;46(Suppl 1):S254-66.
24. Dickens LT, Thomas CC. Updates in Gestational Diabetes Prevalence, Treatment, and Health Policy. Curr Diab Rep. 2019;19(6):33.
25. Mathus-Vliegen EMH. Obesity and the elderly. J Clin Gastroenterol. 2012;46(7):533-44.
26. Kyaw TM, Ismail Z, Selamat MI, Nawawi H, MyHEBAT investigators. Obesity and its associated factors among older adults: MyHEBAT (Malaysian HEalth and Well-Being AssessmenT) study. Health Sci Rep. 2022;5(4):e668.
27. Singh P, Kapil U, Dey AB. Prevalence of overweight and obesity amongst elderly patients attending a geriatric clinic in a tertiary care hospital in Delhi, India. Indian J Med Sci. 2004;58(4):162-3.
28. Swami HM, Bhatia V, Gupta AK, Bhatia SPS. An epidemiological study of obesity among elderly in Chandigarh. Indian J Community Med. 2005;30(1):11-3.
29. Mathus-Vliegen EM; Obesity Management Task Force of the European Association for the Study of Obesity. Prevalence, pathophysiology, health consequences and treatment options of obesity in the elderly: a guideline. Obes Facts. 2012;5(3):460-83.
30. Kennedy RL, Malabu U, Kazi M, Shahsidhar V. Management of obesity in the elderly: too much and too late? J Nutr Health Aging. 2008;12(9):608-21.
31. Diabetes Prevention Program Research Group, Crandall J, Schade D, Ma Y, Fujimoto WY, Barrett-Connor E, et al. The influence of age on the effects of lifestyle modification and metformin in prevention of diabetes. J Gerontol A Biol Sci Med Sci. 2006;61(10):1075-81.
32. Bales CW, Buhr G. Is obesity bad for older persons? A systematic review of the pros and cons of weight reduction in later life. J Am Med Dir Assoc. 2008;9(5):302-12.
33. Davidson LE, Hudson R, Kilpatrick K, Kuk JL, McMillan K, Janiszewski PM, et al. Effects of exercise modality on insulin resistance and functional limitation in older adults: a randomized controlled trial. Arch Intern Med. 2009;169(2):122-31.
34. Goisser S, Kiesswetter E, Schoene D, Torbahn G, Bauer JM. Dietary weight-loss interventions for the management of obesity in older adults. Rev Endocr Metab Disord. 2020;21(3):355-68.
35. Witham MD, Avenell A. Interventions to achieve long-term weight loss in obese older people: a systematic review and meta-analysis. Age Ageing. 2010;39(2):176-84.
36. Weinheimer EM, Sands LP, Campbell WW. A systematic review of the separate and combined effects of energy restriction and exercise on fat-free mass in middle-aged and older adults: implications for sarcopenic obesity. Nutr Rev. 2010;68(7):375-88.
37. Jain SS, Ramanand SJ, Ramanand JB, Akat PB, Patwardhan MH, Joshi SR. Evaluation of efficacy and safety of orlistat in obese patients. Indian J Endocrinol Metab. 2011;15(2):99-104.
38. Zamboni M, Rubele S, Rossi AP. Sarcopenia and obesity. Curr Opin Clin Nutr Metab Care. 2019;22(1):13-9.
39. Roh E, Choi KM. Health Consequences of Sarcopenic Obesity: A Narrative Review. Front Endocrinol (Lausanne). 2020;11:332.
40. Batsis JA, Villareal DT. Sarcopenic obesity in older adults: aetiology, epidemiology and treatment strategies. Nat Rev Endocrinol. 2018;14(9):513-37.
41. Donini LM, Busetto L, Bischoff SC, Cederholm T, Ballesteros-Pomar MD, Batsis JA, et al. Definition and Diagnostic Criteria for Sarcopenic Obesity: ESPEN and EASO Consensus Statement. Obes Facts. 2022;15(3):321-35.
42. Wei S, Nguyen TT, Zhang Y, Ryu D, Gariani K. Sarcopenic obesity: epidemiology, pathophysiology, cardiovascular disease, mortality, and management. Front Endocrinol (Lausanne). 2023;14:1185221.

43. Wang M, Tan Y, Shi Y, Wang X, Liao Z, Wei P. Diabetes and Sarcopenic Obesity: Pathogenesis, Diagnosis, and Treatments. Front Endocrinol (Lausanne). 2020;11:568.
44. Ma R, Zou Y, Wang W, Zheng Q, Feng Y, Dong H, et al. Obesity management in polycystic ovary syndrome: disparity in knowledge between obstetrician-gynecologists and reproductive endocrinologists in China. BMC Endocr Disord. 2021;21(1):182.
45. Liu J, Wu Q, Hao Y, Jiao M, Wang X, Jiang S, et al. Measuring the global disease burden of polycystic ovary syndrome in 194 countries: Global Burden of Disease Study 2017. Hum Reprod. 2021;36(4):1108-19.
46. Azziz R, Carmina E, Chen Z, Dunaif A, Laven JS, Legro RS, et al. Polycystic ovary syndrome. Nat Rev Dis Primers. 2016;2:16057.
47. Messinis IE, Messini CI, Anifandis G, Dafopoulos K. Polycystic ovaries and obesity. Best Pract Res Clin Obstet Gynaecol. 2015;29(4):479-88.
48. Skubleny D, Switzer NJ, Gill RS, Dykstra M, Shi X, Sagle MA, et al. The Impact of Bariatric Surgery on Polycystic Ovary Syndrome: a Systematic Review and Meta-analysis. Obes Surg. 2016;26(1):169-76.
49. Escobar-Morreale HF, Botella-Carretero JI, Alvarez-Blasco F, Sancho J, San Millán JL. The polycystic ovary syndrome associated with morbid obesity may resolve after weight loss induced by bariatric surgery. J Clin Endocrinol Metab. 2005;90(12):6364-9.
50. Saleem F, Rizvi SW. New Therapeutic Approaches in Obesity and Metabolic Syndrome Associated with Polycystic Ovary Syndrome. Cureus. 2017;9(11):e1844.
51. Oxford Research Encyclopedias, Global Public Health (2020). Menopause. [online] Available from https://oxfordre.com/publichealth/display/10.1093/acrefore/9780190632366.001.0001/acrefore-9780190632366-e-176?print=pdf [Last accessed October, 2023].
52. Chopra S, Sharma KA, Ranjan P, Malhotra A, Vikram NK, Kumari A. Weight Management Module for Perimenopausal Women: A Practical Guide for Gynecologists. J Midlife Health. 2019;10(4):165-72.
53. Lumsden MA. The NICE Guideline—Menopause: diagnosis and management. Climacteric. 2016;19(5):426-9.
54. Davis SR, Castelo-Branco C, Chedraui P, Lumsden MA, Nappi RE, Shah D, et al. Understanding weight gain at menopause. Climacteric. 2012;15(5):419-29.
55. Knight MG, Anekwe C, Washington K, Akam EY, Wang E, Stanford FC. Weight regulation in menopause. Menopause. 2021;28(8):960-5.
56. Dubnov G, Brzezinski A, Berry EM. Weight control and the management of obesity after menopause: the role of physical activity. Maturitas. 2003;44(2):89-101.

CHAPTER 10

Future Directions and Research

Key Highlights

- *Personalized pharmacogenetics*: Genetic variants influencing drug response in diabetes treatment enable tailored therapies for improved safety and efficacy.
- *Precision medicine*: Tailoring diabetes care based on genetics and characteristics, spanning type 1 and type 2 diabetes mellitus (T1DM and T2DM) for personalized diagnostics, treatments, and prevention.
- *Genetic influence*: Genetic mutations impact disease and treatment responses in neonatal diabetes mellitus (NDM) and maturity-onset diabetes of the young (MODY), driving individualized care.
- *Obesity prevention*: Environmental changes through policies, such as food labeling, trans fat bans, and family-based interventions offer effective approaches for obesity prevention.
- *Traffic light diet*: Family-based dietary intervention using the traffic light system (green, yellow, and red) guides healthier food choices.
- *Maternal obesity*: Targeted interventions for maternal obesity include counseling, home visits, and nutritional guidelines for healthier pregnancies.
- *Future promise*: Precision medicine's potential in diabetes care is evolving, with genetics, technology, and collaboration reshaping diagnostics, treatments, and prevention.

INTRODUCTION

Obesity

Obesity is an increasingly concerning global public health challenge, being categorized as a nationwide epidemic. Its impact is felt by a significant portion of the population, affecting approximately one out of every three adults and one out of every six children in the United States. Numerous countries across the globe have observed a striking rise, often two- to threefold, in obesity prevalence over the past three decades. This surge can be attributed to factors such as urbanization, sedentary lifestyles, and the heightened consumption of calorie-dense processed foods. The particularly distressing surge in childhood obesity serves as a stark indicator of the forthcoming burden on future public healthcare systems, necessitating substantial efforts in chronic disease prevention. The prevention of obesity assumes paramount importance in the management of obesity-related noncommunicable diseases (OR-NCDs). These encompass conditions such as insulin resistance/metabolic syndrome, characterized by hyperinsulinemia, type 2 diabetes mellitus (T2DM), hyperlipidemia, hypertension, and coronary artery disease.[1]

A global study has projected a concerning future scenario: If significant improvements are not made in prevention, treatment, and support, over half of the world's population will be grappling with overweight and obesity within the next 12 years. The recently published World Obesity Atlas 2023 by the World Obesity Federation offers insights into this potential crisis. The study forecasts that if current measures for prevention and treatment do not witness enhancement, the economic repercussions of overweight and obesity will escalate to a staggering $4.32 trillion annually by 2035. This figure, equivalent to nearly 3% of the global GDP, mirrors the economic impact of the coronavirus disease 2019 (COVID-19) pandemic in 2020.[2,3]

According to these projections, a substantial 51% of the global populace, surpassing 4 billion individuals, could be dealing with either overweight or obesity by 2035, if prevailing trends persist. The prevalence of obesity itself is anticipated to afflict 1 in 4 people, amounting to almost 2 billion individuals. Remarkably, childhood obesity might experience an alarming increase, potentially more than doubling from 2020 levels. Among boys, rates are forecasted to double to 208 million (a 100% rise), and among girls, they are projected to more than double to 175 million (a 125% surge). Notably, this surge among children is outpacing the rate of increase among adults. The implications of these forecasts are profound: If transformative action is not undertaken, over 1.5 billion adults and nearly 400 million children could be living with obesity in just over a decade.[2,3]

While obesity has often been associated with high-income countries, the report highlights an alarming trend: Low- and lower-middle-income countries, which often face challenges in responding effectively to obesity and its consequences, are experiencing the most rapid rise in obesity levels. Nations with substantial populations and lower-middle income status, like India, Pakistan, Indonesia, and Nigeria, could potentially mirror the trajectory of upper-middle-income countries such as Mexico, Brazil, and Turkey, where obesity prevalence has surged, especially among young individuals. Among the 10 countries projected to experience the most significant increases in obesity rates globally, nine belong to low- or lower-middle-income categories, predominantly hailing from Asia and Africa.[2,3]

The findings of the World Obesity Federation's research highlight the multiple obstacles faced by individuals living with obesity when seeking medical care. These hurdles encompass challenges such as difficulties in obtaining a formal diagnosis due to the nonclassification of obesity as a disease. Furthermore, they encounter obstacles in accessing necessary treatments from well-informed and trained healthcare providers (HCPs). Compounding these issues, individuals often find themselves burdened by significant out-of-pocket expenses required for appropriate medical care. A survey conducted by Leach et al. in 2020 shed light on the primary barriers that were commonly reported. These include a "lack of political will or interest," a scarcity of adequately trained professionals and available training, the financial strain of high out-of-pocket payments, limited health literacy, suboptimal behavior patterns, the absence of recognition of obesity as a disease, and the pervasive influence of an "obesogenic environment" (as illustrated in **Fig. 1**).[3,4]

There are significant differences between regions and levels of economic development that require urgent and tailored action to address obesity and reduce the prevalence. Action on obesity is commonly siloed and fragmented, and obesity remains under-prioritized within global health and NCD strategies as a risk factor rather than a disease in its own right. False trade-offs are often seen between prevention and treatment, when the reality is population-level prevention strategies need to be complemented with action within health systems.

Diabetes

Diabetes continues to be a significant concern within the realm of public health. The majority of diabetes cases fall under T2DM, a condition that can be largely averted and, in certain instances, even reversed when detected and addressed

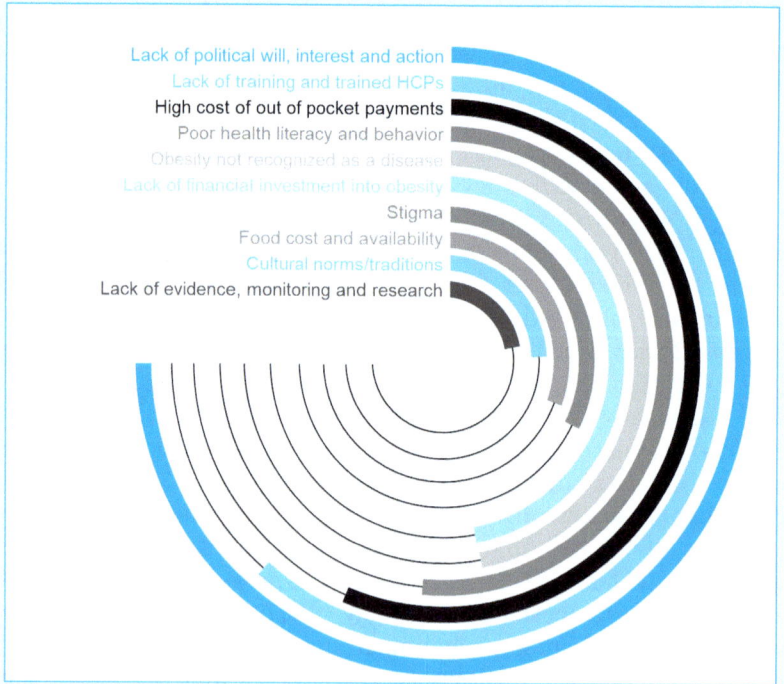

FIG. 1: Based on findings from over 274 obesity specialists from 68 countries. *(For color version, see Plate 5)*

(HCPs: healthcare professionals)

Source: With permission from Leach RJ, et al. (2020).[4]

during its initial stages. Despite this potential, the global prevalence of diabetes is unequivocally on the rise, predominantly attributed to the escalating rates of obesity stemming from a variety of contributing factors. The ongoing struggle to prevent and manage T2DM persists as a formidable challenge. An imperative step is to gain deeper insights into the discrepancies present in risk factor profiles and the burden of diabetes across diverse populations. This understanding is pivotal in devising effective strategies aimed at curbing diabetes risk factors, within the intricate framework of multifaceted and interrelated drivers.[5]

Diabetes imposes a significant load on healthcare systems, as per data from the International Diabetes Federation (IDF), which indicates that in 2021, approximately 537 million individuals globally were afflicted by diabetes. This has led to healthcare expenditures amounting to $966 billion on a global scale, a figure anticipated to surge beyond $1054 billion by 2045. The Global Burden of Disease Study 2021, through meticulous analysis, reported that there were 529 million people worldwide living with diabetes. The standardized diabetes prevalence across the globe stood at 6.1% during this period. In 2021, a substantial portion of disability-adjusted life years (DALYs), amounting to 58.9 million, or 76.5% specifically attributed to T2DM, were linked to risk factors.[5]

Among the array of 16 risk factors evaluated, a heightened body mass index (BMI) emerged as the predominant risk factor contributing to T2DM on a global scale, accounting for 52.2% of the total DALYs associated with this condition. The overall prevalence of diabetes, particularly among the elderly population, predominantly manifests as T2DM. In 2021, this type encompassed 96.0% of diabetes cases and 95.4% of diabetes-related DALYs across the world.[5]

Projections into the future indicate an escalating diabetes scenario, with an estimated 1.31 billion individuals expected to be affected by diabetes by 2050. Age-standardized total diabetes prevalence is forecasted to exceed 10% in two major regions: 16.8% in north Africa and the Middle East, and 11.3% in Latin America and the Caribbean. By 2050, a notable 89 out of 204 countries and territories are projected to have an age-standardized prevalence rate surpassing the 10% threshold.[5]

Currently, the customization of treatment through molecular testing remains a challenge of significant magnitude. Moreover, employing a uniform therapeutic algorithm for diabetes treatment often results in inadequate outcomes, accompanied by a range of diabetic complications. As technology progresses, the emergence of high-throughput sequencing methods facilitates the accumulation of comprehensive "omics" data, encompassing genomics, transcriptomics, proteomics, and metabolomics, enabling a comprehensive analysis of health and disease at a global level. The integration of extensive data sets, including clinical and laboratory information, can pave the way for tailored therapeutic strategies, employing personalized approaches to diabetes management.[6]

NEW THERAPEUTIC TARGETS AND APPROACHES

New Therapeutic Targets in Obesity

The management of obesity continues to present challenges, particularly when compared to other chronic conditions such as hypertension and T2DM.

Unlike these diseases, obesity has limited pharmacological options available for treatment, placing a significant reliance on lifestyle changes and surgical interventions. On one hand, the fundamental approach to treatment remains rooted in dietary adjustments and physical activity, sometimes accompanied by structured behavioral therapy. Despite being considered a foundational strategy, this approach's effectiveness is constrained, repeatedly failing to adequately address the diverse requirements of most individuals with obesity.[7]

On the other hand, bariatric surgery stands out for its remarkable success in achieving substantial weight loss and resolving associated complications such as diabetes, obstructive sleep apnea, and even reducing mortality from cardiovascular issues and cancer, particularly in women. However, the widespread application of bariatric surgery is impractical due to logistical constraints, preventing it from meeting the needs of the entire population. It is important to note that both lifestyle changes and surgical interventions often lead to weight regain over time.

Given this context, there exists a compelling rationale for the exploration and development of effective pharmacological treatments to bridge this gap. The demand for solutions that can more comprehensively and sustainably address the complex nature of obesity underscores the necessity for advancements in pharmacotherapy.[7]

Amidst a series of setbacks, several prominent therapeutic targets have garnered significant attention within the scientific community (depicted in **Table 1**). These targets exemplify the current pinnacle of identifying and progressing novel drug candidates into human trials. Notably, four focal areas—leptin, ghrelin, mitochondrial uncouplers, and growth differentiation factor 15 (GDF15)—were initiated and advanced with a primary therapeutic aim of addressing obesity. In contrast, research involving incretins, particularly glucagon-like peptide-1 (GLP-1), as well as amylin, was primarily centered around diabetes. This research path evolved through concurrent empirical observations of their efficacy in lowering body weight. The progression of incretin biology has led to the emergence of late-phase antiobesity medication (AOM) candidates that robustly activate glucagon-like peptide-1 receptor (GLP-1R) and/or glucose-dependent insulinotropic polypeptide receptor (GIPR), establishing a significantly elevated and new standard for performance. This advancement marks a noteworthy evolution in therapeutic potential.[8]

Numerous drugs in the development pipeline are presently undergoing investigation as potential AOMs. With the exception of sodium-glucose cotransporter-2 (SGLT-2) inhibitors, vitamin E, and gladribin analogs, the remaining drugs exert their effects centrally by diminishing appetite and enhancing the feeling of satiety (**Table 2**).[8]

Incretin-based Therapy

Glucagon-like peptide-1-related drug candidates: Advancements in the realm of incretin biology have led to the creation of a group of registered GLP-1R agonist drug candidates. These developments were, in part, spurred by the successful outcomes of oral dipeptidyl peptidase-4 (DPP-4) inhibitors, which indirectly elevate levels of endogenous GLP-1 and GIP to enhance glycemic control without posing a risk of hypoglycemia. Utilizing parenteral administration of bioactive hormone

TABLE 1: Weight loss drugs in clinical development.

Preclinical			Phase I			Phase II			Phase III		
	Company	Indication	GLP-1/glucagon dual agonists	Company	Indication	GLP-1/glucagon dual agonists	Company	Indication	GIP/GLP-1 dual agonists	Company	Indication
GIPR agonists											
ZP-6590	ZP	Obesity	OXM	EL	T2DM	Cotadutide (MEDI0382)	AZ	T2DM, NASH	Tirzepatide	EL	Obesity, T2DM
GLP-1R agonists			GIP/GLP-1 dual agonists			BI 456906	BI	Obesity, T2DM	GLP-1R agonists		
Celastrol	Academic	Obesity, T2DM	GIP/GLP-1	EL	T2DM	Efinopegdutide	HP	NASH	Efpeglenatide	HP	T2DM
Amylin analogs			GIP/GLP-2	EL	T2DM	GIP/GLP-1/ glucagon triagonists			Rybelsus	NN	Obesity
ZP-8396	ZP	Obesity	GIP/GLP-1/ glucagon tri-agonists			HM15211	HP	NASH			
Drugs targeting the ghrelin pathway			GGG triagonist	EL	T2DM	GLP-1R agonists					
Nox-B11	NP	Obesity	GIPR agonists			Danuglipron	Pfizer	Obesity, T2DM			
Mitochondrial uncoupler			GIPR agonist long acting	EL	T2DM	Y2R agonists					
BAM15	CBio	Obesity, NASH	GLP-1R agonists			NNC0165-1875 + semaglutide	NN	Obesity, T2DM			
			GLPR-NPA	EL	T2DM	Amylin analogs					
			PF-07081532	Pfizer	T2DM	Cagrilintide	NN	Obesity, T2DM			
			Glucagon analog								
			HM15136	HP	Obesity						

Continued

Continued

Preclinical			Phase I			Phase II			Phase III		
GIPR agonists	Company	Indication	GLP-1/glucagon dual agonists	Company	Indication	GLP-1/glucagon dual agonists	Company	Indication	GIP/GLP-1 dual agonists	Company	Indication
			Leptin sensitizers								
			Withaferin A	Academic	Obesity, T2DM						
			Y2R agonists								
			PYY analog	EL	T2DM						
			NN 9748 (NN 9747)	NN	Obesity, T2DM						
			Amylin/calcitonin dual agonists								
			KBP-089	NB	T2DM						
			Drugs targeting the ghrelin pathway								
			CYT009-GhrQb	CB	Obesity						
			Other appetite suppressants								
			GDF15	NN	Obesity						
			LY3463251	EL	T2DM, obesity						
			JNJ-9090/CIN-109	J & J	Obesity						

(GDF15: growth differentiation factor 15; GIP: glucose-dependent insulinotropic polypeptide; GLP-1: glucagon-like peptide-1; GLP-1R: glucagon-like peptide-1 receptor; GLPR-NPA: GLP-1 receptor nonpeptidic agonist; NA: not applicable; NASH: nonalcoholic steatohepatitis; OXM: oxyntomodulin; PYY: peptide tyrosine-tyrosine; T2DM: type 2 diabetes mellitus; Y2R: neuropeptide Y receptor type 2)

(Company name: EL: Eli Lilly; NN: Novo Nordisk; CB: Cytos Biotechnology; CBio: Continuum Biosciences; NP: Noxxon Pharma; J & J: Jansenn; ZP: Zealand Pharma; NB: Nordic Biosciences; HP: Hanmi Pharmaceutical; BI: Boehringer Ingelheim; AZ: AstraZeneca)

TABLE 2: Antidiabetic agents, associated genes, and variant characteristics.

Antidiabetic drug class	Gene and SNPs	Action	Variant characteristics
Sulfonylureas	• *KCNJ11* Glu23Lys (rs5219) • 3p+215 G>A (rs5210)	• Subunits of the K_{ATP} channel • Metabolism of glucose can affect ATP levels and thereby function of K_{ATP} channel	K-allele carriers show higher decrease in HbA1c compared with EE homozygotes. Significantly associated with decrease in FPG
	• *ABCC8* Ser1369Ala (rs757110) *Exon* 163 C>T (rs1799854) rg1273Arg (rs1799859)	Potentiation activity of the K_{ATP} channel	Lower FPG: Wild-type CC genotype shows significantly lower HbA1c levels compared to TT genotype
	TCF7L2 rs7903146 C>T rs12255372 G>C	Potentiation activity of the K_{ATP} channel	Significant reduction in HbA1c and FPG in CC genotype compared to the CT and TT genotype
	CYP2C9 *3(Ile359Leu) (rs1057910); *2 (Arg144Cys) (rs1799853); *3 (Ile359Leu) (rs1057910)	Oral clearance of tolbutamide	• Carriers of *3 allele required lower doses of tolbutamide • Decreased clearance and increased plasma drug exposure
Metformin	*SLC22A1* gene coding the OCT1 protein transporter • Site: Hepatocytes, enterocytes	Mediates metformin uptake, accumulation and pharmacological action in the liver (AMPK activation)	• Decreased hepatic and intestinal metformin uptake Decreased AMPK activation • Increased plasma glucose levels • Lower insulin levels
	SLC22A2 gene coding the OCT2 protein transporter • Site: Renal distal tubule	Facilitate urinary elimination of metformin	• Decreased metformin clearance • Increased plasma concentration
	SLC47A1 gene coding the MATE1 transporter • Sites: Bile canaliculi, renal epithelium	Metformin secretion in bile and urine	May effect glucose lowering effect of metformin
	SLC47A2 gene coding the MATE2K1 transporter • Site: Renal epithelium	Excretion of metformin	Metformin excretion in urine is decreased

Continued

Continued

Antidiabetic drug class	Gene and SNPs	Action	Variant characteristics
Thiazolidinediones	*PPARG* gene Pro12Ala	Energy Intake/expenditure, lipid metabolism	• Loss-of-function mutations in PPARγ are associated with severe IR and DM • Polymorphism Pro12Ala significantly greater decrease in FPG and HbA1c
	Uncoupling protein 2 (UCP2)	Gene of metabolic disorders; it negatively regulates glucose-stimulated insulin secretion	Strong association between rosiglitazone treatment success and UCP2-866 G>A polymorphism
	OATP1B1, CYP2C8	Hepatic uptake of TZDs is and metabolism	• Homozygous carriers of the gain-of-function allele for CYP2C8, CYP2C8*3 coding for the Arg139Lys and Lys399Arg amino acid substitutions have lower rosiglitazone plasma concentrations • Lower efficacy
Dipeptidyl peptidase 4 (DPP-4) inhibitors	*KCNJ11* gene	Regulates one of the pancreatic K^{ATP}	Subjects with KCNJ11 rs2285676 (genotype CC) are more likely to response to DPP-4 inhibitor treatment
	TCF7L2 gene	Incretin secretion from intestinal endocrine L cells and the proliferation of pancreatic β cells	TCF7L2 variants are associated with diminished pancreatic islet cell responsiveness to incretins
	CTRB1 and *CTRB2*	Both encode chymotrypsin, in the regulation of the incretin pathway	Reduced response to treatment with DPP-4 inhibitors
Sodium-glucose cotransporter-2 (SGLT-2) inhibitors	*SGLT-2* gene (*SLC5*)	Inhibits reabsorption of glucose in renal proximal tubule, increasing urinary glucose excretion and decreasing glucose levels	Nonsense and missense mutations in the *SLC2A5* gene that result in the loss of SGLT-2 function cause familial renal glycosuria and are associated with the reduced circulating glucose levels

(AMPK: 5′ AMP-activated protein kinase; DM: diabetes mellitus; FPG: fasting plasma glucose; HbA1c: glycated hemoglobin; IR: insulin resistance; K_{ATP}: adenosine triphosphate-sensitive potassium; PPAR: peroxisome proliferator-activated receptor; SNPs: single nucleotide polymorphisms; TZDs: thiazolidinediones) paralogs and synthetic analogs resulted in heightened drug concentrations within circulation. This, in turn, led to improved glycemic control and a heightened recognition of the inherent capability of GLP-1R agonism to lower body weight. Initial clinical trials employing GLP-1R agonists revealed a modest reduction in weight, aligning closely with the observations made with other gut hormones. However, these pharmacological findings were accompanied by substantial impacts on gastrointestinal motility. This aspect posed challenges in accurately assessing the extent to which weight reduction resulted from adverse local gastrointestinal effects that served to diminish appetite.[8]

In response, the emergence of peptide analogs with extended and consistent pharmacokinetics, coupled with refined dosing strategies that mitigated adverse gastrointestinal effects, paved the way for more sustained and potent treatment approaches. These measures solidified the metabolic and weight-lowering benefits associated with GLP-1R agonism. The intricate mechanism of action involves multiple factors with enhancements in gut, brain, and systemic insulin sensitivity collectively contributing to its overall efficacy. Currently, a range of additional peptide and small-molecule GLP-1R agonists is undergoing clinical development including formulations designed for oral administration. Notably, an oral GLP-1 receptor nonpeptidic agonist (GLPR-NPA) is presently in phase II clinical trials at Eli Lilly.[8]

Glucose-dependent insulinotropic polypeptide-related drug candidates: The utilization of GIPR agonism as a therapeutic approach for obesity and T2DM is met with considerable skepticism due to the diminished insulinotropic effect of GIP in individuals with T2DM. Furthermore, substantial preclinical evidence suggests that GIPR antagonism has the potential to enhance overall energy and glucose metabolism, potentially by bolstering central leptin sensitivity. In a comprehensive assessment, prolonged-acting GIPR agonists have demonstrated the ability to reduce body weight and enhance glucose regulation across a series of preclinical investigations. Presently, a long-acting GIPR agonist is undergoing phase I clinical trials as a prospective treatment for T2DM.[8]

Pharmacotherapies in the Pipeline based on Gut Hormone Combinations with GLP-1

Dual-agonism GLP-1 and GIP

Glucose-dependent insulinotropic polypeptide is a hormone secreted by the jejunum in response to food consumption. It triggers the release of insulin, amplifies glucagon secretion, and enhances the lipid-buffering capability of adipose tissue. In preclinical models, the concurrent activation of GLP-1 and GIP receptors resulted in superior effects on weight loss and glucose reduction compared to the activation of each receptor in isolation. This outcome has heightened interest in the development of unimolecular agonists targeting both GLP-1 and GIP receptors.[9]

One such notable advancement is tirzepatide. It stands as the inaugural dual GLP-1 and GIP receptor agonist sanctioned for the management of T2DM. Administered subcutaneously on a once-weekly basis in doses of 5, 10, and 15 mg, its approval was founded on the comprehensive findings of the SURPASS program. Analysis of the SURPASS program data revealed that tirzepatide yielded substantial reductions in mean glycated hemoglobin (HbA1c), ranging from 1.87 to 2.59% across different dosages. Additionally, a noteworthy proportion of patients, specifically between 62 and 86%, achieved the target HbA1c level of ≤6.5%. The higher doses of tirzepatide (10–15 mg) also yielded significant weight loss, ranging from 9.5 to 12.9 kg. Impressively, a considerable percentage of patients, ranging from 40 to 69%, achieved a weight loss of ≥10%. It is noteworthy that these outcomes were achieved without any supplementary support for lifestyle interventions as part of the SURPASS program.[9]

Dual Agonism with Amylin

Amylin, a hormone cosecreted alongside insulin from pancreatic β-cells in response to food consumption, plays a pivotal role in regulating satiety by exerting its effects within the brain. Additionally, it contributes to improved glycemic control by retarding gastric emptying and suppressing glucagon secretion.[9]

Cagrilintide, an extended-release analog of amylin, is administered subcutaneously once a week. In a phase II trial spanning 26 weeks, various doses of cagrilintide, up to 4.5 mg, exhibited more substantial weight loss compared to a placebo in individuals with obesity (6.0–10.8% vs. 3.0%). Notably, at the 4.5 mg dosage, cagrilintide outperformed liraglutide 3 mg in terms of weight loss (10.8% vs. 9.0%).[9]

The weight loss induced by GLP-1R agonists and amylin analogs arises from both distinct and overlapping mechanisms. Consequently, the combination of these therapies holds potential for synergistic effects, further reducing appetite and enhancing weight loss. A phase Ib study involving individuals with obesity explored the pairing of cagrilintide 2.4 mg with semaglutide 2.4 mg, administered once a week (referred to as CagriSema). Remarkably, this combination yielded a weight loss of 17.1% over 20 weeks, surpassing the 9.8% weight loss observed with a placebo plus semaglutide 2.4 mg, all while maintaining tolerability.[9]

Dual Agonism with Glucagon

Glucagon, emanating from pancreatic α-cells, is released in response to diminished blood glucose levels. While it contributes to heightened blood glucose through hepatic glucose production, it also exerts influence over diverse metabolic pathways. These include a reduction in food intake, an elevation in energy expenditure, and the promotion of hepatic fatty acid oxidation. The potential synergy of glucagon with GLP-1 actions presents an opportunity to enhance weight loss while safeguarding against the diabetogenic risks that glucagon agonism might entail. Encouraging initial outcomes from animal studies spurred the development of several GLP-1/glucagon coagonists. In the context of early-phase clinical trials involving humans, these coagonists have exhibited varying levels of effectiveness in inducing weight loss.[9]

Notably, efinopegdutide (JJ-64565111; HM12525A) yielded promising results. In a phase II trial encompassing individuals with obesity and T2DM, efinopegdutide led to dose-dependent, placebo-adjusted weight loss of up to 7.2% over a 12-week treatment period. However, it is important to note that there was no improvement observed in HbA1c levels. For individuals with obesity (without diabetes), the highest dosage of efinopegdutide led to a placebo-adjusted weight loss of 10% after a 26-week duration. These findings underscore the potential of GLP-1/glucagon coagonists in tackling weight-related challenges.[9]

Triple Agonism (GLP-1/GIP/Glucagon)

Given the notable effectiveness and advantages observed with the dual GLP-1/GIP receptor agonist tirzepatide, as well as the dual GLP-1/glucagon receptor agonists, the pursuit of a triple agonist capable of targeting all three receptors (GLP-1/GIP/glucagon) holds the potential for even greater weight loss and enhanced glycemic control when compared to dual agonists.[9]

LY3437943 (retatrutide), an innovative triple agonist, has displayed superior weight loss outcomes in comparison to tirzepatide during preclinical investigations. Furthermore, it exhibited improvements in glucose profiles. In a phase Ib trial involving individuals with T2DM, subcutaneous administration of retatrutide once weekly for 12 weeks resulted in a placebo-adjusted reduction in HbA1c of up to 1.6%. Remarkably, the highest dosage group experienced a dose-dependent placebo-adjusted weight loss of up to 8.96 kg. The safety profile of LY3437943 was found to be comparable to that of other incretin medications. With a recently completed phase II trial (NCT04881760), a phase III program is poised to commence later in 2023. This progression signifies a promising step forward in harnessing the potential of a triple agonist to address weight loss and glucose control challenges.[9]

GIP Antagonists in Combination with GLP-1R Agonists

Interestingly, the impact on weight loss is not limited to GIP receptor agonism; intriguingly, GIP receptor antagonism has emerged as a potential avenue for obesity treatment. Preclinical investigations have indicated that blocking this receptor can lead to improvements in the metabolic profile and a reduction in food intake. The underlying molecular mechanisms that elucidate the similar effects of GIP receptor agonists and antagonists are currently subjects of research.[9]

This effect becomes even more potent when combining a GIP receptor antagonist with a GLP-1R agonists. Consequently, the development of AMG-133, an injectable formulation intended for monthly subcutaneous administration, was initiated. A phase I study of AMG-133 revealed a noteworthy mean weight loss ranging from 7.2 to 14.5% after a 12-week period for individuals with obesity (without diabetes). Although the main side effects observed were nausea and vomiting, these effects diminished within 48 hours. Presently, a phase II trial is in progress (NCT05669599), marking a significant stride toward exploring the potential of this combined treatment approach.[9]

Emerging Therapies

Fibroblast Growth Factor 21

Fibroblast growth factor 21 (FGF21) is a hormone which is present in circulation, is triggered by fasting, and plays a significant role in the metabolic response during periods of fasting. Numerous investigations involving FGF21 and its analogs have showcased robust control over glucose levels and substantial reductions in body weight in preclinical studies.[10]

In clinical trials, the administration of the FGF21 analog LY2405319 to individuals with obesity and T2DM resulted in a decrease in body weight; however, there was no notable alteration in glycemia over a 28-day period. Another FGF21 analog, pegbelfermin, which boasts long-acting properties, was administered once daily at doses of 10 or 20 mg for 16 weeks to overweight or obese individuals with nonalcoholic steatohepatitis (NASH). Remarkably, this treatment led to a reduction in hepatic steatosis without causing changes in body weight or bone mineral density. The development of a unimolecular, long-acting GLP-1/FGF21 coagonist yielded even more promising outcomes. This coagonist demonstrated a greater reduction in both glycemia and body weight compared to individual agonists, all while circumventing the occurrence of fasting-associated hypoglycemia.[10]

Ghrelin Antagonism

Ghrelin stands as the solitary recognized orexigenic peptide hormone, exerting its influence by triggering neuropeptide Y neurons and suppressing hypothalamic proopiomelanocortin (POMC) neurons to induce feelings of hunger. Given its role in appetite stimulation, targeting the ghrelin receptor emerges as an appealing strategy in the pursuit of obesity treatment. Significant potential lies in ghrelin receptor antagonists and vaccines, both of which have displayed promise in preclinical investigations. These interventions have demonstrated the ability to curtail food intake and reduce body weight, underlining their viability as potential therapeutic approaches for combating obesity.[10]

Growth Differentiation Factor 15

Elevated levels of GDF15 in the bloodstream have been proven to lead to a reduction in food consumption and a decrease in body weight. This effect is achieved by activating the hindbrain receptor known as glial-derived neurotrophic factor receptor α-like, as demonstrated in both rodent and nonhuman primate studies.[10]

New Therapeutic Targets in Diabetes

Given the intricate nature of T2DM, there is a notable surge in interest to formulate novel pharmaceutical therapies for diabetes management. The United States Food and Drug Administration (FDA) has granted approval to a diverse array of drug treatments that tackle various biological systems and mechanisms associated with the disease. In this rapidly evolving field of pharmacology, numerous compounds with antihyperglycemic properties have emerged through natural discovery or synthesis, and many of these are presently undergoing clinical evaluations. Moreover, a multitude of agents are in varying stages of clinical development, targeting both established pathways and innovative mechanisms for potential antidiabetic drugs (as depicted in **Fig. 2**).[11]

CHAPTER 10: Future Directions and Research

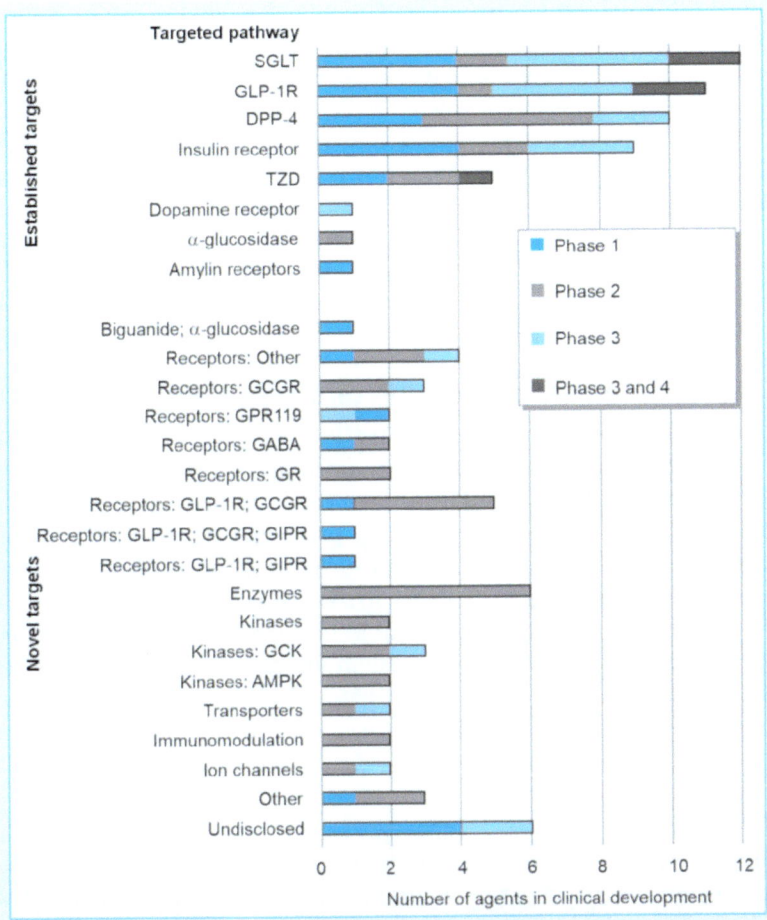

FIG. 2: The molecular targets of the 99 antidiabetic agents in clinical trials. The phase status is the highest clinical phase each agent has achieved. A surprising number clinical agents—nearly half—target novel molecular targets or combination regimens. Novel targets or pathways are those that have not yet been validated through approval of an FDA-approved drug for treatment of diabetes. Approximately half of the agents target already established pathways, i.e., molecular targets that have been validated through the FDA-approval of an agent targeting that pathway for the treatment of diabetes. Six of the agents had an undisclosed mechanism of action.

(AMPK: 5' AMP-activated protein kinase; DPP-4: dipeptidyl peptidase-4; FDA: Food and Drug Administration; GCGR: glucagon receptor; GCK: glucokinase; GIPR: gastric inhibitory polypeptide receptor; GLP-1R: glucagon-like peptide-1 receptor; GPR119: glucose-dependent insulinotropic receptor; GR: glucocorticoid receptor; SGLT-2: sodium-glucose cotransporter-2; TZD: thiazolidinediones)

Established Target

Sodium-glucose Cotransporter and Dual SGLT-1 and SGLT-2 Inhibitors

Sodium-glucose cotransporters (SGLTs) play a pivotal role in regulating the transport of sodium and glucose across cell membranes. Among humans, six SGLT isoforms have been identified, with pharmacotherapy in T2DM primarily focusing on inhibiting SGLT-1 and SGLT-2. Recent pharmacological investigations have indicated that simultaneous inhibition of both SGLT-1 and SGLT-2 yields notable reductions in postprandial glucose levels, while also increasing endogenous GLP-1 levels and promoting urinary glucose excretion. A pioneering dual inhibitor of SGLT-1 and SGLT-2, known as sotagliflozin, has been developed. Notably, it exhibits a 20-fold higher selectivity for SGLT-2 over SGLT-1, demonstrating efficacy comparable to dapagliflozin and canagliflozin in SGLT-2 inhibition, while surpassing them by over 10-fold in SGLT-1 inhibition potency. Clinical trials conducted in phases II and III have highlighted sotagliflozin's ability to enhance glycemic control, diminish postprandial glucose spikes, reduce insulin requirements, curb appetite, and facilitate weight loss in both T1DM and T2DM patients.[12]

Peroxisome Proliferator-activated Receptor α/γ/δ Pan-agonists

Peroxisome proliferator-activated receptors (PPARs), ligand-activated transcription factors among nuclear hormone receptors, encompass PPAR-α (expressed in liver, muscle, and heart), PPAR-γ (found in adipose tissue and vascular endothelial cells), and PPAR-δ (with widespread whole-body presence). These subtypes intricately regulate energy metabolism, where PPAR-δ governs energy expenditure and PPAR-γ oversees energy storage. A novel PPAR-α/γ/δ pan-agonist, chiglitazar, has undergone phase III multicenter, randomized, double-blind, and placebo-controlled trials. Over 24 weeks, both chiglitazar doses demonstrated superior HbA1c reduction compared to placebo, and these effects were sustained for 52 weeks. Specifically, the mean change in HbA1c from baseline was −0.45% ± 1.22% for placebo, −1.30% ± 1.07% for chiglitazar 32 mg, and −1.52% ± 1.19% for chiglitazar 48 mg.[12]

Glimins

Imeglimin, a novel oral antidiabetic drug (OAD) of the "glimins" class, has undergone extensive investigation in landmark clinical trials, showcasing a unique mechanism that enhances glucose-dependent insulin secretion and reduces insulin resistance through mitochondrial oxidative phosphorylation inhibition. This multifaceted approach addresses various metabolic disruptions in T2DM, promoting insulin signaling, β-cell sensitivity, curbing gluconeogenesis, preserving β-cell viability, and potentially offering cardioprotective benefits. Imeglimin's sustained hyperglycemia improvement without severe hypoglycemia or significant side effects, combined with its ability to lower HbA1c and fasting plasma glucose levels in combination therapies, underscores its promising role in the future of T2DM treatment. Its favorable safety profile positions it as a valuable addition to the pharmacotherapeutic arsenal for managing T2DM and potentially offering cardioprotection.[12]

Novel Targets

Over 40% of the agents currently under investigation in clinical trials are directed toward novel therapeutic molecules or combinations of targets (**Fig. 2**). The primary focus lies on receptors and enzymes, constituting the largest categories of novel targets. This is followed by transporters and ion channels, further exemplifying the diverse avenues of exploration in therapeutic research.[11]

Receptors

The pivotal role of glucose protein-coupled receptor 119 (GPR119) in glucose homeostasis is underscored by its expression in pancreatic β-cells and enteroendocrine cells. Prior investigations have revealed that GPR119 agonism elicits insulin and incretin secretion, mirroring the mechanisms of incretin effects in glucose metabolism. The second-generation GPR119 agonist, DA-1241, is presently undergoing phase I trials, with hopes of providing diabetic patients substantial glucose-lowering benefits coupled with improved safety profiles.

Gastric inhibitory polypeptide, an incretin hormone akin to GLP-1, stimulates insulin secretion from pancreatic β-cells in response to glucose levels. Tirzepatide, a dual agonist, is currently advancing through clinical trials (phase III), engaging both the GLP-1 and gastric inhibitory polypeptide receptor. A study involving gastric inhibitory polypeptide receptor has demonstrated reductions in body weight and HbA1c.[11]

While thyroid hormone receptors (THRs) have traditionally been targeted for treating metabolic disorders, recent insights suggest their potential in diabetes management. THR agonism studies conducted in mice have yielded increased energy expenditure, enhanced insulin sensitivity, and lowered glucose concentrations. Notably, a THR agonist named TRC150094, functioning as a functional analog of iodothyronines, is actively progressing through phase III clinical trials. These trials seek to assess its safety in reducing cardiovascular risk among patients with diabetes.[11]

Enzymes in General[11]

- *DGAT inhibitors*: Diacylglycerol acyltransferase (DGAT) is crucial for triacylglycerol synthesis. DGAT-deficient mice resist obesity due to increased energy expenditure and improved insulin sensitivity. Selective DGAT inhibitors like IONIS-DGAT2Rx have completed phase II trials, offering potential for obesity and T2DM management.
- *Kallikrein-kinin system (KKS)*: The KKS shows promise in diabetes treatment. Bradykinin (BK) stimulates glucose uptake and insulin sensitivity via BK2R signaling. Human tissue *kallikrein 1* gene treatment in diabetic mice has positive effects. DM199, a recombinant human tissue kallikrein 1 protein, is under phase II trials for diabetes treatment.
- *FBP1 inhibition*: Fructose-1,6-bisphosphatase 1 (FBP1) plays a role in gluconeogenesis and glucose homeostasis. VK 0612, an investigational agent directly inhibiting FBP1, has completed successful phase II trials.
- *MetAP2 inhibitors*: Methionine aminopeptidase 2 (MetAP2) inhibitors offer potential for obesity and diabetes treatment. Inhibition of MetAP2 results in reduced blood glucose and increased weight loss. ZGN-1061, a MetAP2 inhibitor, shows promise in preclinical and phase II trials.
- *ANGPTL3 inhibition*: Angiopoietin-related protein 3 (ANGPTL3) impacts glucose metabolism by inhibiting lipoprotein lipase. Inhibition of ANGPTL3 holds promise as a strategy and potential drug target for T2DM and metabolic disorders. ISIS-703802, an ANGPTL3 inhibitor, has recently completed phase II trials for hypertriglyceridemia, T2DM, and nonalcoholic fatty liver disease.

- *Glucokinase* (GK/GCK) is a key enzyme in maintaining glucose homeostasis by initiating gluconeogenesis. Activating GK through small molecule therapeutics could enhance insulin secretion, liver glycogen synthesis, and reduce hepatic glucose output. Early GK activators showed promise but led to negative effects. Renewed interest in next-generation glucokinase activators (GKAs) like dorzagliatin and TTP399 has emerged, with dorzagliatin in phase III trials.
- 5' AMP-activated protein kinase (AMPK) regulates energy levels and glucose metabolism. Lifestyle factors and certain antihyperglycemic drugs indirectly activate AMPK. Direct AMPK activators like PXL770 and PBI-4050 have completed phase II trials.
- Fructokinase (FK) activation depletes phosphates, leading to inflammation and insulin resistance. Inhibiting FK, as seen with PF-06835919 and tolimidone (MLR-1023) in phase II trials, offers a promising approach to hyperglycemia treatment.
- Tolimidone stimulates Lyn protein tyrosine kinase, vital for insulin sensitivity. It lowers blood glucose similarly to metformin without hypoglycemia and enhances insulin sensitivity.

Transporters

MSDC-0602K, a promising compound, functions as a modulator of mitochondrial membrane transport proteins, enhancing insulin sensitivity. The link between impaired mitochondrial function and diabetes development is well-established. Representing the second generation of insulin sensitizers, MSDC-0602K is anticipated to offer improved safety compared to its predecessors. Phase III clinical trials for MSDC-0602K are scheduled to commence in 2022.[11]

PERSONALIZED MEDICINE AND PRECISION HEALTH

Personalized Medicine

Personalized medicine in diabetes (PMID) encompasses four key domains: (1) identifying individual risk factors, (2) optimizing resource allocation, (3) tailoring specific therapies, and (4) monitoring treatment efficacy through circulating biomarkers. Genetic variations like single nucleotide polymorphisms (SNPs) in genes such as *ABCC8*, *SLC22A1*, *SLC22A2*, and *PPARG* play a role in modulating responses to OADs. Beyond addressing clinical and laboratory aspects, personalized diabetes care extends to considering the psychological and social well-being of individuals with diabetes. Furthermore, the integration of digital health initiatives and computational platforms with omics data, including genomics, proteomics, metabolomics, and transcriptomics, has revolutionized the landscape of PMID management.[13]

Genetic mutations and polymorphisms introduce a remarkable degree of diversity into the characteristics of diseases and the response to treatments, both in type 1 diabetes mellitus (T1DM) and T2DM. Candidate gene analysis and genome-wide scanning have unearthed molecular markers that illuminate the susceptibility, progression, and potential therapeutic outcomes in diabetes. T1DM is marked by an autoimmune-driven loss of β-cells within the pancreas. Individuals bearing glutamic acid decarboxylase or islet autoantibodies, as well as those with a familial history of T1DM, face an elevated risk of developing the condition. Notably, >40 genetic loci associated with autoimmunity and β-cell viability have been identified in T1DM. These encompass the HLA class II genes, encoding polymorphic antigen-presenting proteins, which confer nearly 50% of the genetic susceptibility to T1DM. Additional genes, including INS, PTPN22, ERBB3, CCR5, IL7R, IL2RA, and PRKCQ, also play roles in this intricate landscape. Distinct human leukocyte antigens (HLA) class II alleles and haplotypes correspond to various disease progressions, outlining acute-onset, fulminant, and slowly progressive variants of the disorder. Furthermore, genetic variations elucidate the varying demands for immunosuppression strategies in T1DM.[13]

In T2DM, the intricacies of insulin secretion and responsiveness are shaped by genetic determinants. Approximately 23 genes associated with T2DM harbor variants that could potentially influence diagnostic approaches, therapeutic interventions, prognosis, and treatment choices. Genes implicated in reduced β-cell mass (*HHEX, CDKN2A/CDKN2B*), β-cell dysfunction (*KCNJ11, TCF7L2*), insulin resistance (*PPARG, ADAMTS9*), and altered BMI (*FTO*) have been pinpointed. Notably, polymorphisms within the transcription factor 7-like 2 (*TCF7L2*) gene are correlated with an escalated susceptibility to T2DM. This intricate genetic landscape offers a deeper understanding of the complex interplay between genetics and diabetes pathophysiology, paving the way for more targeted and precise therapeutic approaches.[13]

The landscape of personalized medicine in T2DM has experienced a gradual shift from solely characterizing subgroups based on molecular architecture to encompassing differential treatment responses. Incorporating straightforward clinical information like age, gender, BMI, and glomerular filtration rate has enabled the calculation of the likelihood of glycemic response to antidiabetic medications. This approach can be further enriched by incorporating additional biomarkers such as C-peptide or omics data like pharmacogenomics, facilitating predictions about specific classes of OADs or their safety profiles. Gender and BMI, for instance, have been instrumental in stratifying responses to thiazolidinediones (in obese females) and sulfonylureas (in slim males). Recent breakthroughs have defined novel subgroups of T2DM using data-driven cluster analysis involving six variables for newly diagnosed diabetes individuals. These clusters, termed severe autoimmune diabetes (SAID), severe insulin-deficient diabetes (SIDD), severe insulin-resistant diabetes (SIRD), mild obesity-related diabetes (MOD), and mild age-related diabetes (MARD), exhibit distinct characteristics and risks of diabetic complications.[13]

Neonatal diabetes mellitus (NDM) is a rare form of diabetes diagnosed within the first 6 months of life, characterized by insulin-sensitive hyperglycemia. It encompasses transient neonatal diabetes mellitus (TNDM), which remits before 1 year but may relapse later, and permanent neonatal diabetes mellitus (PNDM). Around 10% of NDM cases are associated with syndromes and pancreatic aplasia. Genetic factors play a significant role, with mutations identified in genes such as *KCNJ11, ABCC8, IDDM2, PTF1A*, and *FOXP3*, influencing aspects like insulin production, β-cell function, and immune response control. The Madras Diabetes Research Foundation (MDRF) highlights common mutations in the SUR (*ABCC8*) and *KCNJ11* genes, showing excellent glucose control with high-dose sulfonylureas without added hypoglycemic risks. Patients with TNDM and a 6q24 methylation defect respond to low-dose sulfonylureas. Genetic screening in India revealed improved glucose and HbA1c levels when switching from insulin to oral sulfonylurea in cases carrying KCNJ11 and ABCC8 mutations.[13]

Maturity-onset diabetes of the young (MODY) constitutes 5% of diabetes cases, typically manifesting before age of 25 years with autosomal dominant inheritance. MODY is often manageable without insulin initially, but insulin therapy becomes necessary after about 5 years. Characterized by impaired insulin secretion due to an autoimmune response to β cells, MODY is primarily monogenic. Key *MODY* genes include GCK, hepatic nuclear factor 1α (HNF1α), and hepatic nuclear factor 4α (HNF4α). GCK-MODY maintains high fasting glucose levels, while HNF1α, HNF4α, and HNF1β demonstrate progressive glucose deterioration but respond to low-dose sulfonylurea. HNF1β-MODY involves β-cell development defects and necessitates insulin treatment. GCK-MODY accounts for 5% of gestational diabetes cases and holds clinical significance in management. The MDRF and Christian Medical College in India have contributed substantially to MODY research, uncovering various MODY subtypes and novel genetic mutations including NKX6-1. Genomic analysis highlights common MODY genes, while next-generation sequencing (NGS) offers effective mutation screening. Collaborative efforts reveal insights into MODY's genetic basis and its implications for pregnancy-related diabetes.[13]

The effectiveness of diabetes treatment is influenced by patients' genetic makeup. Pharmacogenetic studies seek to identify biomarkers that predict treatment response. Genetic variations, particularly SNPs, contribute to differences in drug metabolism and action among diverse patient groups. Genes coding for drug targets, transporters, and metabolizing enzymes for oral hypoglycemic agents can affect therapy outcomes. A comprehensive understanding of these genetic factors and their influence on drug metabolism enables personalized treatment approaches for optimized effectiveness and safety **(Table 3)**.[13]

Precision Health

Precision diabetes diagnostics encompasses both phenotypic and genetic classification of the disease. Deutsch et al. present two complementary strategies: a phenotypic approach utilizing clinical variables like autoantibodies, BMI, and HbA1c, and a genetics-based approach considering single-gene mutations, genetic variants, and polygenic scores. These methods reveal clusters of individuals with distinct clinical phenotypes, facilitating a more accurate classification of disease development, progression, and treatment. Building upon this, Herder and Roden explore how stratified subgroups are linked to diverse trajectories in disease progression and the onset of diabetes-related complications. They further delve into tailoring prevention and treatment approaches for precision diabetology.[14] Additionally, Bonnefond and Semple provide an illustration of applying precision care to monogenic insulin-deficient and insulin-resistant diabetes, showcasing how this approach can be applied to disorders with a simpler genetic basis and potentially serving as a proof of concept.[15]

TABLE 3: Newer anti-obesity medicines.

Antiobesity medication	Drug class	Trial status	% of weight loss	Population achieving >10%	Population achieving ≥15%
Cagrisema	Amylin analog GLP-1RA(I)	Phase II in T2DM with BMI ≥27 kg/m²	15.6	• Cagrisema: 71% • Cagrilintide: 14% • Semaglutide: 23%	• Cagrisema: 54% • Cagrilintide: 7% • Semaglutide: 0%
Survodutide	GCGE and GLP-1R agonist	Phase II in people with BMI ≥27 kg/m²	19	Not available	Not available
Orforglipron	Nonpeptide GLP-1RA	Phase II in people with BMI ≥30 kg/m² or ≥27 kg/m² with one weight-related condition	14	• Orforglipron: 75% • Placebo: 9%	• Orforglipron: 43% • Placebo: 1%
Ecnoglutide	GLP-1RA	Phase II in people with BMI ≥30 kg/m² or ≤40 kg/m²	14.7	Not available	Not available
Retatrutide	GIP/GLP-1/GCG	Phase II in people with BMI ≥30 kg/m² or ≥27 kg/m² with one weight-related condition	24.2	• Retatrutide: 93% • Placebo: 9%	• Retatrutide: 83% • Placebo: 2%
Tirzepatide	GIP and GLP-1RA	Phase III in people with BMI ≥27 kg/m² with HbA1c 7–10%	22.5	• Tirzepatide: 65% • Placebo: 9%	• Tirzepatide: 48% • Placebo: 8.8%
Oral semaglutide	GLP-1RA	Phase III in people with BMI ≥30 kg/m² or at least 27 kg/m² with one weight-related complications	17.8	• Oral semaglutide: 75% • Placebo: 12%	• Oral semaglutide: 58% • Placebo: 5%

(BMI: body mass index; GLP-1: glucagon-like peptide-1; GLP-1R: glucagon-like peptide-1 receptor; GLP-1RA: glucagon-like peptide-1 receptor agonist; HbA1c: glycated hemoglobin)

Precision medicine extends its potential to precision prevention as well. Wareham highlights the need to tailor the generalized advice currently offered to individuals at high risk of developing T2DM, suggesting various ways to personalize T2DM prevention strategies.[16] Recognizing the diverse responses individuals have to prevention measures, Sørensen et al. delve into the role of gene-environment interactions in T2DM prevention, shedding light on how these interactions inform precision prevention approaches.[17] While some level of personalization already exists in prevention efforts, finding a balanced approach that effectively addresses T2DM as a widespread public health concern poses a challenge. Gestational diabetes, a prevalent endocrinopathy during pregnancy, amplifies the risk of complications for both mother and offspring.[18] Sparks and Ghildayal et al. analyze commonly utilized preventive measures and underscore the factors that facilitate the precise tailoring of lifestyle interventions to avert gestational diabetes.[19]

Precision medicine, which heavily relies on advanced diagnostic techniques, holds significant promise for delivering direct clinical advantages to patients while simultaneously optimizing resource utilization for society by avoiding inefficient treatment approaches. The case of monogenic diabetes, as exemplified by HNF1A-MODY, as explored by Bonner and Saponaro, highlights the potential for tailoring therapies to individuals with distinct mutations in the *HNF1A* gene.[20] However, the application of pharmacological precision medicine to T2DM remains largely unfulfilled, as meticulously detailed by Florez and Pearson. This challenge is rooted in the intricate and heterogeneous nature of T2DM, where current treatment decisions often prioritize factors such as comorbidities, cost, or side effects, rather than addressing the unique underlying pathophysiology in each patient—a fundamental tenet of precision diabetes medicine.[21] Similarly, Jordi Merino delves into the realm of precision nutrition within the context of diabetes, shedding light on how genetic variations, gut microbiome diversity, and other clinical and lifestyle variables can distinctly influence an individual's response to specific dietary interventions.[22] Further expanding the horizon, Charlotte Ling introduces us to the emerging field of pharmacoepigenetics in T2DM, where the perturbation of epigenetic enzymes in tissues of individuals with this condition offers intriguing prospects for potential epigenetic therapies to be harnessed for diabetes treatment.[23]

Precision medicine holds the potential to revolutionize the clinical management of T1DM as well. While considerable strides have been made in enhancing the categorization of various manifestations of T2DM, the accuracy of diagnosis remains a challenge for T1DM. Surprisingly, up to one in three adults initially receive a misdiagnosis of T2DM when they actually have T1DM. Carr et al. underscore the advancements achieved in refining devices, insulin formulations, and delivery systems to optimize the clinical care of T1DM.[24] Yet, they emphasize that a more comprehensive exploration of the intricate pathogenesis of T1DM is warranted. Such an in-depth comprehension could potentially pave the way for groundbreaking advancements in disease-modifying treatments and strategic interventions, ultimately aiming at preventing or even reversing the pathogenic processes underlying T1DM.

PUBLIC HEALTH STRATEGIES AND POLICY RECOMMENDATIONS

Public Health Policy and Environmental Changes

Promoting environmental changes stands as a paramount approach in tackling the obesity burden, with far-reaching impact. Several key public policy measures can drive these transformative shifts:[1,25]

- Implementation of stringent food labeling regulations by the FDA, mandating comprehensive calorie and nutrition information on all food products
- Official prohibition of trans fats in foods sold across restaurants and grocery stores, as enforced by the FDA
- Channeling obesity prevention efforts toward children, especially within schools, fostering healthy habits. Local governments should restrict commercial permits for fast-food establishments within 0.5 miles of schools, while encouraging the establishment of health-conscious food vendors
- Elevation of physical education standards within schools, while promoting active commuting such as walking or biking
- Implementation of impactful taxation on unhealthy foods coupled with subsidies for healthier options, despite ethical considerations. Various jurisdictions have introduced taxes on sugar-sweetened beverages, exemplifying this strategy.
- Focused public health policies that prioritize creating activity-supportive communities including the development of dedicated bike lanes and pedestrian pathways
- Provision of meals adhering to national nutritional standards, aligning with guidelines such as the US dietary guidelines
- Establishment of minimum and maximum calorie thresholds for school breakfast and lunch, tailored to specific age groups
- Elimination or controlled access to sugar-sweetened beverages within school premises
- Ensuring easy availability of drinking water for students in dining areas and throughout the school day
- Mandatory daily physical education for students from grades K-12
- Prescription of a total of 150 minutes of weekly physical education in elementary school and 225 minutes in middle and high schools
- Collaboration with local communities to optimize the utilization of school and community spaces for physical activities during and beyond school hours

Family-based Interventions

Utilizing a family-based approach stands out as the most effective strategy for achieving lasting weight loss and maintaining a healthy weight in individuals with overweight or obesity. The presence of family support becomes crucial for overweight individuals aiming to make lifestyle changes. Various studies have demonstrated the efficacy of a low-fat diet rich in protein and low in glycemic index for ensuring sustained weight maintenance and preventing weight regain.[1]

A practical and user-friendly tool within the realm of family-based dietary interventions is the "traffic light diet," a classification system categorizing foods as green, red, or yellow. In matters of food selection, the traffic light system employs three designations: GREEN signifies "GO," YELLOW signifies "SLOW," and RED signifies "WHOA." The categorization of foods into these three groups may exhibit minor variations across the programs that developed or adopted this concept. GREEN, denoted as GO foods, is recommended as the primary choice when making dietary decisions. These foods contain fewer than 2 g of fat and boast rich nutrient content and/or fiber. The majority of fruits and vegetables fall under the GREEN category, along with whole wheat bread, oatmeal, fat-free or 1% low-fat milk, grilled fish and shellfish, as well as skinless chicken or turkey. YELLOW, categorized as SLOW foods, should be the secondary option when determining what to eat. These foods contain between 2 and 5 g of fat. Examples include 2% milk, 100% fruit juice, sports drinks, white grains, such as bread, rice, and pasta, granola, ham, and peanut butter. RED, representing WHOA foods, should be consumed sparingly. These items offer minimal nutritional value while being high in fat, sugar, and calories. WHOA foods contain 5 or more grams of fat. Common examples encompass whole milk, standard hot dogs, french fries, butter, chocolates, cream cheese, sugary cereals, muffins, and soft drinks.[26]

Weight Bias in Healthcare

The weight bias in the healthcare system can be explicit (consciously expressed) or implicit (involuntarily expressed). Implicit weight bias is not rare to see among HCPs. Society's negative biases toward overweight or obesity often are shared and exhibited by the HCP. The weight bias by the healthcare team can impair the patient's healthcare quality. Most HCPs believe in the energy balance theory of weight control, which encourages the thinking of obesity issues being a personal responsibility and limiting the scope of appropriate counseling. The following interventions could help in reducing the weight bias in health practice.[1]

- To educate the healthcare professionals about the complex etiology of obesity including genetic, metabolic, and social factors.
- To make providers aware of the fact that the weight bias could influence the quality of the care.
- To train the medical trainees how to communicate without implicit bias.
- Another strategy is to expose counter-stereotypical exemplars of people with obesity who are successful and intelligent.
- HCPs should address the overall health and the patient's understanding of obesity-associated comorbidities along with weight loss management.
- HCPs should be encouraged to use people-first language, e.g., patients with obesity instead of obese patients. Also, using terminology like high BMI instead of morbid obesity will help in motivating the patient.

Current Policy, Financial, and Programmatic Gaps to Prevent, Screen, and Manage Maternal Obesity

In the context of India, the *Poshan Abhiyaan* (2018–2022), a government initiative, emphasizes intersectoral collaboration, behavior change communication, and counseling to provide health and nutrition services for children, pregnant, and postpartum women. However, maternal obesity reduction is not a primary focus in national policy targets. A proposed nutrition service package aims to integrate nutrition into routine antenatal care services. This package includes five key actions: (1) nutritional assessment, (2) classification of nutritional risk, (3) supplementation, (4) referral/management, and (5) counseling. Recommendations for managing maternal obesity entail personalized counseling on its implications during pregnancy, dietary and exercise guidelines, regular home visits to monitor compliance with care services, and information about healthy meal planning. The service package was piloted in eight states/union territories (Bihar, Delhi, Haryana, Jharkhand, Karnataka, Madhya Pradesh, Telangana, and Uttar Pradesh), and maternal nutrition guidelines were implemented in four states (Bihar, Delhi, Jharkhand, and Madhya Pradesh). Challenges faced include the absence of gestational weight gain charts and optimal weight gain recommendations, limited integration of nutrition norms in the service delivery system, lack of budget allocation for implementation, inadequate private sector engagement, missed targets for maternal obesity in the Poshan Abhiyaan, and the absence of tracking and review indicators in the government's health information management system.[27]

REFERENCES

1. Tiwari A, Balasundaram P. Public Health Considerations Regarding Obesity. In: StatPearls [Internet]. Treasure Island (FL): StatPearls Publishing; 2023.
2. Worldobesity. (2023). Economic impact of overweight and obesity to surpass $4 trillion by 2035. [online] Available from https://www.worldobesityday.org/assets/downloads/World_Obesity_Atlas_2023_Press_Release.pdf [Last accessed October, 2023].
3. World Obesity Federation. (2023). World Obesity Atlas 2023. [online] Available from https://www.worldobesityday.org/assets/downloads/World_Obesity_Atlas_2023_Report.pdf [Last accessed October, 2023].
4. Jackson Leach R, Powis J, Baur LA, et al. Clinical care for obesity: A preliminary survey of sixty-eight countries. Clin Obes. 2020;10(2):e12357.
5. GBD 2021 Diabetes Collaborators. Global, regional, and national burden of diabetes from 1990 to 2021, with projections of prevalence to 2050: a systematic analysis for the Global Burden of Disease Study 2021. Lancet. 2023;402(10397):203-34.
6. Venkatachalapathy P, Padhilahouse S, Sellappan M, Subramanian T, Kurian SJ, Miraj SS, et al. Pharmacogenomics and Personalized Medicine in Type 2 Diabetes Mellitus: Potential Implications for Clinical Practice. Pharmgenomics Pers Med. 2021;14:1441-55.
7. Finer N. Future directions in obesity pharmacotherapy. Eur J Intern Med. 2021;93:13-20.
8. Müller TD, Blüher M, Tschöp MH, DiMarchi RD. Anti-obesity drug discovery: advances and challenges. Nat Rev Drug Discov. 2022;21(3):201-23.
9. Melson E, Miras AD, Papamargaritis D. Future therapies for obesity. Clin Med (Lond). 2023;23(4):337-46.
10. Abdel-Malek M, Yang L, Miras AD. Pharmacotherapy for chronic obesity management: a look into the future. Intern Emerg Med. 2023;18(4):1019-30.
11. Dahlén AD, Dashi G, Maslov I, Attwood MM, Jonsson J, Trukhan V, et al. Trends in Antidiabetic Drug Discovery: FDA Approved Drugs, New Drugs in Clinical Trials and Global Sales. Front Pharmacol. 2022;12:807548.
12. Shah N, Abdalla MA, Deshmukh H, Sathyapalan T. Therapeutics for type-2 diabetes mellitus: a glance at the recent inclusions and novel agents under development for use in clinical practice. Ther Adv Endocrinol Metab. 2021;12:20420188211042145.
13. Mohan V, Das AK, Mukherjee JJ, Seshadri K, Jha S, Kalra S. From Individualized to Personalized Medicine in Diabetes: An Expert Overview. J Assoc Physicians India. 2019;67(9):78-82.

14. Deutsch AJ, Ahlqvist E, Udler MS. Phenotypic and genetic classification of diabetes. Diabetologia. 2022;65(11):1758-69.
15. Herder C, Roden M. A novel diabetes typology: towards precision diabetology from pathogenesis to treatment. Diabetologia. 2022;65(11):1770-81.
16. Bonnefond A, Semple RK. Achievements, prospects and challenges in precision care for monogenic insulin-deficient and insulin-resistant diabetes. Diabetologia. 2022;65(11):1782-95.
17. Wareham NJ. Personalised prevention of type 2 diabetes. Diabetologia. 2022;65(11):1796-803.
18. Sørensen TIA, Metz S, Kilpeläinen TO. Do gene-environment interactions have implications for the precision prevention of type 2 diabetes? Diabetologia. 2022;65(11):1804-13.
19. Sparks JR, Ghildayal N, Hivert MF, Redman LM. Lifestyle interventions in pregnancy targeting GDM prevention: looking ahead to precision medicine. Diabetologia. 2022;65(11):1814-24.
20. Bonner C, Saponaro C. Where to for precision treatment of HNF1A-MODY? Diabetologia. 2022;65(11):1825-9.
21. Florez JC, Pearson ER. A roadmap to achieve pharmacological precision medicine in diabetes. Diabetologia. 2022;65(11):1830-8.
22. Merino J. Precision nutrition in diabetes: when population-based dietary advice gets personal. Diabetologia. 2022;65(11):1839-48.
23. Ling C. Pharmacoepigenetics in type 2 diabetes: is it clinically relevant? Diabetologia. 2022;65(11):1849-53.
24. Schaefer-Graf U, Napoli A, Nolan CJ; Diabetic Pregnancy Study Group. Diabetes in pregnancy: a new decade of challenges ahead. Diabetologia. 2018;61(5):1012-21.
25. HARVARD T. H. CHAN, School of Public Relation. School Obesity Prevention Recommendations: Complete List. [online] Available from https://www.hsph.harvard.edu/obesity-prevention-source/obesity-prevention/schools/school-obesity-prevention-recommendations-read-and-print/ [Last accessed October, 2023].
26. Brown RD. The traffic light diet can lower risk for obesity and diabetes. NASN Sch Nurse. 2011;26(3):152-4.
27. Chopra M, Kaur N, Singh KD, Maria Jacob C, Divakar H, Babu GR, et al. Population estimates, consequences, and risk factors of obesity among pregnant and postpartum women in India: Results from a national survey and policy recommendations. Int J Gynaecol Obstet. 2020;151 Suppl 1(Suppl 1):57-67.

CHAPTER 11

Conclusion

SUMMARY AND IMPLICATIONS FOR CLINICAL PRACTICE

Summary

Over 90% of individuals with diabetes are affected by overweight or obesity, exacerbating insulin resistance, while weight reduction helps mitigate the progression of diabetes-related complications. Given the heightened risk of complications in obese diabetic patients, healthcare providers must possess a comprehensive understanding of addressing obesity within diabetic populations. This involves delivering counseling, behavioral interventions, referrals to weight loss programs, and judicious medication management.[1]

Unquestionably, the epidemiological data presented in Chapter 1 highlights an indisputable trend: a consistent rise in the obesity and type 2 diabetes mellitus (T2DM) population. However, proactive strategies to prevent and combat obesity hold the potential to alleviate the future burden of T2DM. The intricate interplay in the pathogenesis of obesity and T2DM predominantly centers on the amplifying effects of obesity on genetic susceptibility and environmental factors. To elaborate, obesity triggers significant metabolic microenvironmental changes that drastically impair insulin signaling, fostering a gradual elevation in blood glucose levels. This arises from the detrimental overaccumulation of specific nutrients and metabolites, heightened low-grade inflammation, disrupted autophagy processes, and energy imbalances resulting from dysregulation of the microbiome–gut–brain axis. These alterations are chiefly propelled by the extensive ectopic expansion of adipose tissue, which not only instigates systemic immunometabolic reprogramming but also inflicts local toxicity on the pancreas, ultimately depleting functional beta cell numbers. Given these intricate relationships, the available treatments for obesity and T2DM exert mutual influences on each other. Future endeavors must prioritize collaborative multidisciplinary work to meticulously track prevalence, unravel the underlying biological mechanisms, enhance diagnostic precision, and optimize treatment efficacy. This entails exploring advanced therapeutic modalities while ensuring their widespread accessibility, minimizing potential side effects, and complications to markedly benefit patient outcomes.[2]

It is crucial to underscore that prevention remains the most cost-effective and enduring approach to addressing obesity and T2DM. Collective, resolute action is imperative to finally achieve tangible progress in this long-standing challenge that has eluded us for decades.

Implications for Clinical Practice

When addressing the diagnosis of obesity, clinicians must exhibit sensitivity and awareness. Research underscores that individuals with obesity often encounter diminished respect compared to those with normal weight, and such biased interactions detrimentally influence weight-related behaviors like binge-eating, weight trajectory, and overall health outcomes. Employing the 5 As model for behavior change during discussions about weight loss has demonstrated substantial benefits. This model enhances patients' motivation for weight loss and amplifies their success in achieving it. Regardless of whether clinicians directly offer weight loss support or facilitate referrals to weight loss programs, the 5 As framework remains a pivotal tool.[1]

The 5 As model for behavior change and its application in weight management practice is described as follows:[3]

1. *Assess*:
   - Evaluate patients for obesity or overweight in the presence of metabolic risk factors.
   - Determine patients' readiness and capacity for change at the current moment.
2. *Advise*:
   - Counsel patients on the heightened cardiovascular disease risks linked to excess adiposity.
   - Inform patients about the health advantages associated with weight loss and adopting a healthier lifestyle.
3. *Agree*:
   - Collaborate with patients to establish a concrete and attainable weight loss objective that will yield health benefits (e.g., aiming to lose 5% of initial body weight within 6 months).
4. *Assist*:
   - Aid patients in devising a comprehensive weight management strategy, which could involve in-practice weight loss counseling or directing them to a specialized weight loss program.
5. *Arrange*:
   - Organize follow-up sessions to establish a structured framework for accountability and to provide feedback on progress.

The initial treatment goal recommends a weight loss of 5–10% of baseline body weight, which correlates with a reduction of 0.6–1.0% in glycated hemoglobin (HbA1c) levels and various other health enhancements. A sustained 7% weight loss yields broader benefits for individuals with diabetes and overweight/obesity, encompassing improved fitness, reduced waist circumference, lowered blood pressure, enhanced sexual functioning, and alleviated peripheral neuropathy symptoms. While guiding patients toward healthier lifestyles, clinicians play a crucial role in medication management when treating T2DM and obesity.[1]

Clinicians are advised to consider utilizing specific glucose-lowering medications that either maintain weight neutrality or potentially foster weight loss. Notably, metformin, pramlintide, glucagon-like peptide 1 (GLP-1) receptor agonists, dipeptidyl peptidase 4 (DPP-4) inhibitors, and sodium-glucose cotransporter-2 (SGLT-2) inhibitors fall within this category. Metformin, for instance, has demonstrated a correlation with a 3-kg reduction in weight. Pramlintide, apart from a 3.7-kg weight loss, can also decrease daily insulin requirements in patients utilizing insulin therapy. GLP-1 receptor agonists exhibit a 5.3-kg weight loss effect. While DPP-4 inhibitors are generally weight neutral, SGLT-2 inhibitors offer a potential weight loss of 2.4 kg and a decrease in insulin requirements.[1]

Simultaneously, clinicians should steer clear of diabetes medications that tend to induce weight gain (such as sulfonylureas, thiazolidinediones, and insulin). Additionally, a thorough assessment of other medications linked to weight gain is recommended. Whenever feasible, clinicians should endeavor to reduce or identify alternatives for common medications known to increase appetite and contribute to weight gain. These include sedating antihistamines, steroids, certain selective serotonin reuptake inhibitors, beta blockers, and a majority of antipsychotic agents.[1]

The Pharmacist's Role

Pharmacists play a pivotal role in enhancing treatment strategies for individuals managing diabetes alongside concurrent obesity. A comprehensive assessment of the patient's medication regimen, spanning both antidiabetic and nonantidiabetic medications, is imperative to identify potential contributors to weight gain (e.g., antipsychotics, insulin, corticosteroids). Given that the impact of most antidiabetic medications on weight loss hinges on dosage, meticulous attention must be paid to proper titration to optimize treatment benefits. A focused counseling session should be conducted to ensure patients are well-informed about potential adverse effects associated with these medications.[4]

It is noteworthy that gastrointestinal discomfort is a frequent occurrence; patients should be educated on strategies to alleviate such events (e.g., taking metformin with meals) to enhance treatment tolerability. Vigilant monitoring and consistent follow-up are paramount to fine-tune treatments, and any indications of adverse effects should be promptly reported. Pharmacists should underscore that medications exhibit their utmost efficacy when used alongside dietary adjustments and lifestyle modifications. Therefore, educational initiatives centered on fostering healthy eating habits and designing physical activity plans are integral to achieving optimal patient outcomes. Should medication interventions and lifestyle changes prove insufficient to support the patient's weight loss objectives, pharmacists should consider the prospect of referring the patient for metabolic surgery, provided the requisite criteria are met.[4]

CHALLENGES AND OPPORTUNITIES FOR THE FUTURE

Challenges in Management of Obesity with Diabetes

Physicians often lack comprehensive education on obesity and its management during their training, resulting in inadequate knowledge in this area. Personal biases, whether explicit or implicit, have been identified among physicians, potentially influencing the care they provide. Additionally, physicians frequently express challenges related to their busy schedules, which can impede the amount of time they allocate for addressing obesity-related concerns. It is common to find primary and secondary care facilities lacking essential resources such as dietitians, educators, and psychologists who possess expertise in obesity management.[5]

Many patients are unaware that obesity is a chronic condition requiring lifelong intervention and tend to associate its treatment solely with weight loss. However, given the common occurrence of weight regain, strategies to prevent such regain are crucial. Long-term commitment to dietary and physical activity changes may be difficult for some obese individuals to realize or accept, possibly due to a reluctance to implement substantial lifestyle alterations. This may lead to poor compliance with prescribed pharmacological interventions.[5]

Patients from low socioeconomic backgrounds encounter various barriers, including higher costs of healthier foods, easier access to inexpensive yet less nutritious options, and limited opportunities for physical activity. Access to healthcare advice and the cost of medication can also serve as significant obstacles. There can also be a cultural acceptability of obesity within certain socioeconomic groups, possibly due to associations between weight loss and illnesses like tuberculosis that are prevalent in these communities. Furthermore, time constraints can hinder the adoption of healthier habits, such as planning and cooking nutritious meals instead of resorting to calorie-dense fast food options. Social and professional obligations, such as the consumption of alcohol alongside unhealthy foods, can also pose challenges to maintaining a healthier lifestyle. Effective support from family and friends is essential for sustaining weight loss efforts, particularly considering that many individuals seeking obesity treatment may also grapple with mental health issues such as depression, anxiety disorders, and eating disorders.[5]

Disrupted or inadequate sleep patterns, often associated with conditions like obstructive sleep apnea, can contribute to obesity by hampering physical activity and compliance with weight loss strategies. Obesity-related health issues, including osteoarthritis and cardiovascular conditions, may also limit a person's ability and motivation to engage in physical activity and adopt healthier lifestyles. Insulin resistance conditions like T2DM and polycystic ovary syndrome can complicate weight loss efforts due to their influence on metabolism and appetite regulation. Lastly, awareness and access to surgical treatments for obesity remain limited, and concerns about potential complications, cost, and the nature of pharmacological therapy may deter patients from seeking treatment options.[5]

In Youth-onset Type 2 Diabetes Mellitus

Youth-onset T2DM has a more extreme metabolic phenotype than adult onset T2DM, with greater insulin resistance and more rapid deterioration of beta cell function; intermediate complications often develop in late childhood or early adulthood, and end-stage complications, including kidney failure, develop in midlife. Owing to limited efficacy and safety data, several drugs that are available for the treatment of adults with T2DM have not been approved for the treatment of youth, which reduces the options that are available to normalize glycemia in these patients. Managing youth-onset T2DM and mitigating the risk of microvascular and macrovascular complications require the development of more effective interventions as well as strategies to overcome barriers to adherence that are not typically encountered in adult patients.[6]

Opportunities for the Future

The coming decade holds the promise of a significantly expanded arsenal of therapies for T2DM. Nearly 300 companies are actively engaged in developing drugs dedicated to T2DM, with ongoing efforts in the development of oral GLP-1 agonists. An example of this progress is semaglutide, initially administered as a weekly injection, showing remarkable potential in its once-daily oral formulation for effective glucose reduction and weight loss. This oral variant is currently advancing through its development stages.[7]

Innovations on the horizon include the potential introduction of oral insulin, contingent upon the resolution of challenges posed by stomach digestive juices. Another breakthrough, "smart insulin" or glucose-responsive insulin, holds the capability to activate when blood sugar reduction is needed and deactivate when safe levels are achieved. Furthermore, a novel injectable nano-network, comprising nanoparticles housing a solid insulin core, modified dextran, and glucose oxidase enzymes, has shown promise.[8]

Despite novel treatment methods such as islet cell transplantation, gene therapy, and stem cell therapy primarily targeting type 1 diabetics, there exists potential for their application in T2DM as well. Notably, the artificial pancreas or bionic pancreas system, which employs continuous glucose monitoring and algorithm-driven subcutaneous insulin and glucagon delivery, originally designed for type 1 diabetics, may find utility in select T2DM cases.[9]

A groundbreaking medication, utilizing engineered polymeric nanoparticles for controlled delivery of a Notch signaling inhibitor directly to white fat cells, is under development. In a mouse model, this nanoparticle, composed of a polymer known as PLGA and containing the drug dibenzazepine, disrupted Notch signaling, leading to the creation of brown fat cells.[10]

Recent research has unveiled the intricate connection between the gut microbiome and the development of T2DM and obesity. Numerous mechanisms link microbiota to insulin resistance and diabetes onset, encompassing alterations in bowel permeability, endotoxemia, bile acid interactions, changes in brown adipose tissue proportion, and effects related to drug usage like metformin.

Presently, the utilization of pro- and prebiotics, alongside novel techniques like gut or fecal microbiota transplantation, demonstrates potential as valuable tools in modulating obesity and insulin resistance through dietary intervention.[11]

Anticipated advancements also extend to medications targeting another defect in diabetes pathophysiology: the heightened rate of glucose absorption from the digestive system.[12]

The ideal antidiabetic medication should possess a range of features such as long-term effectiveness in lowering high blood sugar without hypoglycemic risk; the ability to mitigate the natural progression of the disease; the capacity to slow and halt disease advancement; suitability for use in renal and hepatic impairment, at any stage of the disease, and in combination with other comorbidities; durability; simplicity of administration; contribution to weight reduction; improvement of lipid disorders, hypertension, and cardiovascular outcomes; exceptional safety profile without adverse effects; and affordability and tolerability.

REFERENCES

1. Bramante CT, Lee CJ, Gudzune KA. Treatment of Obesity in Patients with Diabetes. Diabetes Spectr. 2017;30(4):237-43.
2. Ruze R, Liu T, Zou X, Song J, Chen Y, Xu R, et al. Obesity and type 2 diabetes mellitus: connections in epidemiology, pathogenesis, and treatments. Front Endocrinol (Lausanne). 2023;14:1161521.
3. Gudzune K. Dietary and Behavioral Approaches in the Management of Obesity. Gastroenterol Clin North Am. 2016;45(4):653-61.
4. Barlow B, Barlow A. Management of Obesity in Patients with Diabetes. US Pharm. 2021;46(11):31-42.
5. S VM, Nitin K, Sambit D, Nishant R, Sanjay K; (on behalf of Endocrine Society of India). ESI Clinical Practice Guidelines for the Evaluation and Management of Obesity In India. Indian J Endocrinol Metab. 2022;26(4):295-318.
6. Bjornstad P, Chao LC, Cree-Green M, Dart AB, King M, Looker HC, et al. Youth-onset type 2 diabetes mellitus: an urgent challenge. Nat Rev Nephrol. 2023;19(3):168-84.
7. Davies M, Pieber TR, Hartoft-Nielsen ML, Hansen OKH, Jabbour S, Rosenstock J. Effect of Oral Semaglutide Compared with Placebo and Subcutaneous Semaglutide on Glycemic Control in Patients with Type 2 Diabetes: A Randomized Clinical Trial. JAMA. 2017;318(15):1460-70.
8. Gu Z, Aimetti AA, Wang Q, Dang TT, Zhang Y, Veiseh O, et al. Injectable nano-network for glucose-mediated insulin delivery. ACS Nano. 2013;7(5):4194-201.
9. Ang KH, Tamborlane WV, Weinzimer SA. Combining glucose monitoring and insulin delivery into a single device: current progress and ongoing challenges of the artificial pancreas. Expert Opin Drug Deliv. 2015;12(10):1579-82.
10. Jiang C, Cano-Vega MA, Yue F, Kuang L, Narayanan N, Uzunalli G, et al. Dibenzazepine-Loaded Nanoparticles Induce Local Browning of White Adipose Tissue to Counteract Obesity [published correction appears in Mol Ther. 2022;30(1):502]. Mol Ther. 2017;25(7):1718-29.
11. Muñoz-Garach A, Diaz-Perdigones C, Tinahones FJ. Gut microbiota and type 2 diabetes mellitus [published correction appears in Endocrinol Diabetes Nutr. 2017;64(9):514]. Erratum to: Microbiota y diabetes mellitus tipo 2 [published correction appears in Endocrinol Diabetes Nutr. 2017;64(9):514]. Endocrinol Nutr. 2016;63(10):560-8.
12. Chen L, Tuo B, Dong H. Regulation of Intestinal Glucose Absorption by Ion Channels and Transporters. Nutrients. 2016;8(1):43.

Index

Page numbers followed by *b* refer to box, *f* refer to figure, *fc* refer to flowchart, and *t* refer to table.

A

Abetalipoproteinemia 183
Absolute skeletal muscle mass 230
Acarbose 151
Acetonic breath 80
Acetyl coenzyme A 27
Activator protein 1 31
Acute angle-closure glaucoma 160
Acyl-CoA A dehydrogenase 103
Adenocarcinoma, esophageal 201
Adenosine
 diphosphate 143
 monophosphate 25, 141, 143
 triphosphate 79, 123, 143, 146, 152, 250
Adipocytes 25*f*
Adipocytokines 46, 47
Adipokine 193, 194, 202
Adiponectin 47
Adipose tissue 27*f*, 28, 32*f*, 34*f*, 35*b*, 37*fc*, 39*fc*, 46, 256
 hormones 46
 macrophage 27, 33
 role of 29
Adiposity 26, 121
 abdominal 57
 high 61
Advanced glycation end products, formation of 175
Air displacement plethysmography 90
Airway
 obstruction 197
 pressure, positive 168, 199
Alanine
 aminotransferase 183
 transaminase 190
Albright hereditary osteodystrophy 63, 66
Albuminuria 186
Alcohol 105, 122
 consumption, excessive 183
Aldehyde dehydrogenase-2 172
Aldolase-B 123
Alleviated peripheral neuropathy symptoms 269

Alogliptin 150
Alpha-1 antitrypsin deficiency 183
Alpha-cells 39*fc*, 44, 45
Alpha-glucosidase inhibitors 141, 151
Alpha-melanocyte stimulating hormone 43, 67
Alstrom syndrome 65
American Academy of Sleep Medicine 197, 199
American Cancer Society 202
American College of Sports Medicine 226
American Diabetes Association 122, 145, 184, 186, 210, 217*fc*
Amino acids 37*fc*
Amitriptyline 168
Ammonia 41*f*
AMP-activated protein kinase 38, 250
Amphetamine-regulated transcript neurons 67
Amphetamines 159
Amylin 163, 252
 analogs 247
 mimetic drugs 141
Anabolic hormones, secretion of 12
Anamorelin 231*f*
Angiopathies 80
Angiopoietin-related protein 3 257
Angiotensin-converting enzyme 224
 inhibitors 168, 183, 187
Angiotensin-receptor blockers 168, 183, 187
Ankle reflexes, examination of 175
Anorectic peptides 47
Anorexigenic functions 46
Anterior tibial electromyogram 199
Anthocyanins 102
Anthropometry 88
Antidepressants 160, 161, 165, 178
 medications 165
Antidiabetic 165
 agents 151
 oral 140
 drugs 249
 general mechanism of action of 143*f*
 medications 151, 165, 272
Antiepileptic 165
 medications 165

Antihistamines 165
  medications 165
Antihypertensives 165
  medications 165
Anti-obesity drugs 158f, 211, 261
  development of 164
  newer 261t
  pate-phase 246
  use of 227
Antioxidants 133
  role of 131
Antipsychotics 165, 269
  medications 165
Antiretroviral 165
  medications 165
Anxiety 111
Apnea reduction, stimulation therapy for 201
Apoptosis 37f
Apoptotic pathways 193
Appetite 76
  stimulation 254
  suppresses 211
Arcuate nucleus 43, 126
Arterial hyalinization 182f
Artery disease, coronary 171, 243
Ascorbate 102
Aspartate aminotransferase 183
Atherosclerosis
  development of 14
  progression of 171
Automated insulin delivery systems 215
Autophagy 36

B

Back pain 76, 160
Bacterial translocation triggers 40
Bardet–Biedl syndrome 63, 65
Bariatric surgery 153, 212, 227, 228, 235, 246
Basal metabolic rate 49
Behavioral modification 108, 224
Behavioral risk factor surveillance system 222
Behavioral therapy 238
Berlin questionnaire 198
Beta-blockers 183
Beta-cell 24f, 39fc
  accelerated loss of 39fc
  dysfunction 13, 37fc, 40
  function 147
  mass, reduced 259
Biguanides 140, 141
Bile acid 41, 141
Bilevel positive airway pressure 199
Biliopancreatic diversion 209
Bioelectric impedance analysis 90, 230

Biopsy-proven nonalcoholic steatohepatitis 191
Blood
  glucose 107
    control of 105
    fasting 16, 107, 220
    homeostasis, regulating 148
    monitoring 210t, 217
    self-monitoring of 210, 220, 221
  lipid profiles 118
  pressure 123, 168, 190
    control 187
    diastolic 102, 186, 190
    systolic 102, 171, 186
    target 185
Bloodstream 28
Blount's disease 209
Body
  energy status 125
  fat 75
  mass index 1, 6, 7f, 22, 54, 70, 85f, 87, 89, 94,
    169, 186, 208, 209, 221, 224, 230, 235, 261
    elevated 139
  weight 121, 254
Bone
  marrow lesions 194
  morphogenetic protein 182
Botulinum toxin type A 179
Brachial artery flow-mediated dilation 103
Brain-derived neurotropic factor 65, 67
Brainstem 125
  regulating appetite 42
Branched-chain amino acid 38, 125, 126f
Breast cancer 202
  postmenopausal 201
Breath, shortness of 79
Bupropion 156, 157, 160, 161, 238

C

Cagrilintide 252
Cagrisema 261
Calcium 134, 232
  channel
    alpha-2-delta ligands 168
    blockers 183
Caloric restriction 99, 231
Canadian Diabetes Association 122
Canadian Pain Society 176
Canagliflozin 151, 152
Cancer 169
  cells 202
  colorectal 201
  endometrial 201
  prostate 92, 201
  renal 201
  types of 88, 201

Candida albicans 80
Cannabinoids 179
Carbohydrates 105, 120, 121, 155, 238
   diet, moderately low 118
   simple 123
Carbon oxide 41*f*
Carbonic anhydrase 159
Carboxypeptidase 64
Cardiometabolic health 125
Cardiomyopathy 171
   diabetic 171
Cardiovascular complications 98
Cardiovascular disease 54, 75, 98, 123, 133, 147, 170, 171, 183
   atherosclerotic 142
Cardiovascular health 139
Cardiovascular mortality, higher risk of 180
Carnitine palmitoyltransferase 1 124
Catalase 103
Catechin 103
Catecholamines 79
Catechol-O-methyltransferase 103
Celastrol 247
Cellular stress 27*f*, 37*fc*
Cellulitis 76
Central nervous system 62, 147
Chemocytokines 31*fc*
Chemokine ligand 182
Cholecystokinin 41, 43, 66, 126
Cholesterol 76, 210
   oxidation products 194
   total 102, 103, 194
Chromium 134
Chronic exercise enhances insulin sensitivity 106
Chronic kidney disease 147, 186
   causes of 180
   epidemiology collaboration equation 184
Cocaine 67
Cognitive behavioral therapy 109, 200
Cohen syndrome 63, 66
Complex syndrome 175
Computerized tomography 91
Constipation 159, 160, 162
Continuous positive airway pressure 199
Corticosteroids 269
Cortisol 79
   hyperproduction of 50
Cough 160
C-reactive protein 103, 129
   high-sensitivity 189
Cross-sectional electronic health survey 18
Curb appetite 256
Cushing's syndrome 49
Cyclic adenosine monophosphate 25
Cyclooxygenase 103, 176
Cytokine 29
   production 193

D

Dapagliflozin 152
De novo lipogenesis 36, 123
Dehydration 80
Dementia 169
Dendritic cells 41*f*
Densitometry 90
Deoxyribonucleic acid 153
Depression 111
   treatment of 160
Depressive disorders 111
D-glyceraldehyde 123
Diabetes 1, 2, 7, 10, 83, 99, 115, 117, 156, 206, 222, 244, 254
   adolescent 212, 213
   burden of 10, 11
   complications 169, 267
   control and complications trial 83
   diagnosis of 83*b*
   distress 111
   endocrine cause of 49
   family history of 16
   global trend of 3
   higher prevalence of 8
   incidence of 15
   management 108, 118, 130, 140, 168, 227
   mellitus 38, 75, 79*f*, 82*fc*, 154*fc*, 171, 209, 250, 259
   gestational 83, 206, 216, 219, 219*f*, 221
   impact of 139
   management of 108
   nature of 140
   non-insulin-dependent 78
   pathogenesis of 32
   prognosis of 153
   risk factor 10, 11*t*, 97
   treatment 131, 141, 149
   type 1 3, 109, 130, 180, 210, 212, 258
   type 2 3, 6, 9*f*, 10*t*, 17*t*, 18, 22, 23, 24*f*, 32, 34*f*, 38, 39*fc*, 41*f*, 44, 45*f*, 54, 86, 98, 100, 106, 104*f*, 105*t*, 108, 115, 116, 118*f*, 119*f*, 121*t*, 123, 139, 140, 142*t*, 169, 183, 198*f*, 207, 209, 217, 243, 248, 267, 271
   mild obesity-related 259
   pathophysiology 22
   pediatric 212, 213
   pharmacotherapy for 138
   prevalence of 6, 169

Prevention Program 98, 99, 110, 225
psychological support of 109
regional prevalence of 3
self-management education 216
severe insulin-deficient 259
significant impact of 213
signs of 75
symptoms of 75
treatment of 255f
type of 214
Diacylglycerol 31, 125
 acyltransferase 257
Diarrhea 159, 162
Dietary
 antioxidants 133
 cholesterol 122
 eating patterns 121
 fats 123
 fiber 122
 management 238
 modification 188
 reference intake 208
 sodium 185
  restriction 187
Digital tools 108
Dihydroxyacetone phosphate 123, 124
Dilution method 91
Dipeptidyl peptidase 142, 143, 149, 150, 154, 224, 255
 inhibitors 141, 145, 150, 151, 246, 250, 269
Disability-adjusted life years 245
Distal foot 175
Distress, psychological 109
Dizziness 159, 160
Docosahexaenoic acid 118
Dopamine 159
Dorsal motor nucleus 43
Dorsal vagal complex 42, 43
Dorsomedial hypothalamus 43
Down syndrome 66
Drosophila homolog-1, single-minded 64
Dry mouth 159, 160
Dry skin 76
Dual-energy X-ray absorptiometry 91
Duodenal switch 209
Dysfunctional mitochondria 176f
Dyslipidemia 13, 88, 139, 156, 169, 172, 180, 193, 194, 194f, 209
Dysmotility 80

E

Ecnoglutide 261
Ectopic bone formation 194
Edema 147

Edmonton obesity staging system 85, 86t
Efinopegdutide 252
Eicosapentaenoic acid 118
Electrocardiogram 199
Empagliflozin 152
Endocrine disorders 48
Endocrinotropic drugs, weight impact of 165
Endoplasmic reticulum 31, 38, 39, 172
 stress 26, 32f
Endoscopic interventions 224, 227
Endothelial nitric oxide synthase 103
Energy
 balance 42, 43f, 121
 consumption 2
Enteroendocrine cells 41f, 42
Enzymes 257
 activity of 79
Epworth Sleepiness Scale 198
Estimated glomerular filtration rate 142, 187
European Association for Study of Diabetes 145, 186
European Association for Study of Obesity 229
European Medicines Agency 157t, 158f, 177
European Society for Clinical Nutrition and Metabolism 229
European Society of Cardiology 145
Exercise 100, 107
Extracellular matrix 24, 32
Extracellular signal-regulated kinase 25, 176
Extrapancreatic organs 28

F

Family behavior therapy 111
Fasting blood glucose 16, 107, 220
 impaired 81-83
Fasting glycemia, impaired 10
Fasting plasma glucose 81, 83, 104f, 214, 217, 250
Fat 105, 120, 123, 155
 foods 2
 mass 230
Fatigue 79, 160
 general 214
Fatty acid 38
 excessive influx of 27f
 homeostasis, dysregulation of 32f
 metabolism 27f
 oxidation 46
 transport proteins 26
Fatty liver disease 40
 metabolic dysfunction with 168, 188, 189
 nonalcoholic 38, 169, 188, 209, 257
Federal Trade Commission 74
Federation of Neurological Societies 176

Fibers 105
  function 175
  role of 131
Fibroblast growth factor 125, 126, 182, 253
Fluid intake 76
Follicle-stimulating hormone 49
Food and Drug Administration 255
Fragile X syndrome 63, 65
Free fatty acids 30f, 32, 38, 123, 172, 193
Fructokinase activation depletes phosphates 258
Fructosamine 130
Fructose 79, 122
  1,6-bisphosphatase 1 257
  6-phosphate 25
  metabolism 123
Fruity odor 80

G

Gamma-aminobutyric acid 41
Gamma-glutamyl transferase 190
Gastric inhibitory
  peptide 150
  polypeptide 257
    receptor 255
Gastroesophageal reflux disease 92, 209
Gastrointestinal disorders 162
Gastrointestinal tract 43
Genetic variants 69
  carrier 11
Genome-wide association studies 71f
Gestational diabetes mellitus 83, 206, 219, 219f, 221
  diagnosis of 84b
  prevalence of 216
  weight management of 216
Ghrelin 164
  antagonism 254
  neutralizing molecules 164
  O-acyltransferase, inhibitors of 164
  pathway 247
  producing cells 47
  receptor 67
    emerges 254
Gila monster lizard, venom of 149
Gladribin analogs 246
Glibenclamide 141
Gliclazide 141
Glimepiride 141, 146
Glimins 256
Glitazones 146
Global nutrient database 119
Glomerular filtration rate 186, 196
Glomerular thylakoid cell hypertrophy 182f

Glomerulopathy, diabetic 182f
Glomerulus, pathology of 182f
Glucagon 37fc, 45, 79, 163, 252
  inhibition 150
  receptor 255
  secretion 46
Glucagon-like peptide 41, 43, 44, 66, 126, 141, 143, 149, 150, 154, 158, 165, 217, 248, 261
  actions of 45f
  agonists 145, 148
  receptor 248, 255, 261
    agonist 143, 168, 173, 183, 224, 261, 269
Glucagonoma 50
Glucocorticoid receptor 255
Glucokinase 255, 258
Glucolipotoxicity 39fc
Gluconeogenesis 37f, 153
Glucose 23
  6-phosphate 25, 27
  dependent insulinotropic polypeptide 41, 43, 44, 45f, 126, 174, 246, 248, 255
  homeostasis 161
  intolerance 22
  levels 148, 210
  load test 84
  lowering effects 148
  metabolism disorders 81
  monitoring, continuous 210
  protein-coupled receptor, pivotal role of 257
  reabsorption 182f
  responsive insulin 271
  stimulated insulin secretion 38
  storage of 28
  translocation of 26
  transporter 25, 27, 30, 103, 104, 147, 149, 150, 152
Glutamate receptors 159
Glutathione peroxidase 103
Glycated hemoglobin 82, 102, 110, 130, 145, 154, 186, 210, 217, 250, 261
Glycemic control 99, 111
Glycemic index 121, 127
Glycemic load 121, 127
  concept of 127
Glycogen 28
  synthesis 26, 27f
Glycosuria 76, 78
Gonadotropins 49
Gonads 49
Granulocyte-macrophage colony-stimulating factor 34
Growth
  differentiation factor 248, 254
  factor receptor-bound protein 25
  hormone 12, 49, 79

Gut microbiota 48
Gut peptide
  hormone co-agonists 163
  role of 47

H

Headache 151, 160
Healthcare
  professionals 264
  systems 92
  weight bias in 264
Heart disease
  coronary 207
  diabetic 171, 172*f*
  ischemic 78, 172
  valvular 160
Heart failure 141, 152, 171
  congestive 92, 142
Hemochromatosis 183
Hemoglobin 107
  glycated 82, 102, 110, 130, 145, 154, 184, 186, 210, 217, 250, 261
Hepatic autophagy 37*f*
Hepatic fatty acid oxidation 252
Hepatic glucose production 23
Hepatic glycogenolysis 153
Hepatic insulin signaling 25
Hepatic nuclear factor 4 alpha 260
Hepatitis
  B 183
  C 183
Hepatotoxicity 159
Hexosamine pathway 176*f*
High-density lipoprotein 13, 148, 210
  cholesterol 76, 102, 103, 194
High-fat feeding 40
High-fructose corn syrup 123
High-glycemic index 116
Homeostatic model assessment 129
Homolog 32, 71
Hormonal imbalances 35, 44
Hormone 66
  counterregulatory 45
  incretin 44
  production 40
  sensitive lipase 25
Host's glucose metabolism 40
Human glucagon-like peptide 1 161
Hunger, feeling of 254
Hydrogen sulfide 41*f*
Hydrometry 91
Hydroxy fatty acid, branched fatty acid esters of 31

Hydroxytryptamine 41
Hydroxytyrosol 103
Hypercortisolism 48
Hyperglycemia 27*f*, 31*fc*, 37*fc*, 44, 50, 75, 79, 83, 176*f*, 182*f*, 218, 219
  activates numerous metabolic pathways 176*f*
  chronic 44
  development of 41*f*
  management of 187
  persistent 78
  postprandial 148, 221
  symptoms of 214
Hyperinsulinemia 27*f*, 37*fc*, 132, 202, 243
Hyperlipidemia 11, 243
Hyperosmotic hyperglycemic nonketotic state 217
Hypertension 11, 15, 54, 76, 117, 139, 156, 169, 170, 172, 180, 188, 209, 243
  family history of 16
  gestational 218
  glomerular 180
Hypertriglyceridemia 257
Hypoglycemia
  fasting-associated 254
  post-bariatric 151
  risk of 147, 151
Hypogonadism 49
Hypokalemia 153
Hyposalivation 80
Hypotension 80
Hypothalamic arcuate nucleus 127
Hypothalamic-pituitary
  gonadal axis 49
  thyroid 48
Hypothalamus 43, 67*f*, 159
  nuclei in 42
  ventromedial 42, 43
Hypothyroidism 48
Hypoxia 26
  inducible factor-1 alpha 32
  intermittent 198*f*

I

Immune
  cells, role of 35*b*
  system 32
Immunity
  adaptive 32, 34*f*, 35*b*
  innate 32, 34*f*, 35*b*
Immunoglobulin G 34, 35
Impaired glomerular filtration rate 180
Impaired glucose tolerance 10, 49, 82, 83, 139, 221

Inducible nitric oxide synthase 176
Infections 80
Inflammation 30, 202
  chronic low-grade 32
  synovial 193
Inflammatory cells, renal infiltration of 182*f*
Inflammatory cytokines 106
Inflammatory pathways 180, 197
Injury, vascular 180
Insulin 46, 66, 269
  action 25*f*
  activates 25
  administration of 24*f*
  analogues 153
  deficiency, combination of 79
  effects of 23
  facilitates 153
  hyposecretion 80
  impact 43
  like growth factor 1 38, 49, 126, 202
  preparations, types of 155*t*
  producing cells 38
  pump settings, modifying 215
  receptor 67
    isoform 25
    substrate 23, 27
  resistance 23, 26, 29, 35*b*, 38, 98, 123, 125,
      175, 194, 202, 243, 250
    development of 32, 33
    score, homeostasis model assessment of
      190
  secretagogues 146
  secretion 46, 141, 150
  sensitive hyperglycemia 259
  sensitivity 123, 147, 210
    vital for 258
  sensitizing drugs 106, 236
  signaling 23
  smart 271
  stimulates adipogenesis 26
  therapy 140, 153
Intensive glycemic control 187
Intercellular adhesion molecule 1 103, 182
Interferon regulatory factor 3 31
Interleukin 32, 34, 102, 172, 176
International Agency for Research into Cancer
    201
International Association for Study of Pain 175
International Association of Diabetes and
    Pregnancy Study Groups 219
International Diabetes Federation 4*f*, 169, 245
International Obesity Task Force 207
Intestinal glucose absorption 151
Intestinal microbiota 135

Intra-articular corticosteroid 196
Intra-articular hyaluronate 196
Intracellular metabolism 182*f*
Intracranial hypertension, idiopathic 209
Iodine 134
Iron 134
Irritability 159
Ischemic heart disease 78, 172
  development of 76
Islet autoimmunity, development of 213
Isoleucine 128

J

Joint damage, structural 193

K

Kallikrein
  elevate plasma levels of 180
  gene treatment 257
  kinin system 257
Kallmann syndrome 66
Ketoacidosis, diabetic 142, 217
Ketohexokinase 123, 124
Ketone bodies 80
Kidney 170
  disease
    chronic 147, 186
    diabetic 152, 180
    improving global outcomes 186
    risk of end-stage 184
  failure 133
Kussmaul respiration 80

L

Lactate dehydrogenase 143
Lactic acidosis 151
Laparoscopic adjustable gastric band 209
Learning disabilities 135
Leptin 46, 64
  pathway 67*f*
  receptor 64, 67
  sensitizers 248
Leucine 125
Leukemia 202
Ligand-activated transcription factors 256
Linagliptin 150, 151
Linolenic acid 118
Lipase inhibitor 236
Lipids 121
  homeostasis 42
  levels, reduced 105

management 186, 188
metabolism 23, 43, 123
Lipodystrophy 26, 153, 165, 183
Lipogenesis 37f, 153
  activates 25
  hepatic 27f
Lipolysis 153, 198f
Lipolytic regulatory proteins 26
Lipopolysaccharide 41
Lipoprotein
  low-density 13, 122, 148
  very low-density 36, 123
Liraglutide 156, 157, 161, 168, 238, 239
Liver
  biopsy 183
  disease 147
    fatty 40
    steatotic 191
  enzymes aspartate aminotransferase 190
  steatosis 183
Long-chain
  fatty acid 125f
  specific acyl-CoA dehydrogenase 124
Lorcaserin 156, 157, 159, 160
Low glycemic index diets 102
Low-density lipoprotein 13, 122, 148
  cholesterol 102, 103, 186, 194, 210
Low-gastrointestinal diet 118, 130
Luteinizing hormone 49

M

Macronutrient balance and caloric intake 119
Macronutrient distribution 105, 121
  range 121
Macrophage 41f
  colony-stimulating factor 182
  inflammatory protein-1 182
  migration inhibitory factor 182
Magnesium 134
Magnetic resonance imaging 91
Major integrated health system 92
Malignancy 201
Malignant melanoma 202
Mandibular repositioning devices 200
Manganese 134
Mass lesions 183
Matrix metalloproteinase 194
  production 194
Maturity-onset diabetes of young 260
Maxillomandibular advancement 201
Medical nutrition therapy 225
Mediterranean diet 102, 118
Medium-chain fatty acid 124

Medullary thyroid carcinoma 217
Meglitinides 145, 148
  advantages of 148
  disadvantages of 148
Melanocortin
  pathway 67f
  receptor 64
Membrane cofactor protein-1 172
Menopause 4, 236, 237
  transition 237
Messenger ribonucleic acid 147
Metabolic 180
  abnormalities 44
  adaptation 139
  cardiomyopathy 172
  complications
    prevention of 101
    treatment of 101
  disease 198f
  disorders 23, 98, 182f, 257
  disturbances 12
  dysfunction 168, 188, 189
    management of 191
  dysregulation 27f, 35
  energy, storage of 35
  health 128, 131
  osteoarthritis, pathophysiology of 193
  syndrome 98, 101fc, 102t, 165, 218, 243
    risk of 218
    treatment of 102t
  treatment 104
Metformin 141, 143f, 144, 151, 153, 236, 249, 269
Metoprolol 162
Microbiome-gut-brain axis dysfunction 40
Micronutrient 105, 133
  deficiencies 134f
  role of 131
  supplements 122
Microvascular complications 170, 184
Miglitol 151
Minerals 133
Mitochondria fatty acid oxidation 229fc
Mitochondrial dysfunction 27f, 32f, 194
Mitochondrial electron transport chain 124
Mitochondrial oxidative stress 194
Mitogen-activated protein kinase 25, 103
Molecular patterns, damage-associated 180
Molecule, breakdown of 155
Monocyte
  chemoattractant protein-1 103
  chemotactic protein-1 30f, 32
Monounsaturated fatty acid 31, 122
Motivational enhancement therapy 200

Multicomponent training exercise program 226
Multiple endocrine neoplasia 217
Multiple myeloma 202
Muscle
  activity 197
  tissue 106
Myeloma 202
Myocardial dysfunction 172*f*
Myostatin inhibitors 231*f*

N

Naltrexone 156, 157, 160, 238
Nasopharyngitis 160
National Academy of Sciences Institute of Medicine 74
National Glycohemoglobin Standardization Program 83
National Health and Nutrition Examination Survey 14, 229
National Health Service 7*f*, 109, 110
National Institute for Health and Care Excellence 109, 176, 186
  guidelines 237
National Institutes of Health 74
Natural killer cells 27, 32
Nausea 159, 160, 162
Nephrolithiasis 159
Nephrology referral criteria 186
Nephropathy 174, 177
  diabetic 133, 175, 177, 180
  management 184
Nephrotoxicity 159
Nerve damage 133
Nervous system 170
Neuralgia, trigeminal 179
Neuroendocrine tumors 50
Neuroleptic malignant syndrome 160
Neuronal dysfunction 176*f*
Neuronal pathways 62
Neurons 44, 127
  expressing melanocortin 4 receptor 127
Neuropathic pain 175, 179
  pharmacotherapy for 178
Neuropathy 80, 174
  diabetic 175, 176*f*
  peripheral 133
  treatment of 187
Neuropeptide Y 43, 67
  receptor type 2 248
Neurotensin 47
Neurotrophic tyrosine kinase receptor type 2 64

Nicotinamide adenine dinucleotide 143
  phosphate 133, 182
Nitric oxide 41*f*, 103
Nocturia 214
Noncommunicable diseases 16, 243
Non-Hodgkin's lymphoma 202
Nonsteroidal anti-inflammatory drugs 168, 177, 196
Normoglycemia 101
Nuclear factor kappa B 27, 31, 32*f*, 34, 172, 182
Nuclear hormone receptors 256
Nucleus tractus solitaries 43
Nutrient absorption 150
Nutrition 115, 208
  management 215
  parental 183
  therapy 121*t*
  transition 116

O

Obesity 1, 2, 5*f*, 18, 22, 24*f*, 26, 27*f*, 32, 32*f*, 34*f*, 37*fc*, 39*fc*, 40, 41*f*, 47, 54, 60, 65*t*, 68, 69, 78*t*, 87, 87*fc*, 99, 115, 117, 130, 138, 169, 180, 201, 208, 222, 229*fc*, 242, 243, 245
  abdominal 57, 202
  adolescent 206, 208, 209*fc*
  assessment of 83
  cardiomyopathy 172
  central 58
  childhood 72
  classification of 62
  comorbidities 88
  complications 169, 223
  consequences of 23, 223
  development of 37*fc*
  diagnosis of 268
  encompasses, severe 208
  endocrine cause of 48
  epidemic 3*b*, 207
  family history of 16
  genetics of human 54
  global trend of 4
  heritability of 55
  hypogonadism 49
  management of 168, 243, 245, 270
  maternal 264
  molecular pathways linking 29
  monogenic forms of 62, 63
  nonsyndromic 63
  parental 62
  pathophysiology 22
  pediatric 206, 208

pharmacotherapy for 138
polygenic forms of 62, 68
prevalence of 6, 88, 169, 192, 222
prevention 263
regional prevalence of 5
sarcopenic 228, 229, 229fc, 230, 231f
severe 211, 212
signs of 75, 77f
symptoms of 75, 77f
syndromic 63
treatment of 83, 238
triggers inflammation 32f
Obeticholic acid 192
Obstructive sleep apnea 88, 139, 196, 198f, 200fc
 development of 197
 diagnosis of 198
 management of 199
 severe 209
 surgical treatment of 201
Olmesartan 187
Omega-3 fatty acids 122
Opioids 179
 strong 179
Oral antidiabetic drug, novel 256
Oral glucose tolerance test 81-84, 217, 221
Oral hyperglycemic therapy dosage 144t
Orforglipron 261
Orlistat 156, 157, 159, 211, 227, 236, 238
Osteoarthritis 88, 92, 168, 192, 194, 195
 obesity-related 195
 slow-acting drugs of 196
Overnight polysomnography 198
Overnutrition 38
Overweight 202, 268
 classification of 85f
 global trend of 4
 regional prevalence of 5
 treatment of 83
Oxidative stress 26, 133, 172f, 182f, 198f, 202
Oxygen saturation 199
Oxyntomodulin 126, 163, 248

P

Pain, neuropathic 175, 179
Painful diabetic neuropathy 175, 179
Pancreas 66
Pancreatic alpha-cells 44, 252
Pancreatic autophagy 37fc
 dysregulation of 37fc
Pancreatic beta-cell 27f, 106, 146f, 148, 252
 function 106
 mass 27f

Pancreatic islets 39fc
Pancreatitis 151, 159
Paraventricular nucleus 43, 126, 127
Peptide
 hormone 45
 tyrosine tyrosine 126, 163, 248
 YY 66
Perimenopause 237
Peroxisome proliferator-activated receptor 250, 256
 alpha 147
 gamma 103, 147
Pharmacotherapy 211, 227
Phentermine 139, 156, 157, 159, 160, 238
Pheochromocytoma 50
Phosphatidylinositol
 3-kinase 25, 27, 30f, 38, 103
 4,5-bisphosphate 25
Phosphodiesterase 103
Phosphoenolpyruvate carboxykinase 27
Phosphofructokinase 79
Phosphoinositide dependent kinase 1 25
Phosphorus 134
Phosphorylation 27, 31
Phosphotyrosine binding proteins 23
Pickwickian syndrome 76
Placebo plus semaglutide 252
Plasma
 glucose 83, 146f
  fasting 81, 83, 104f, 214, 217, 250
 high-sensitivity C-reactive protein level 190
 insulin, higher 35
 lipid levels 132
 membrane 24
 triglycerides 14, 190
Plasminogen activator inhibitor 1 103, 176
Platelet derived growth factor 182
Podocytosis 182f
Polycystic ovarian syndrome 169, 206, 221, 233-235, 270
 treatment of 234
Polydipsia 78, 214
Polygenic obesity 68
Polyol pathway 175
Polyphagia 76, 79
Polysomnography 198-200
Polyunsaturated fatty acids 31, 103, 122, 191
Polyuria 76, 78, 214
Poshan Abhiyaan 264
Postprandial glucose
 levels 45f
 spikes 256
Potential antidiabetic drugs, mechanisms for 254

Prader–Willi syndrome 63, 65
Pramlintide 269
Prebiotics 191
Prediabetes 7, 16, 83, 83b, 97, 98
　prevalence of 8
Pregnancy 218
Probiotics 191
Pro-inflammatory
　cytokines 29, 32f
　T helper 1 33
Pro-opiomelanocortin 43, 64, 67, 126, 158
　activity of 161
　deficiency 164
Proprotein convertase 67
Protein 105, 120-122, 125, 126f
　diets, moderate-high 102
　kinase 25-27, 27f, 38, 103, 141, 172, 175, 176f
　orexigenic agouti-related 127
　proportion of 238
　synthesis 153, 225
Proteinuria 180, 182f
Proteolysis 153
Proton pump inhibitor 196
Proximal tubule 152f
Pruritus 153
Psychodynamic therapy 111
Public Health Policy and Environmental
　　Changes 263
Public Health Strategies and Policy
　　Recommendations 263
Public Healthcare Systems 243

Q

Quantitative sensory testing 175
Quercetin 103

R

Random plasma glucose 214
Randomized controlled trial 100, 104, 128
Rapamycin 125
　complex, mechanistic target of 24, 38
　mammalian target of 182
Rapid heart rate 80
Reactive oxygen species 27, 38, 124, 125, 172, 182
　generation of 175
Renal disease
　end-stage 188
　moderate-to-severe 151
Renal glomeruli 152f
Renin–angiotensin–aldosterone system 182
　inhibitor 186
Repaglinide 148

Resistin 47
Resmetirom 192
Resveratrol 103
Retatrutide 253, 261
Retina 170
Retinopathy 174
　diabetic 133, 184
Ribosomal S6 kinase 1 126
Rosiglitazone 147
Roux-en-Y gastric bypass 151, 209

S

Sarcopenic obesity 228, 229fc, 230, 231f
　assessment of 230fc
　management of 229, 231f
　screening for 230
Satiety, feeling of 246
Saturated fatty acid 31
Saxagliptin 150
Selective androgen receptor modulators 231f
Selenium 134
Semaglutide 150, 157, 161, 163
　disadvantages of 150
　oral 261
Sensory symptoms 175
Setmelanotide 157
Sex hormones 202
　binding globulin 49
　secretion of 49
Short-chain fatty acid 41, 124
Single nucleotide polymorphism 70, 250, 258
Sitagliptin 150
Skeletal muscle 27f, 153, 229fc
Skinfold thickness 90
Sleep
　apnea 76, 198, 198f
　disorder questionnaire 198
　fragmentation 198f
　management 211
　physiological parameters during 199
　scoring of 199
　time, total 199
Slipped capital femoral epiphysis 209
Small dense low density lipoprotein particles 102
Smith–Magenis syndrome 66
Sociodemographic index 120
Sodium 105, 122
Sodium-glucose cotransporter 142, 143, 152f, 154, 165, 182, 255
　inhibitors 151, 162, 168, 174, 183, 246, 255, 269
　upregulation of 180

Somatostatin analogs 50
Somatostatinoma 50
Sorbitol dehydrogenase 172
Sotagliflozin 256
Starvation 183
Steatohepatitis, non-alcoholic 38, 165, 209, 248
Steatotic liver disease 191
  metabolic dysfunction with 188, 189
Sterol regulatory element-binding protein 25, 103, 126
Stroke
  family history of 16
  higher risk of 207
Sucrose 122
Sulfonylurea 140-142, 144, 249
  mechanism of action of 146f
Superoxide dismutase 103
Suppressing hypothalamic proopiomelanocortin neurons 254
Surgery
  pancreatic 50
  post-bariatric 165
Survodutide 261
Sympathomimetic amine 159, 211
Synbiotics 191

T

Tachycardia 80
T-cells 33
  regulatory 35
Tesofensine 162
Testosterone 49, 231f
Thermogenesis 139
Thiazolidinediones 141-144, 146, 236, 250, 255, 269
  insulin sensitizers, glycemic mechanism of action of 147f
Thrifty phenotype 55
Thrombin 180
Thylakoid stromal deposition 182f
Thyroid 49
  disorders 50
  hormone 48
    receptors 257
    secretion of 48
  tumors 202
Thyrotropin-releasing hormone 48
Tirzepatide 261
Tissue inflammation, chronic 31
Tocopherol 103
Tolbutamide 141
Tolerance test 210

Tolimidone stimulates Lyn protein tyrosine kinase 258
Tolzamide 141
Topiramate 139, 156, 157, 159, 160, 238
Total skeletal muscle mass 230
Trans fat 122
Transforming growth factor-beta 176
Triacylglycerol synthesis 257
Tricyclic antidepressants 168
Triglyceride 31, 46, 102, 125, 172, 193, 194, 210
  levels 76
Trisphosphate 24
Tropomyosin-related kinase B 68
Truncal musculature 88
Tubular epithelial atrophy 182f
Tubular glomerular feedback mechanism 180
Tubulobulbar feedback balance 182f
Tumor necrosis factor 182
  alpha 30f, 32, 34, 102, 103, 172
Twin cycle hypothesis 36fc
Tyrosine
  kinase 103
    receptor 67
    phosphorylation 30

U

Upper respiratory tract infections 151
Urination, excessive 214
Urine albumin excretion 186

V

Valine 125
Vascular cell adhesion
  molecule-1 182
  protein 1 103
Vascular endothelial cells 147, 256
Vascular growth factor 182
  production 202
Vascular smooth muscle 172
Venous thrombosis embolus 76
Vertical sleeve gastrectomy 209
Very low-carbohydrate ketogenic diet 104f
Very low-density lipoprotein 36, 123
Vildagliptin 150
Visceral fat deposition 123
Vitamin 105, 133
  A 133
  B12 133
  C transporters, sodium-dependent 103
  D 133, 231f, 232
  E 191, 246
Vomiting 159

W

WAGR syndrome 65
Waist circumference 87, 89, 94, 230, 269
Waist-to-hip ratio 89
Weight
  for-height Z-score values 207
  loss 106, 128, 129, 139, 166f, 172, 185, 187, 208, 252, 256, 268
    benefits 156
    dietary strategies for 99
    diet-induced 106
    drugs 247t
    efforts, complement 238
    medications 153
    sudden 79
    sustain 106
    therapies 231f, 232
    unexplained 214
  management 128, 206, 219, 234, 238
    apps 109
    long-term 139
  reduction, management strategies for 238
White adipose tissue 43
Whole-body vibration therapy 232
Wilson's disease 183
World Cancer Research Fund 201
World Health Organization 83

Z

Zinc 134